Nutrition and Diet in Health

Nutrition and diet play a crucial role in sustaining good health throughout human lives. Food provides us with essential nutrients involved in many physiological activities and biological processes in the body, including growth and development, metabolism, immune function, and overall well-being. *Nutrition and Diet in Health: Principles and Applications* reviews and discusses the issues related to the roles of nutrition and diet in human health and diseases.

The book contains two sections: one section features principles; the other covers applications. Part I provides information on sustainable use of nutrition and diets in health and diseases; advanced biotechnological approaches to improve nutritional content of food; trace elements in nutrition; drug and nutrient interactions; functional foods and nutraceuticals in health maintenance; and biomarkers of functional foods and nutraceuticals in health maintenance. Part II discusses the significance of nutrition in selected human diseases, including cardiovascular diseases, cancer, infection, neurodegenerative diseases, and metabolic co-morbidities. It also discusses optimal nutrition for wellness, fitness, pregnancy, mental health, aging, and longevity.

FEATURES

- Molecular and cellular-based research findings on the principles and applications of nutrition and diets in health.
- Roles of nutritional agents in the pathogenesis of human diseases.
- Underlying mechanisms that govern activities and strategies to prevent pathological conditions using nutritional agents.

Nutrition and Diet in Health: Principles and Applications is suitable for academia and scientists, and it enhances knowledge of students in healthcare and areas of biological sciences.

Adenike Temidayo Oladiji is a professor of nutritional biochemistry and the current Dean of the Faculty of Life Sciences, University of Ilorin.

Johnson Olaleye Oladele is a lecturer at the Department of Chemical Sciences, Faculty of Science, Kings University, Nigeria.

Ebenezer I. O. Ajayi is a lecturer at the Biochemistry Department, College of Science, Engineering and Technology, Osun State University, Osogbo, Nigeria.

Nutrition and Diet in Health
Principles and Applications

Edited by
Adenike Temidayo Oladiji,
Johnson Olaleye Oladele, and Ebenezer I. O. Ajayi

CRC Press
Taylor & Francis Group
Boca Raton London New York

CRC Press is an imprint of the
Taylor & Francis Group, an **informa** business

First edition published 2024
by CRC Press
2385 NW Executive Center Drive, Suite 320, Boca Raton FL 33431

and by CRC Press
4 Park Square, Milton Park, Abingdon, Oxon, OX14 4RN

CRC Press is an imprint of Taylor & Francis Group, LLC

© 2024 Taylor & Francis Group, LLC

ISBN: 978-1-032-42171-1 (hbk)
ISBN: 978-1-032-71885-9 (pbk)
ISBN: 978-1-003-36149-7 (ebk)

DOI: 10.1201/9781003361497

Typeset in Times LT Std
by Apex CoVantage, LLC

Contents

PART I   Principles

PART II   Applications

Preface

Nutrition and diet play a crucial role in sustaining good health throughout human lives. Food provides us with essential nutrients such as vitamins, minerals, protein, carbohydrates, and fats that are necessary for our bodies to function properly. These nutrients are involved in many processes, including growth and development, metabolism, immune function, and overall well-being. The type and quantity of food we consume can have a significant impact on our health. Indeed, beyond what we eat, we are what we absorb. As such, by extension, poor nutrition can lead to various health problems, including obesity, heart disease, certain types of cancer, stroke, high blood pressure, type 2 diabetes, and malnutrition. Furthermore, a diet high in processed foods, refined carbohydrates, and unhealthy fats can lead to health problems such as weight gain, high blood pressure, high cholesterol, and other chronic diseases. Consuming excessive amounts of added sugars, saturated and trans fats, and sodium can also increase the risk of developing these health problems.

A balanced and varied diet that includes lean protein, whole grains, vegetables, fruits, and healthy fats can help prevent these health problems, manage these diseases, and improve overall health outcomes. Moreover, proper nutrition is essential for different stages of life, such as infancy, childhood, adolescence, and adulthood. During pregnancy, proper nutrition is vital for the healthy growth and development of the foetus. In older adults, good nutrition can help maintain muscle mass, bone density, and cognitive function, which are critical for healthy aging.

This book is a collection of several chapters that review and discuss the current level of knowledge and information on certain issues related to the roles of nutrition and diets in human health and diseases. The contents of this book are sectioned into two parts: Part I, "Principles" and Part II, "Applications". Part I provides information on the sustainable use of nutrition and diets in health and diseases, advanced biotechnological approaches in improving food nutrients, trace elements in nutrition, drug and nutrient interaction, functional foods and nutraceuticals in health maintenance, and markers of functional foods and nutraceuticals in health maintenance, while Part II discusses the significance of nutrition in some selected human diseases, such as cardiovascular diseases, cancer, infection, neurodegenerative diseases, metabolic co-morbidities, and in wellness, fitness, pregnancy, mental health, aging, and longevity.

The importance of diet in health is further emphasized by the dietary guidelines developed by various health organizations, notably the World Health Organization and the U.S. Department of Agriculture. These guidelines provide evidence-based recommendations on the types and amounts of food that should be consumed to maintain optimal health and prevent chronic diseases. Overall, a healthy and balanced diet is essential for maintaining good health throughout life. By consuming a variety of nutrient-rich foods and limiting processed foods and unhealthy fats, we can promote optimal health and reduce the risk of chronic diseases.

This book presents comprehensive information on the aetiology and pathogenesis of selected human chronic diseases; the role of nutrition and diet in the treatment of these diseases highlights molecular and cellular events that occurred between nutrients, phytochemicals, and cellular macromolecules and depicts the nature of interactions and underlying mechanisms that govern the activities of nutritional agents.

Adenike Temidayo Oladiji, PhD
Johnson Olaleye Oladele, PhD
Ebenezer I. O. Ajayi, PhD
Editors

Editors

Adenike Temidayo Oladiji, Ph.D., is a professor of nutritional biochemistry and the current Vice Chancellor of the Federal University of Technology, Akure, Nigeria. Prior to this, she held various positions and served on university committees as chairman and member. She served as the Dean of the Faculty of Life Sciences, University of Ilorin, Director of Administration of Association of West African Universities, Advisory Board Member of CG Bhakta Institute of Biotechnology, Uka Tarsadia University, Bardoli, India, and Director of Central Research Laboratories, University of Ilorin. She is an editorial board member of many scientific journals and has authored 150 research articles and contributions to book series publications. Professor Oladiji has received many awards and recognitions for her achievements and associated organizations, including Fellow of the Nigerian Academy of Science, Fellow of the Nigeria Society of Biochemistry and Molecular Biology, among others.

Johnson Olaleye Oladele, Ph.D., is a Director at Royal Scientific Research Institute, Osun State, Nigeria, and a lecturer at the Department of Chemical Sciences, Faculty of Science, Kings University, Nigeria. He earned a bachelor's degree (B.Sc. [Hons]) in biochemistry and a certificate in entrepreneurial education from Osun State University. He completed his postgraduate studies at University of Ibadan, where he earned his master's degree (M.Sc.) in biochemistry and molecular toxicology, and he earned his Ph.D. (biochemistry) from University of Ilorin. He completed his postdoctoral studies in toxicology at Texas A&M University, College Station, Texas, USA. He has also completed online modules program at Wicking Dementia Research & Education Centre, University of Tasmania, Australia, and Griffith University, Queensland, Australia. Dr. Oladele belongs to a number of national and international professional associations. He has authored many research articles published in peer-reviewed journals and chapters in book series. He serves as a reviewer for a number of journals hosted by Elsevier and Springer and as an editorial board member of two learned peer reviewed journals. Dr. Oladele has vast experience in both teaching and research. As a research fellow and seasoned facilitator, he has presented papers and oral presentations in a number of seminars, workshops, and conferences. He has also received awards and honours in recognition of his efforts, distinguished services, and contributions to his career and associated organizations.

Ebenezer I. O. Ajayi is a Lecturer at the Department of Biochemistry, Faculty of Basic and Applied Sciences, College of Science, Engineering and Technology, Osun State University, Osogbo, Nigeria. He is a former sub-dean of Student's Affairs, College of Science, Engineering and Technology. He received his B.Sc. (2004) from the University of Ado Ekiti, M.Sc. (2008), and Ph.D. (2015) from the University of Ibadan, Nigeria. He has published 32 scientific papers, reviews, and book chapters and has served as reviewer for reputable journals. He is a recipient of many grants and awards, the most recent being a three-year postdoctoral fellowship by the Argentinian Ministry of Science, Technology, and Productive Innovation. He is the leader of the Computational Membrane Biochemistry and Bionanotechnology group with research interests in diabetes complications and infectious diseases involving wound healing using biophysical, nanotechnology and microfluidics tools.

Contributors

Alaba A. Adebayo
Department of Microbiology
Faculty of Science
Ekiti State University
Ado-Ekiti, Nigeria

Stephen Adeniyi Adefegha
Functional Foods and Nutraceuticals Unit
Department of Biochemistry
School of Sciences
Federal University of Technology Akure
Akure, Ondo State, Nigeria

Omowumi O. Adewale
Department of Biochemistry
Osun State University
Osogbo, Nigeria

Taiwo Scholes Adewole
Department of Chemical Sciences
Kings University
Odeomu, Nigeria

Titilayo Oluwaseun Agunbiade
Department of Chemical Sciences
Oduduwa University
Ipetumodu, Nigeria

Ebenezer I. O. Ajayi
Diabesity Complications and Other Neglected
    Infectious Diseases Group
Department of Biochemistry
Osun State University
Osogbo, Nigeria

Taoheed Olawale Bello
Department of Natural Sciences and
    Mathematics
College of Arts and Sciences
William V. S. Tubman University
Harper, Liberia
and
Department of Biochemistry
University of Ilorin
Ilorin, Nigeria

Monica Butnariu
Chemistry and Biochemistry
    Discipline
University of Life Sciences "King Mihai I"
    from Timisoara
Timis, Romania

Stanley Chukwuejim
Department of Biochemistry
Federal University
Oye-Ekiti, Nigeria

Aderonke E. Fakayode
Bioinformatics and Molecular Biology
    Unit
Department of Biochemistry
Federal University of Technology
    Akure
Akure, Nigeria

Idowu Yetunde Fakolujo
Department of Biochemistry
University of Ilorin
Ilorin, Nigeria

John Adeolu Falode
Department of Biochemistry
Federal University
Oye-Ekiti, Ekiti State, Nigeria

Oluwafisayo Modupe Gbadeyan
Department of Biochemistry
University of Ilorin
Ilorin, Nigeria

Fatima Alaba Ibrahim
Department of Biochemistry
University of Ilorin
Ilorin, Nigeria

Adenike Kuku
Department of Biochemistry and Molecular
    Biology
Obafemi Awolowo University
Ile-Ife, Nigeria

Olorunfemi R. Molehin
Department of Biochemistry
Faculty of Science
Ekiti State University
Ado-Ekiti, Nigeria

Abraham Nkumah
Phytochemistry and Phytomedicine
    (Molecular) Unit
Department of Pharmacognosy
Faculty of Pharmacy
University of Ibadan
Ibadan, Nigeria

Mariam A. Odebode
Department of Science Laboratory Technology
Faculty of Science
Ekiti State University
Ado-Ekiti, Nigeria

Gbenga Emmanuel Ogundepo
Department of Biochemistry and Molecular
    Biology
Obafemi Awolowo University
Ile-Ife, Nigeria

Adeniyi S. Ohunayo
Department of Science Laboratory Technology
Faculty of Science
Ekiti State University
Ado-Ekiti, Nigeria

Jacinta O. Okonkwo
Department of Biochemistry
University of Port Harcourt
Rivers State, Nigeria

Johnson Olaleye Oladele
Biochemistry Unit
Department of Chemistry
Kings University
Odeomu, Osun State, Nigeria
and
Phytochemistry and Phytomedicine Research
    Unit
Royal Scientific Research Institute
Osun State, Nigeria

Oluwaseun Titilope Oladele
Department of Biochemistry
Osun State University
Osogbo, Nigeria

Adenike Temidayo Oladiji
Department of Biochemistry
University of Ilorin
Ilorin, Nigeria

Olabimpe Olayinka
Phytochemistry and Phytomedicine
    (Molecular) Unit
Department of Pharmacognosy
Faculty of Pharmacy
University of Ibadan
Ibadan, Nigeria

Rukayat A. Oyegoke
Department of Biochemistry
University of Ilorin
Ilorin, Nigeria

Nisha Rana
Central Research and Incubation Centre
Swami Vivekanand Subharti University
Meerut (U.P.), India

Vartika Singh
Central Research and Incubation Centre
Swami Vivekanand Subharti
    University
Meerut (U.P.), India

Part I

Principles

1 Sustainable Uses of Diets and Nutrition in Human Health

Johnson Olaleye Oladele

1.1 INTRODUCTION

Nutrition is a vast and essential field that deals with the study of the relationship between food and the human body's overall health and well-being. It is a complex and interdisciplinary science that encompasses a broad range of topics such as biochemistry, physiology, and psychology. The field of nutrition plays a crucial role in helping people maintain a healthy lifestyle, prevent diseases, and manage chronic conditions. Nutrition is a field that has been extensively researched in recent years, and the findings have led to a better understanding of the relationship between diet and health. For instance, one of the critical areas of research in nutrition is the role diet plays in managing and preventing chronic illnesses like obesity, diabetes, and heart disease. A Mediterranean diet, which is high in fruits, vegetables, whole grains, lean protein, and healthy fats, was linked to a lower risk of several chronic diseases, according to a systematic review and meta-analysis report (Dominguez et al., 2021).

One of the essential aspects of nutrition is understanding the role of different nutrients in the body. Another important aspect of nutrition is the understanding of the relationship between diet and chronic diseases including obesity, diabetes, and heart diseases. Research has shown that poor dietary habits such as consuming foods high in sugar, salt, saturated fats, and trans fats may facilitate the risk of developing these chronic diseases. Contrarily, a diet abundant in fresh produce, lean protein, whole grains, healthy fats, fruits, and vegetables can help prevent and manage these conditions.

Nutrients such as carbohydrates, proteins, fats, vitamins, and minerals are crucial for various bodily functions, including energy production, cell growth, and repair. The balance of these nutrients in the diet is essential to maintaining good health. Another area of research in nutrition is the effect of specific nutrients on health outcomes. It has been documented that a high intake of dietary fibre was associated with a lower risk of cardiovascular disease and all-cause mortality (McRae, 2017). Furthermore, larger intakes of omega-3 fatty acids were linked to a lower risk of cardiovascular disease and mortality from all causes, according to a systematic review (Ong et al., 2023).

Nutrition also plays a critical role in sports performance. Athletes require a specific balance of nutrients to fuel their bodies and help them recover from intense training sessions. Sports nutritionists work with athletes to develop personalized nutrition plans that optimize their performance. A study reported that a high-protein diet was beneficial for athletes looking to build muscle and improve performance (Tipton, 2011). Furthermore, a systematic review and meta-analysis of 17 studies found that caffeine ingestion improved endurance exercise performance (Wang et al., 2022).

In recent years, there has been a growing interest in alternative diets, such as veganism and the ketogenic diet. A study documented that a plant-based diet was connected with a lower risk of chronic diseases, including diabetes, cardiovascular disease, and certain types of cancer (McMacken and Shah, 2017). However, another study reported that a low-carbohydrate, high-protein diet was associated with a higher risk of cardiovascular disease (Tingting et al., 2020).

Nutrition is a field that has seen significant advancements in recent years, and the findings have led to a better understanding of the role of diet in health outcomes. By understanding the role of different nutrients in the body and developing healthy dietary habits, individuals can improve their overall well-being and quality of life. Research has shown that a diet rich in fruits, lean protein,

DOI: 10.1201/9781003361497-2

vegetables, whole grains, and healthy fats can help prevent chronic diseases. However, it is essential to understand the potential risks and benefits of alternative diets and to ensure that all necessary nutrients are included in the diet. This chapter focuses on the sustainable uses of diet and nutrition in human health.

1.2 CLASSIFICATION OF NUTRIENTS

The division of nutrients into macronutrients, micronutrients, and non-nutrients is a classification used to characterize animal nutrient demands. When taken in relatively substantial amounts (grams or ounces), macronutrients (carbohydrates, fats, proteins, and water) are largely utilized to produce energy or to integrate into tissues for development and maintenance.

Micronutrients have subtle biochemical and physiological roles in cellular processes including vascular function and nerve conduction; they are required in lower amounts (milligrams or micrograms). A deficiency state is caused by insufficient levels of necessary nutrients as well as disorders that interfere with absorption. This places development, survival, and procreation in danger. Consumer dietary nutrient intake recommendations, such as the United States Dietary Reference Intake, are based on the consequence of inadequacy and issue macronutrient and micronutrient guidelines for both minimum and maximum intake limits. Many countries' regulations mandate that large amounts of macronutrients and micronutrients be displayed on food labels. Nutrients can be detrimental if consumed in excess of what the body requires. Polyphenolic compounds are non-nutrient substances, and thousands of distinct phytochemicals emerge, each with its own chemical structure and function. Polyphenols account for a significant fraction of these compounds. Some of these compounds have basic structures, such as phytate, while others, like polyphenols, have more complicated shapes.

1.2.1 MACRONUTRIENTS

Carbohydrates, lipids, and proteins are all macronutrients that occur as polymers or long chains. They offer energy in the form of kilocalories (kcal) as well as few other human-specific components (ADA, 2006). Lipids and carbs supply most of the energy, with proteins supplying a smaller proportion. Carbohydrates and lipids originating from plants and animals account for about 85% of the energy (measured in kilocalories or kilojoules) ingested by humans in the developed world, and probably up to 90% or more in other regions of the world (ADA, 2006). Protein provides most of the additional energy required daily. Proteins are vital because they offer nitrogen, which is required for the production of genetic code and associated molecules, in complement to their corresponding amino (ADA, 2006; Oladiji and Oladele, 2023).

1.2.2 MICRONUTRIENTS

Micronutrients include vitamins and minerals, which play particular roles in metabolism. Micronutrients must be consumed in modest quantities throughout the day. Water-soluble vitamins and lipid-soluble vitamins are the two types of vitamins. The solubility of these two types of vitamins in water or organic solvents such as lipids distinguishes them. Several cellular and extracellular chain reactions need vitamins. Lipid-soluble vitamins, such as vitamins A and D, are examples. Vitamin A supports development and eyesight, whereas vitamin D supports calcium metabolism and can be absorbed from diet or created when subjected to sunshine.

Minerals are employed in chemical reactions and as structural constituents in body tissues. Calcium, for example, is required for the formation of hard structures such as osseous tissue and dentition as well as a range of other functions. Macrominerals must be ingested in amounts exceeding 100 milligrams daily. Microminerals should be taken daily in amounts below 100 milligrams. Minerals are usually related with water.

1.2.3 NON-NUTRIENT PHYTOCHEMICAL

Phytochemical or phytomolecules are molecules obtained from plants (Oladele et al., 2020, 2021). Only plant-based foods include phytochemicals. Phytochemicals are manufactured by plants to conduct a variety of tasks. Fibre, for example, is a structural constituent of plant cell walls and supplies stiffness to plant tissues. It is also referred to as dietary fibre in human nutrition (ADA, 2003).

Phytochemicals play an essential function in sustaining human health but do not supply humans with energy (in the form of calories) (Ajayi et al., 2021). Fibre molecules, for example, play a significant role in human gastrointestinal tract health (ADA, 2003). Other phytochemicals protect cells from oxidative stress radicals and highly reactive compounds created by cell metabolic pathways by acting as antioxidants. The idea that all phytochemicals are good to human health is false, since phytochemicals are manufactured by plants to fulfill their own demands instead of the needs of humans. Some phytochemicals are actually poisonous and must be avoided (ADA, 2006).

1.3 FUNCTION OF NUTRIENTS

We eat grains, lentils, vegetables, fruits, dairy products, proteinous food, sugar, fat, oils, and other things on a daily basis. Nutrients are chemical components found in a range of diets. The chemical makeup of these is used to classify them. Each dietary class has a specialized role, but for the nutrients to be beneficial, they must perform together (Mudambi and Rajagopal, 2007). Foods contain carbohydrates, proteins, lipids, minerals, vitamins, and water, among other components (Mudambi and Rajagopal, 2007). Fibre is also an integral part of our diet. The following are the listed functions of the nutrient.

1.3.1 CARBOHYDRATES

Starches, which can be found in cereals and sugar, which can be found in sugarcane and fruits, are examples of carbohydrates in diets. The major function of carbohydrates is to supply energy to our bodies. The carbohydrates that are not utilized right away are deposited as glycogen or turned to lipid and stored, ready to be used for energy production when necessary (Mudambi and Rajagopal, 2007).

1.3.2 FATS

Seed oils, butter from dairy products, and lard from animals are examples of fats present in diets. Fats are a source of vital fatty acids as well as a high-energy fuel and transporter of fat-soluble vitamins. Surplus fats in the food are retained in the body as fat reserves. Excess energy is reserved as fat in our body if it is ingested in excess of the body's demands (Mudambi and Rajagopal, 2007).

1.3.3 PROTEINS

Casein from dairy products such as milk, albumin from egg white, globulins from the bean family, and gluten from cereal are all examples of proteins found in diets. Protein's key role is to aid in the development of new tissues, including the maintenance and repair of existing ones. Food proteins are also involved in the production of regulatory and protective chemicals, which include enzymes, hormones, and immunoglobulin. Proteins in food contribute roughly 10% of total energy. Protein taken in surplus of the body's demand is transformed to carbs and lipids, which are then reserved in the body (Mudambi and Rajagopal, 2007).

1.3.4 MINERALS

Macro-elements, and micro-elements in conjunction with organic and inorganic substances, can be found in a wide range of foods. Minerals are needed for bodybuilding, bone and tooth production, and the building elements of soft tissues (Mudambi and Rajagopal, 2007). They also contribute in regulating biological processes like muscular contraction, blood coagulation, and nerve stimulation, among others (Mudambi and Rajagopal, 2007).

1.3.5 VITAMINS

Vitamins A, D, E, and K are referred to as fat soluble because they are soluble in organic solvent as well as water-soluble vitamins B and C, which dissolve in water and are found in foods. These are essential for proper bodily function and processes as well as for proliferation (Mudambi and Rajagopal, 2007).

1.3.6 WATER

Water is present in many of the foods we consume as well as a significant amount of the fresh water we take as water and drinks. Water is a vital part of our biological structure, accounting for roughly 60% of our weight. Water is essential for both the digestion of meals and disposal of food waste in the human body. It controls biological functions like body temperature regulation (Mudambi and Rajagopal, 2007).

To execute the same physical activities, everyone demands equal nutrients. The quantity of each nutrient needed varies depending on age group, size, task, and other factors. Most foods include various levels of the nutrients.

1.4 SUSTAINABLE USES OF DIETS AND NUTRITION IN HUMAN HEALTH AND DISEASES

Numerous studies have been conducted on the role of diet in the etiology of different diseases, and the connection between dietary factors and the onset and progression of many chronic illnesses is strongly supported. For example, a diet high in calories, saturated and trans fats, and added sugar has a significant role in the emergence of obesity. In consequence, obesity raises the risk of developing a number of chronic illnesses, such as type 2 diabetes, heart disease, and even some cancers. This is similar to how high-refined-carbohydrate and added-sugar diets can cause type 2 diabetes, which has reduced glucose tolerance and insulin resistance as its main characteristics.

Additionally, diets high in trans and saturated fats can cause inflammation, which is linked to the emergence of type 2 diabetes. Cholesterol, trans and saturated fats, and sodium-rich diets can encourage hypertension, atherosclerosis, and inflammation, which can all lead to the development of cardiovascular disease. A higher risk of cancer has been associated with a number of dietary factors, including an excessive intake of sugar-sweetened beverages, alcohol, red and processed meat. In both the onset and treatment of inflammatory bowel disease (IBD), diet has a significant role. In contrast to a diet abundant in vegetables, fruits, and whole grains, a diet high in processed foods, sugar, and fats has been related to a higher risk of developing IBD. All of these instances highlight the important role that nutrition can play in the onset and course of various diseases.

We can lower our chance of developing chronic diseases and enhance our general health by choosing a balanced, sustainable diet. Sustainable diets are those that are healthy, affordable, and environmentally sustainable. By promoting sustainable diets, we can help prevent and manage various human diseases while also supporting the health of the planet. For instance, a sustainable diet that is rich in vegetables, healthy fats, lean protein, fruits, and whole grains can help maintain a healthy heart and prevent cardiovascular disease. Similarly, a sustainable diet that is low in added sugars and processed foods but high in fibre-rich whole foods can help prevent and manage type 2 diabetes.

Sustainable diets that are rich in plant-based foods and low in red and processed meats can help prevent certain types of cancer, while those high in nutrient-dense whole foods can help prevent and manage obesity. A diet that is diverse and nutrient-rich can help prevent and manage malnutrition. Interestingly, consuming sustainable sources of protein such as beans, lentils, and nuts can help reduce the environmental impact of the diet. Consumption of sustainably produced whole grains, fruits, and vegetables can help support environmental sustainability and can help support the availability of food for future generations.

1.5 POSSIBLE FUTURE PROSPECTS FOR SUSTAINABLE DIETS IN HUMAN HEALTH

The future prospects for sustainable diets in the prevention and management of human diseases are promising. The following are a few potential areas:

1. Personalized nutrition: Advances in technology and genetics are allowing for personalized nutrition recommendations based on an individual's unique genetic makeup, lifestyle, and environmental factors. This approach can help individuals make more sustainable dietary choices that are tailored to their specific needs and goals.
2. Food systems transformation: As awareness of the impact of food systems on human and environmental health grows, there is potential for food systems transformation toward more sustainable and equitable models. This could include changes in production, distribution, and consumption practices that prioritize sustainable and healthy food options.
3. Digital health tools: The increasing use of digital health tools, such as mobile apps and wearable devices, can help individuals track their dietary habits and make more sustainable choices. These tools can also provide personalized recommendations based on an individual's dietary preferences and health goals.
4. Food labelling and certification: The use of food labelling and certification schemes can help consumers make more informed and sustainable dietary choices. Labels that indicate sustainably produced foods, organic or non-GMO products, and other environmental or health certifications can help consumers make choices that align with their values.
5. Collaboration and education: Collaboration among healthcare providers, food industry stakeholders, and policymakers can help promote sustainable dietary choices and support healthy food systems. Education initiatives that promote sustainable diets can also help raise awareness of the importance of sustainable dietary choices for human and environmental health.

Overall, the future prospects for sustainable diets in the prevention and management of human diseases are promising, and continued efforts in research, education, and collaboration can help promote sustainable dietary choices for a healthier and more sustainable future. By promoting healthy and environmentally responsible dietary choices, we can support both human and planetary health.

REFERENCES

Ajayi E.I.O., Molehin O.R., Adefegha S.A., Fakayode A.E., Oladele J.O., Adewumi S.O. (2021). Nutritional regulation of metabesity. In Nutrition, Food and Diet in Ageing and Longevity. Healthy Ageing and Longevity. 14. Springer International Publishing. doi:10.1007/978-3-030-83017-5_27

American Dietetic Association (ADA). (2003). Position of the American dietetic association and dietitians of Canada. Vegetarian diets. J Acad Nutr Diet. 103:748–765.

American Dietetic Association (ADA). (2006). Position of the American dietetic association: Food and nutrition misinformation. J Acad Nutr Diet. 106:601–607.

Dominguez L.I., Di Bella G., Veronese N., Barbagallo M. (2021). Impact of Mediterranean diet on chronic non-communicable diseases and longevity. Nutrients. 13(6):2028. doi:10.3390/nu13062028

McMacken M., Shah, S. 2017. A plant-based diet for the prevention and treatment of type 2 diabetes. J Geriatr Cardiol. 14(5):342–354. doi:10.11909/j.issn.1671-5411.2017.05.009

McRae M.P. (2017). Dietary fibre is beneficial for the prevention of cardiovascular disease: An umbrella review of meta-analyses. J Chiropr Med. Dec;16(4):289–299. doi:10.1016/j.jcm.2017.05.005. Epub 2017 Oct 25. PMID: 29276461; PMCID: PMC5731843.

Mudambi S.R., Rajagopal, M.V. 2007. Fundamental of Foods, Nutrition and Diet Therapy. New Age International Publisher Limited. 5th Edition. ISBN (13): 978-81-224-2972-5.

Oladele J.O., Ajayi E.I.O., Oyeleke O.M., Oladele O.T., Olowookere B.D., Adeniyi B.M., Oyewole O.I., Oladiji A.T. (2020). A systematic review on COVID-19 pandemic with special emphasis on Curative potentials of medicinal plants. Heliyon. 6:1–17.

Oladele J.O., Oyeleke O.M., Oladele O.T., Oladiji A.T. (2021). Covid-19 treatment: Investigation on the phytochemical constituents of *Vernonia amygdalina* as potential Coronavirus-2 inhibitors. Comput Toxicol. 18.100161. doi:10.1016/j.comtox.2021.100161

Oladiji A.T., Oladele J.O. (2023). Spices as potential human disease panacea. Chapter 16. In Sustainable Uses and Prospects of Medicinal Plants. Eds. L. Kambizi and C. Bvenura. CRC. doi:10.1201/9781003206620-16

Ong K.L., Marklund M., Huang L., Rye K., Hui N., Pan X. et al. (2023). Association of omega 3 polyunsaturated fatty acids with incident chronic kidney disease: Pooled analysis of 19 cohorts. BMJ. 380:e072909. doi:10.1136/bmj-2022-072909

Tingting D., Guo M., Zhang P., Sun G., Chen B. (2020). The effects of low-carbohydrate diets on cardiovascular risk factors: A meta-analysis. PLoS One. 15(1):e0225348. doi:10.1371/journal.pone.0225348

Tipton K.D. (2011). Efficacy and consequences of very-high-protein diets for athletes and exercisers. Proc Nutr Soc. May;70(2):205–214. doi:10.1017/S0029665111000024. Epub 2011 Mar 7. PMID: 21375795.

Wang Z., Qiu B., Gao J., Del Coso J. (2022). Effects of caffeine intake on endurance running performance and time to exhaustion: A systematic review and meta-analysis. Nutrients. Dec 28;15(1):148. doi:10.3390/nu15010148. PMID: 36615805; PMCID: PMC9824573.

2 Advanced Biotechnological Approaches in Improving Food Nutrients

Nisha Rana and Vartika Singh

2.1 INTRODUCTION

Without much room for horizontal development, dwindling cultivable land, and climate uncertainty, feeding the planet's 7.8 billion people now and the predicted 9 billion by 2050 will surely be a challenge (Vemireddy 2014). Worldwide, an estimated 842 million people are considered to be malnourished, and an additional 1 billion people suffer from insidious hunger brought on by a lack of essential micronutrients such as vitamins and minerals in a conventional diet, roughly 97% of whom live in underdeveloped and developing nations (Malik and Maqbool 2020). Acute dietary micronutrient deficiencies can cause a variety of disorders, especially in women and children, like poor vision, hypertension, mental retardation, and immune system disorders, resulting in an elevated risk of contracting infectious diseases (Bhatnagar et al. 2011). Ending food instability, hunger, and malnutrition is an urgent worldwide issue. The nutritional value, safety, and quality of processed foods can all be significantly increased by using biotechnological equipment and methodologies wisely.

Food biotechnology is a rapidly evolving industry, and improvements brought about by ongoing research and development have enhanced the health advantages, shelf life, and yield of food as well as effectively solved issues with food security. Early biotechnology was mostly concerned with enhancing input qualities or agronomic features, such as pest/insect resistance, herbicide tolerance, cytoplasmic male sterility, and yield enhancement, leading to the first generation of transgenic crops. The enhancement of nutritional value, water use efficiency, nitrogen use efficiency, and various biotic and abiotic stress tolerances such as disease tolerance (bacterial, viral, and fungal diseases), salinity tolerance, temperature sensitivity, etc. – features that directly benefit the consumer – are more heavily emphasized in the second generation of transgenic plants (Kalamaki 2010). Precision and speedier genetic manipulation of plants have been made possible by the advent of biotechnological technologies like genetic engineering or transgenic technology, genome editing, genome mapping, molecular marker-assisted breeding (MAB), etc. (Munaweera et al. 2022). Utilizing biotechnological tools and methodologies properly can dramatically enhance the nutrient value, quality, and safety of food products.

2.2 GENETIC TRANSFORMATION

When it comes to satisfying the global demand for wholesome food and offering fresh approaches to address particular requirements, genetically modified (GM) foods can emerge as potent allies to those grown using conventional means. By carefully inserting foreign DNA into an organism's genome, genetic engineering has been utilized to create genetic variants with economic significance. The genes may be altered and placed back into the same species, or they may be separated from one species and transferred to another. In order to create transgenic plants with desirable traits, novel genes – also known as transgenes – are incorporated into a plant through a procedure called transformation. Genetically modified crops can be employed to raise harvests, nutritive values,

DOI: 10.1201/9781003361497-3

vigour, and flavour, extend shelf life, reduce production costs, and even produce crucial biomolecules that are hard to locate or aren't found in nature.

2.2.1 TRANSGENESIS (GENE TRANSFER)

The process of introducing an exogenous gene (known as a transgene) from one organism into the germline of another organism is referred to as transgenesis. The intended outcome is for the transgenic organism to express the gene and display a novel trait that can be passed on to its progeny. Transgenic organisms are able to express transgenes because the genetic code is universal for all organisms. Transgenesis can be performed by using pronuclear injection, plasmid vectors, protoplast fusion, particle bombardment, ballistic DNA injection, etc. It is used to generate crops with ideal traits, high productivity, and high quality. It also serves as a factory for the creation of recombinant proteins, which can be utilized to make antibiotics and vaccines.

2.2.2 CISGENESIS/INTRAGENESIS

Cisgenesis and intragenesis are novel tools of breeding technologies, developing as viable strategies for the future intended to modify crops. Cisgenesis entails genetic modification by the transfer of natural genes with their regulatory components between closely related species, maintaining the genetic diversity of the recipient species, as opposed to intragenesis, which refers to the transfer of novel genetic combinations and regulatory sequences from different genes and loci within a particular species. Thus, genetic expressions can be altered by employing various promoter or terminator regions. The use of cisgenesis and intragenesis as alternatives to traditional transgenesis is restricted to a small number of species, mostly because the necessary regulatory sequences are not well understood. Both cutting-edge innovations are viewed as promising tools for the future that will transform conventional plant breeding, as these techniques can speed up gene transfer without linkage drag. Consumer acceptance and the claim that using DNA from inside cross-compatible species is a safer choice as compared to transgenics are two main justifications for employing these methods in plant breeding (Spinoza et al. 2013; Ahmad et al. 2020).

2.3 GENOME EDITING

Genome editing has emerged as one of the most potent methods for genetic modification, allowing for targeted, precise alterations to genomes (Pixley et al. 2022). It enables the addition, ablation, or correction of genetic material at specific genomic regions. Earlier, hybrid protein-based genome editing tools such as ZFNs and TALENs were common, but the recently developed CRISPR/Cas9 system proved to be a major break-through biological tool that creates precise gene knock-outs, knock-ins, and site-directed mutagenesis. Given that they do away with the restrictions of traditional breeding techniques, genome editing approaches have been receiving a lot of attention. By regulating the expression and altering the roles of genes involved in the pre- and post-metabolic pathways, it will be feasible to vary the build-up of target functional elements while maintaining the other beneficial traits of the host (Nagamine and Ezura 2022).

2.3.1 ZFNs

Zinc finger nucleases (ZFNs) are artificial endonucleases consisting of designed zinc finger DNA-binding proteins (DBPs), attached to the cleavage domain of *Fok*I (a natural IIS restriction enzyme), which are utilized as gene-targeting tools to trigger DNA double-strand breaks (DSBs) at predetermined loci, allowing for selective genome editing (Carroll 2011). Cellular DNA repair mechanisms, viz. NHEJ (non-homologous end joining) and HR (homologous recombination), which are triggered by ZFN-induced DSBs, frequently result in targeted gene substitution as well as targeted mutagenesis. NHEJ mediated by a splitting event brought on by ZFN can result in small deletions or insertions that are equivalent to gene knock-outs in cell lines. Reverse genetics in *Arabidopsis thaliana* has now been established using the NHEJ strategy in an effective manner. If the break is fixed using the HR approach in the presence of promoters or reporters, entire transgenes or minor alterations can be incorporated into the chromosome. This results in gene correction and gene knock-in cell lines, as indicated. Unique alleles in *Nicotiana tabacum* have been created using the HR technique (Urnov et al. 2010). There are certain downsides to ZFN-mediated gene editing, such as the absence of off-target mutations, the building of protein domains for specific genomic loci is expensive and challenging, and there is a chance that single nucleotide changes or faulty domain interactions will result in erroneous cleavage of the target DNA sequence (Abdallah et al. 2016).

2.3.2 TALENs

In 2011, artificial restriction enzymes TALENs (Transcription Activator-Like Effector Nucleases) were generated from TALE (Transcription Activator-Like Effector) proteins secreted by pathogenic bacteria *Xanthomonas*, which turned into the first tool that could be developed reasonably easily to improve the efficiency and precision of genome editing (Abdallah et al. 2016; Nemudryi et al. 2014). TALEs are members of a DNA-binding protein family that can be employed to induce gene expression, consisting of a nuclear localization signal, a domain that triggers the target gene transcription, and a DNA-binding central domain generally having 34 monomeric tandem repeats. In the experimental program, the catalytic domain of *Fok*I restriction endonuclease was fused with appropriate monomers of the DNA-binding domain of the TALE protein to create TALENs (Becker and Boch 2021). Thus, a nuclear localization signal, a synthetic DNA-binding domain, and a *Fok*I catalytic domain make up the finished TALEN nuclease. The binding sites of TALENs are designed to reside on opposing DNA strands and are isolated by a 12–24 bp spacer sequence, as they operate in pairs. The *Fok*I domains dimerize to trigger a double-strand break in the spacer sequence, when artificial nucleases enter the nucleus and attach to specific locations. TALEN has been used to produce genetically determined, disease-resistant lines of different plant species, notably *Nicotiana tabacum* and *Oryza sativa*, by making site-specific mutations. Significant advances in genome editing have been made with TALEN, including the first commercialization of an engineered crop in 2019, and because of its adaptability, it is theoretically possible to target specific DNA sequences, creating a wealth of new possibilities. (Abdallah et al. 2016; Pandey et al. 2019)

2.3.3 CRISPR/Cas9

Clustered, regularly interspaced, short, palindromic repeats (CRISPR)/CRISPR-associated protein 9 (Cas9) technology commissions an RNA-guided Cas9 endonuclease, capable of inciting site-specific DNA double-strand breaks, allowing further genetic manipulation via cellular DNA repair pathways. The use of CRISPR/Cas9 gene-editing tool to obtain genetically modified crops with optimized nutritional traits is still in its infancy, ascribed to insufficient genomic sequence data along with inadequate regeneration and transformational procedures. However, the CRISPR/Cas technology has greatly facilitated the metabolic engineering of food crops owing to its high efficacy, accuracy, simplicity, and feasibility (Es et al. 2019) Precise genetic manipulation has elevated CRISPR-Cas genome editing to a prominent technique, relieving it of the moral dilemmas associated with transgenic crops. Due to its high performance, short cycle, strong consistency, and cost effectiveness, the CRISPR-Cas9 method has been widely used in crop improvement initiatives. The technique is now being used to bio-fortify vegetables like *Solanum lycopersicum* and *Solanum tuberosum* as well as cereal crops like rice, wheat, maize, etc. It has been used to boost the levels of starch, protein, oleic acid, GABA (gamma-aminobutyric acid), gluten, and glycoalkaloid components while also improving the longevity, aroma, and flavour (Kumar et al. 2022).

2.4   MOLECULAR MARKER BASED ASSISTED BREEDING, OR MAB

MAB, or molecular marker-assisted breeding, is an innovative and potent tool of molecular breeding that employs DNA markers to improve the precision and productivity of traditional plant breeding. MAB entails the use of genetic markers, along with genomic maps and sequencing, to modify traits based on genotypic assays. It integrates conventional plant breeding with the methods and findings of molecular and computational biology (Jiang 2015, Nazarul et al. 2021). This chapter discusses some of the modern breeding procedures, theoretical considerations, and practical applications of MAB in plants, including MAS, MABC, and gene pyramiding. The incorporation of MAB into traditional breeding operations is an encouraging approach for crop development and enhancing the genetic makeup of plants in the future. Many molecular markers are now being used in crop production for genetic modification (Table 2.1).

2.4.1   MAS

The practise of employing morphological, biochemical, or DNA/RNA markers to indirectly select significant traits or traits of interest – e.g., disease and pest resistance, yield, quality, biotic and abiotic stress tolerance – in crop breeding is known as marker-assisted selection (MAS). This procedure is used to increase the efficacy and precision of selection and transfer of desirable traits (Ashraf et al. 2012).

2.4.2   MABC

Marker-assisted backcrossing (MABC), which is currently one of the most prevalent and effective strategies in operational molecular breeding, is referred to as the fundamental kind of marker-assisted selection. In order to improve the targeted phenotype, MABC intends to transfer QTLs (quantitative trait loci) or even a single gene of interest from one genetic source of inferior quality (donor parent) into a finer breeding line (recurrent parent) (Perween et al. 2020). The number of

---

TABLE 2.1

Examples of Molecular Markers and Their Target Gene/QTLs for Genetic Modification of Rice, Wheat, and Maize

S. No.	Crop	Trait(s)	Target gene/QTLs	Reference
1.	Rice	Low glutenin content	Lgc1	Chen et al. 2010
		Eating and cooking quality	Waxy	Zhou et al. 2003a
		Quality and bacterial blight	Xa21, xa13	Joseph et al. 2004
		Endosperm amylase and low amylose content	Waxy	Yamanaka et al. 2004; Ayres et al. 1997
2.	Wheat	Processing quality	Glu-A3, Talox-B1	Wang et al. 2009; Geng et al. 2012
		Polyphenol oxidase activity	Ppo-D1	He et al. 2007
		High glutenin	GluA11, GluD1	Radovanovic and Cloutier 2003
		High protein content and disease resistance	Gpc-B1, Yr36	Kidwell et al. 2008
3.	Maize	High lysine and tryptophan	Opaque-2	Babu et al. 2004
		Provitamin A content	PSY1, crtRBI1	Azmach et al. 2013
		A-carotene content	ZmcrtRB3	Zhou et al. 2012
		Oil content	DGAT1-2	Chai et al. 2012

markers employed and their distance from the target locus, the population density for each generation of backcrossing, as well as undesired linkage drag all affect MABC productivity (Jiang 2015). MABC can be used to speed up selection before fruiting and flowering, to enhance the heritability of an inferior trait, to identify diseases and pests so that the appropriate resistance genes can be injected, and it also helps in gene pyramiding. MAB was able to increase soybean yields by integrating yield QTL from a wild variety of soybean into its commercial variety (Perween et al. 2020).

2.4.3 MAGP

When several genes are accumulated for one or more traits into a single genotype to incorporate desirable qualities using traditional breeding or recombinant DNA technology, this process is known as gene pyramiding. Gene pyramiding is attracting a lot of attention, since it results in the simultaneous expression of multiple genes in a variety, which would boost the effectiveness of plant breeding and help in the precise development of broad-range resistance capacities. It has been suggested as a way to improve disease and pest resistance (Shah et al. 2017). Pyramiding, for instance, has been effective in battling rice bacterial blight and stripe rust in barley (Pandey et al. 2019). Pyramiding might be accomplished by regular breeding, but it's generally difficult to spot the plants with numerous genes. Individual plants must be assessed for each of the examined features using standard phenotypic screening. As a result, it could be extremely challenging to evaluate plants based on particular population groups or attributes. Due to the non-destructive nature of DNA marker assays and the ability to test several specific genes using a single DNA sample without phenotyping, DNA markers can significantly aid in selection (Collard and Mackill 2008). One of the most notable techniques for employing DNA markers in plant breeding is marker-assisted gene pyramiding (MAGP). MAGP has made it feasible for the breeder to carry out numerous selection rounds in a season. The integration of gene pyramiding with marker technology and ongoing plant breeding techniques around the globe will enable researchers to discover, transfer, and modify genes with a precision and speed that was unachievable before. The number of genes to be transferred, the distance between the flanking markers and the target genes, the quantity of genotypes chosen in each breeding phase, the type of germplasm, etc., are all important elements that play crucial roles in the success of gene pyramiding (Joshi and Nayak 2010).

2.5 CONCLUSION

The evolution of food and nutrition security will potentially include biotechnology. Molecular techniques are being used today to generate goods with improved breeding efficacy and appropriateness – as well as a stronger insight into the final product – in order to allay public concerns about genetically modified (GM) crops. Transgenic crops and marker-assisted selection used in conjunction with conventional breeding have the potential to significantly boost food production. Recent years have seen an increase in both GM and non-GM genetic improvement innovations, which is an excellent sign for the food biotechnology sector. The industry has advanced through time with a variety of non-GM technologies to speed up product development and avoid the high expenses of regulatory investigations for crops with biotechnological origins. Food-tech businesses all over the world have begun to invest in facilitating platform technologies that would aid in the development of crops via non-GM and GM processes. GMOs and the mighty power of genome editing offer the chance to quickly develop novel variations that have the potential to address issues in the real world. Research needs to take into account a complex milieu of concerns ranging from regulation, intellectual property, cultural preferences, local conditions, and existing market standards in order for the potential of biotechnology to be realized. While some people have expressed worry about the biosafety and health risks linked to GM crops, there is no justification for holding back on eating products that have been intelligently created and rigorously evaluated. The objective of achieving food security for both the present and future generations can be accomplished by integrating contemporary biotechnology with traditional agronomic systems in a responsible way.

REFERENCES

Abdallah, Naglaa A., Channapatna S. Prakash, and Alan G. McHughen. "Genome editing for crop improvement: Challenges and opportunities." GM Crops & Food. 6(4): 183–205, 2016. doi:10.1080/21645698.2015.1129937.

Ahmad, Sarfaraz, M. L. Jakhar, Dalip Jangir, Shivam Maurya, and Hari Ram Jat. "Cisgenesis and Intragenesis in Modern Plant Breeding." Int J Curr Microbiol App Sci 11: 3989–3998, 2020.

Ashraf, M., N. A. Akram, Mehboob-Ur-Rahman, and M. R. Foolad. "Marker-assisted selection in plant breeding for salinity tolerance." Methods Mol Biol. 913: 305–333, 2012. doi:10.1007/978-1-61779-986-0_21.

Ayres, N., A. McClung, P. Larkin, et al. "Microsatellites and a single-nucleotide polymorphism differentiate apparent amylose classes in an extended pedigree of US rice germ plasm." Theoret Appl Genet. 94: 773–781, 1997.

Azmach, G., M. Gedil, A. Menkir, and C. Spillane. "Marker-trait association analysis of functional gene markers for provitamin A levels across diverse tropical yellow maize inbred lines." BMC Plant Biol. 13: 227, 2013.

Babu, R., S. K. Nair, B. M. Prasanna, and H. S. Gupta. "Integrating marker-assisted selection in crop breeding – prospects and challenges." Curr Sci. 87: 607–619, 2004.

Becker, Sebastian, and Jens Boch. "TALE and TALEN genome editing technologies." Gene and Genome Editing. 2, 2021. doi:10.1016/j.ggedit.2021.100007.

Bhatnagar, Madhurima, Pooja Bhatnagar-Mathur, D. Srinivas Reddy, Vanamala Anjaiah, and Kiran K Sharma. "Crop biofortification through genetic engineering: Present status and future directions." In: Genomics and Crop Improvement: Relevance and Reservations, Institute of Biotechnology, Acharya NG Ranga Agricultural University, Hyderabad. 392–407, 2011.

Carroll, Dana. "Genome engineering with zinc-finger nucleases." Genetics. 188(4): 773–782, 2011. doi:10.1534/genetics.111.131433.

Chai, Y., X. Hao, X. Yang, et al. "Validation of DGAT1–2 polymorphisms associated with oil content and development of functional markers for molecular breeding of high-oil maize." Mol Breed. 29: 939–949, 2012.

Chen, Tao, Meng-xiang Tian, Ya-dong Zhang, et al. "Development of simple functional markers for low glutelin content gene 1 (Lgc1) in rice (Oryza sativa)." Rice Sci. 17(3): 173–178, 2010.

Collard, Bertrand C. Y., and David J. Mackill. "Marker-assisted selection: An approach for precision plant breeding in the twenty-first century." Philos Trans R Soc Lond B Biol Sci. 363(1491): 557–572, 2008. doi:10.1098/rstb.2007.2170.

Eş, Ismail, Mohsen Gavahian, Francisco J. Marti-Quijal, et al. "The application of the CRISPR-Cas9 genome editing machinery in food and agricultural science: Current status, future perspectives, and associated challenges." Biotechnol Adv. 37(3): 410–421, 2019. doi:10.1016/j.biotechadv.2019.02.006.

Geng, H., X. Xia, L. Zhang, et al. "Development of functional markers for a lipoxygenase gene on chromosome 4BS in common wheat." Crop Sci. 52: 568–576, 2012.

He, X., Z. He, L. Zhang, et al. "Allelic variation of polyphenol oxidase (PPO) genes located on chromosomes 2A and 2D and development of functional markers for the PPO genes in common wheat." Theoret Appl Genet. 115: 47–58, 2007.

Jiang, Guo-Liang. "Molecular marker-assisted breeding: A plant breeder's review." In: Al-Khayri, J., Jain, S., Johnson, D. (eds), Advances in Plant Breeding Strategies: Breeding, Biotechnology and Molecular Tools. Springer, Cham. 1: 431–472, 2015. doi:10.1007/978-3-319-22521-0_15.

Joseph, M., S. Gopalakrishnan, R. K. Sharma, et al. "Combining bacterial blight resistance and Basmati quality characteristics by phenotypic and molecular marker assisted selection in rice." Mol Breed. 13: 377–387, 2004. doi:10.1023/B:MOLB.0000034093.63593.4c.

Joshi, Raj Kumar, and Sanghamitra Nayak. "Gene pyramiding-A broad spectrum technique for developing durable stress resistance in crops." Biotechnol Mol Biol Rev. 5(3): 51–60, 2010.

Kalamaki, Mary S. "Biotechnological approaches for food quality improvement." JO – Proceedings of the 1st International Conference on Advances in Biotechnology-Industrial Microbial Biotechnology, 2010.

Kidwell, K., D. Santra, V. deMacon, et al. "Precision breeding, wheat research progress report." Washington State University, Agricultural Research Center, 2008.

Kumar, Dileep, Anurag Yadav, Rumana Ahmad, Upendra Nath Dwivedi, and Kusum Yadav. "CRISPR-based genome editing for nutrient enrichment in crops: A promising approach toward global food security." Front Genet. 13, 2022. doi:10.3389/fgene.2022.932859.

Malik, Kausar Abdulla, and Asma Maqbool. "Transgenic crops for biofortification." Front Sustain Food Syst. 4: 1–15, 2020. doi:10.3389/fsufs.2020.571402.

Munaweera, T. I. K., N. U. Jayawardana, Rathiverni Rajaratnam, and Nipunika Dissanayake. "Modern plant biotechnology as a strategy in addressing climate change and attaining food security." Agric & Food Secur. 11: 26, 2022. doi:10.1186/s40066-022-00369-2.

Nagamine, Ai, and Hiroshi Ezura. "Genome editing for improving crop nutrition." Front Genome Ed. 4: 850104, 2022. doi:10.3389/fgeed.2022.850104.

Nazarul, Hasan, Sana Choudhary, Neha Naaz, Nidhi Sharma, and Rafiul Amin Laskar. "Recent advancements in molecular marker-assisted selection and applications in plant breeding programmes." J Genet Eng Biotechnol. 19(1): 128, 2021. doi:10.1186/s43141-021-00231-1.

Nemudryi, A. A., K. R. Valetdinova, S. P. Medvedev, and S. M. Zakian. "TALEN and CRISPR/Cas genome editing systems: Tools of discovery." Acta Naturae. 6(3): 19–40, 2014.

Pandey, Kuldeep, Ravindra Dangi, Uma Prajapati, et al. "Advance breeding and biotechnological approaches for crop improvement: A review." Int J Chem Stud. 7(1): 837–841, 2019.

Perween, Shahina, Anjani Kumar, N. Swathi Rekha, Swapnil, Priyanka Kumari, and Surya Prakash. "Marker assisted backcrossing (MAB) an approach for selection by using molecular markers." In: Recent Advances in Chemical Sciences and Biotechnology. New Delhi Publishers, New Delhi. 161–172, 2020.

Pixley, Kevin V., Jose B. Falck-Zepeda, Robert L. Paarlberg, et al. "Genome-edited crops for improved food security of smallholder farmers." Nat Genet. 54: 364–367, 2022. doi:10.1038/s41588-022-01046-7.

Radovanovic, N., and S. Cloutier. "Gene-assisted selection for high molecular weight glutenin subunits in wheat doubled haploid breeding programs." Mol Breed. 12: 51–59, 2003.

Shah, Liaqat, Asif Ali, Yulei Zhu, Shengxing Wang, Hongqi Si and Chuanxi Ma. "Wheat resistance to fusarium head blight and possibilities of its improvement using molecular marker-assisted selection." Czech J Genet Plant Breed. 53: 47–54, 2017. doi:10.17221/139/2016-CJGPB

Spinoza, C., R. Schlechter, D. Herrera, E. Torres, A. Serrano, C. Medina, and P. Arce-Johnson. "Cisgenesis and intragenesis: New tools for improving crops." Biol Res. 46(4): 323–331, 2013. doi:10.4067/S0716-97602013000400003.

Urnov, Fyodor D., Edward J. Rebar, Michael C. Holmes, H. Steve Zhang, and Philip D. Gregory. "Genome editing with engineered zinc finger nucleases." Nat Rev Genet. 11: 636–646, 2010. doi:10.1038/nrg2842.

Vemireddy, Lakshminarayana R. "Food and nutrition security: Biotechnology intervention." Springer Sci Rev. 2: 35–49, 2014. doi:10.1007/s40362-014-0018-y.

Wang, C. L., Y. D. Zhang, Z. Zhu, et al. "Development of a new japonica rice variety Nanjing 46 with good eating quality by marker assisted selection." Mol Plant Breeding. 7: 1070–1076, 2009.

Yamanaka, Sinsuke, Ikuo Nakamura, Kazuo N. Watanabe, and Yo-Ichiro Sato. "Identification of SNPs in the waxy gene among glutinous rice cultivars and their evolutionary significance during the domestication process of rice." Theoret Appl Genet. 108: 1200–1204, 2004.

Zhou, P. H., Y. F. Tan, Y. Q. He, C. G. Xu, and Q. Zhang. "Simultaneous improvement for four quality traits of Zhenshan 97, an elite parent of hybrid rice, by molecular marker-assisted selection." Theor Appl Genet. 106: 326–331, 2003a.

Zhou, Yi, Yingjia Han, Zigang Li, et al. "ZmcrtRB3 encodes A carotenoid hydroxylase that affects the accumulation of a-carotene in maize kernel." J Integr Plant Biol. 54: 260–269, 2012. doi:10.1111/j.1744-7909.2012.01106.x.

3 Trace Elements in Nutrition

Stephen Adeniyi Adefegha

3.1 INTRODUCTION

Nutrition is an important part of health and development[1]. Good nutrition is related to improved infant, child and maternal health, stronger immune systems, safer pregnancy and childbirth, lower risk of non-communicable diseases (such as diabetes and cardiovascular disease), and longevity[2]. People with adequate nutrition are more productive and can create opportunities to gradually break the cycles of poverty and hunger[3]. Nutrition, coined from the Latin word *nutrire* meaning "to nourish", is defined as the sum of all processes involved in how organisms obtain nutrients, metabolize them, and use them to support all of life's processes[4]. It includes food intake, absorption, assimilation, biosynthesis, catabolism, and excretion[4]. Of great importance is the balance between the nutritional and anti-nutritional factors in food[4,5]. The major nutrients present in edible plants are: carbohydrates, which could be in form of starch and free sugars; proteins; fats and oils; minerals; vitamins and organic acids; and that of anti-nutrients such as phytic acids or phytate, tannic acid/tannin, cyanide, and trypsin inhibitors[6]. Nutrients in foods can be divided into macronutrients and micronutrients. A healthy diet is one in which macronutrients are consumed in appropriate proportions to support energetic and physiologic needs without excess intake while also providing sufficient micronutrients and hydration to meet the physiologic needs of the body[1, 7]. Macronutrients (i.e., carbohydrates, proteins, and fats) provide the energy necessary for the cellular processes required for daily functioning[8, 9]. Micronutrients – otherwise known as trace elements – are required in comparatively small amounts for normal growth, development, metabolism, and physiologic functioning[10]. Trace elements are of utmost significance due to the pivotal role they play in an organism. They belong to the micronutrient group of nutrients. Trace elements – also referred to as trace metals – are elements present in diet, and they constitute a very tiny percentage of an organism's total weight[11]. This percentage is typically below 0.02. They are crucial for the normal growth, development and functionality of an organism. According to WHO, there are nineteen trace elements, which were then grouped into three, primarily on their nutritional significance. They can either be essential, probably essential (indispensable), or elements with potential toxicity. Zinc (Zn), copper (Cu), selenium (Se), chromium (Cr), cobalt (Co), iodine (I), manganese (Mn), and molybdenum (Mo) are classified as indispensable trace elements. Certain trace elements serve as co-factors; some are involved in oxidation-reduction reaction generating energy in the process. Some trace metals are essential in maintaining structural integrity, and others play a key role in regulating important biological processes[9–11]. The body stores some trace elements, while it doesn't store some. Depending on how well the trace elements are absorbed, that determines the availability of the trace elements in the storage site. Essential trace-element anomalies can be risk factors for a variety of diseases of health concern. Due to the fact that specific diseases haven't been associated with these trace elements, diagnosing their deficiencies clinically is difficult. The determination of their deficiencies in humans will necessitate a better understanding of mechanisms of action as well as improved analytical procedures and functional tests[11].

3.2 TRACE ELEMENTS AND THEIR ROLES IN NUTRITION

3.2.1 ZINC

One of the most prevalent trace elements in the human system is zinc. Zinc plays a pivotal role in maintaining the human health. It functions in signaling and transduction, physiological

DOI: 10.1201/9781003361497-4

processes, cell development and differentiation, including metabolism[12]. 11mg and 9mg for adult males and females, respectively, is the recommended dietary intake. Zinc is not one of the trace elements the body stores in excess, and as such, must be supplied through diet regularly. Red meat, fish, and poultry are common sources of Zn in the diet[13, 14]. Because of the positive charge on zinc, many proteins utilize it to maintain their structure as well as for catalytic function. This element plays a significant role in pregnancy development and also growth during adolescent years[15]. Zinc deficiency can result in taste bud, smell, and night vision impairment oligospermia, loss of weight, hyperammonemia, stunted growth, hypogonadism in males, skin conditions, reduced appetite, bullous-pustular dermatitis, diarrhea, anorexia, prolonged wound healing, depression, and alopecia. Severe zinc deficiency can be lethal if not diagnosed and treated[16–18]. Excessive intake of zinc can result in nausea, epigastric pain, vomiting, and tiredness. Copper deficiency can take place when zinc intake is ten to twenty times higher than the daily required quantities, resulting in anemia and neutropenia symptoms[16]. Type 2 diabetes, diarrhea, pneumonia and Wilson's diseases are pathologies that have been reported to yield positive results with zinc supplementation. This suggests that zinc plays a key role in the management of these pathologies[12].

3.2.2 CHROMIUM

Chromium function, in the management of blood sugar and fat levels, is the most significant mineral for people who are overweight. Because chromium is the primary component of Glucose Tolerance Factor (GFT), it aids insulin in lowering blood glucose levels by promoting glucose absorption by muscles and other tissues. Low levels of chromium results in low level of circulating level of (GFT); this reduces the efficacy of insulin in lowering blood sugar. High level of chromium is also detrimental because it increases insulin levels and renders it ineffective. A consistent continuation of this cycle can be a risk factor for insulin resistance – the preconditioning for diabetes and its consequences[19].

Hypoglycemia and mood swings, high blood pressure, heart disease, stroke, and obesity are some of the symptoms linked with chromium deficiency[20].

Consumption of food rich in refined carbohydrates, like white flour, potatoes, pasta, rice, and processed meals, rapidly depletes chromium and can result in its deficiency[21]. Appropriate intake for young men is less than 35 g/day, and that for young women is less than 25g/day[22].

Whole grains, cereals, broccoli and mushrooms, liver, spices, and processed meats are all good sources of chromium.

3.2.3 MANGANESE

Manganese is critical for the metabolism of lipids, proteins, and carbohydrates. It is vital for blood sugar control, energy metabolism, a healthy immune system, reproduction, digestion, and protection from reactive oxygen species (ROS)[12]. Some metalloenzymes require this trace element for their normal functioning. Arginase, phosphoenolpyruvate decarboxylase, glutamine synthetase, and manganese superoxide dismutase are examples of such enzymes[23–25]. Overexposure to manganese, either through diet or inhalation, results in toxicity. This includes oxidative stress, apoptosis, mitochondrial dysfunction, protein misfolding, autophagy dysregulation, endoplasmic reticulum stress, and impairment of other metal homeostasis. However, there are few accounts of manganese deficiency in people, with incidences of transitory dermatitis, hypercholesterolemia, and the development of osteoporosis in women being recorded[12]. Nuts, bread, and cereal items are the main sources of manganese in diet[26]. Adult men and women require 2.3 and 1.8 mg of Mn per day, respectively, with an acceptable upper intake level of 11 mg per day for adults[23].

3.2.4 IODINE

Iodine is critical to the development and normal functioning of thyroid hormone. The importance of thyroid hormones in human growth and development gives iodine a vital role in nutrition. Iodine deficiency disorders (IDD) are currently used to describe the consequences of iodine deficiency on growth and development, which can occur at any stage of development but are most common in the fetus, neonate, and infant[22]. These disorders include hypothyroidism and goiter. Excess iodine intake can, likewise, result in hypothyroidism. Recommended dietary allowance of iodine in adult is 150μg.

Goiter surveys, determining urinary iodine excretion, and measuring thyroid hormone and pituitary thyroid stimulating hormone (TSH) levels can all be used to determine iodine nutritional status[27]. Iodized salt has long been the most prevalent way to ensure appropriate iodine intake. Seafood and foods cultivated on high-iodine soils are also good sources of iodine.

3.2.5 MOLYBDENUM

Most foods contain molybdenum, but the main sources include legumes, dairy products, and meats. This metal is vital because it is part of the molybdenum cofactor complex. It serves as an essential co-factor for three mammalian enzymes xanthine oxidase (XO), aldehyde oxidase (AO), and sulfite oxidase (SO)[28]. These enzymes help the body metabolize sulfites as well as break down waste products and toxins. High intake of molybdenum can be hazardous, resulting in joint discomfort, anemia, and diarrhea. Deficiency is very uncommon. The daily recommended intake for adults is 45 mcg.

3.2.6 COPPER

Copper is one of the most abundant minerals in the human body, with the liver and brain containing the most. This mineral is necessary in the release of energy as well as the formation of key enzymes that help antioxidants scavenge free radicals. Some of the notable functions of copper include the formation and regulation of hormones such as melatonin, the production of neurotransmitters like norepinephrine and other neuroactive substances like catecholamines and enkephalins, the production of collagen and red blood cells, the oxidation of fatty acids, as well as the absorption of iron and proper functioning of vitamin C, to name a few.

Copper's interaction with zinc is one of its most notable properties, which frequently results in deficiency in the body. When the body has a higher quantity of zinc, zinc and copper compete for the same absorption sites in the digestive system, which ultimately prevents adequate copper absorption and results in copper deficiency[29]. This deficiency is often characterized by a significant decrease in the ceruloplsamic activity of the plasma and inhibition of optimal iron release from the liver and other iron-storing tissues like the skeletal muscles, spleen, and bone marrow[22]. Furthermore, the symptoms of copper deficiency are often evidenced in the malfunctioning of systems and metabolic processes that rely on zinc. For instance, zinc deficiency can result in hormonal imbalance due to copper's involvement in several hormonal systems; this means that organs and tissues contained within such systems can become dysfunctional – e.g., dysfunction of the brain, altered level of cholesterol and erythrocytes, and poor bone and joint function due to collagen deficiency[29].

Some of the food sources known to be rich in copper are tuna, liver, lamb, crab, shrimp, olives, nuts, garlic, and carrots. In addition to nutritional sources, copper can also be absorbed through the skin if worn as copper bands. Some people do this to aid in other to supplement their copper levels and aid in the treatment of inflammatory diseases. In fact, cookware, utensils, and copper pipes provide a significant portion of our dietary copper.

3.2.7 SELENIUM

Selenium content within the human body is estimated to be within the ranges of 13–20 mg. Brazilian nuts are reported to possess the highest concentration of dietary selenium, followed by lobster, crabs, tuna, and kidney. Eggs, fish, mushrooms, and cereals are also good sources of selenium[22].

Despite its toxicity in high concentrations, selenium is still required in trace amounts for the cellular functioning of several organisms. Preliminary research into selenium's biological role focused on its activity as a major constituent of thioredoxin reductase and glutathione peroxidase – antioxidant enzymes involved in the reduction of oxidized molecules in living cells. However, new findings purport an interconnected activity between iodine and selenium metabolism, which aids deiodinase (a selenium-containing enzyme) in the conversion of thyroxine to 3,5,3'-triiodothyronine.

3.3 CONCLUSION

The inadequate intake of an essential trace element may decline major biological functions of an organism and increasing the physiological levels of that element will ameliorate or avert the impaired biological function. However, one of the most complicated tasks is to pinpoint trace element deficiencies nutritionally as well as medically. The level of essential trace metals circulating in blood and stored in cells is managed and regulated by an intricate system in the human body. Decline of levels of trace elements might occur when there is impairment in the normal function of the body or when the amount of trace elements in food sources is below the recommended intake.

REFERENCES

[1] Locke A, Schneiderhan J, Zick SM. Diets for health: Goals and guidelines. Am Fam Phys. 2018; 97(11):721–728.
[2] Cena H, Calder PC. Defining a healthy diet: Evidence for the role of contemporary dietary patterns in health and disease. Nutrients. 2020; 12(2):334. doi:10.3390/nu12020334
[3] Echouffo-Tcheugui JB, Ahima RS. Does diet quality or nutrient quantity contribute more to health? J Clin Invest. 2019; 129(10):3969–3970.
[4] Adefegha SA. Functional foods and nutraceuticals as dietary intervention in chronic diseases; Novel perspectives for health promotion and disease prevention. J Diet Suppl. 2018; 15(6):977–1009.
[5] Gibson R. The role of diet and host related factors in nutrient bioavailability. Food Nutr Bull. 2007; 28:S77–100. doi:10.1177/15648265070281S108
[6] Samtiya M, Aluko RE, Dhewa T. Plant food anti-nutritional factors and their reduction strategies: An overview. Food Prod Process and Nutr. 2020; 2:6.
[7] Stark C. Guidelines for food and nutrient intake. In Biochemistry, Physiology and Molecular Aspects of Human Nutrition, 3rd ed.; Stipanuk MH, Caudill MA, Eds.; Elsevier Saunders: St. Louis, MO, USA, 2013; pp. 34–47.
[8] Stipanuk MH, Caudill MA. Structure and properties of the macronutrients. In Biochemistry, Physiology and Molecular Aspects of Human Nutrition, 3rd ed.; Stipanuk MH, Caudill MA, Eds.; Elsevier Saunders: St. Louis, MO, USA, 2013; p. 49.
[9] Stipanuk MH, Caudill MA. The vitamins. In Biochemistry, Physiology and Molecular Aspects of Human Nutrition, 3rd ed.; Stipanuk MH, Caudill MA, Eds.; Elsevier Saunders: St. Louis, MO, USA, 2013; pp. 537–539.
[10] Stipanuk MH, Caudill MA. The minerals and water. In Biochemistry, Physiology and Molecular Aspects of Human Nutrition, 3rd ed.; Stipanuk MH, Caudill MA, Eds.; Elsevier Saunders: St. Louis, MO, USA, 2013; pp. 719–720.
[11] Fairweather-Tait S, Cashman K. Minerals and trace elements. World Rev Nutr Diet. 2015; 111:45–52. doi:10.1159/000362296.
[12] Vinha AF, et al. Trace minerals in human health: Iron, zinc, copper, manganese and fluorine. Int J Sci Res. 2019; 13(3):57–80.
[13] Maham LK, Escott-Stump S, Raymond JL. Krause: Alimentos, Nutrição e Dietoterapia. 13ª edição. Elsevier Saunders: Rio de Janeiro, 2012. ISBN: 978-85-352-5512-6.

[14] Freake HC, Sankavaram K. Zinc: Physiology, dietary sources, and requirements. In H. C. Freake, K. Sankavaram. (eds): Encyclopedia of Human Nutrition, 3rd ed.; Reference Module in Biomedical Sciences. Academic Press: Cambridge, MA, USA, 2013; pp. 437–443. doi:10.1016/B978-0-12-375083-9.00286-5.

[15] Bylund DB. Zinc. In Reference Module in Biomedical Sciences. 2017; pp. 568–572. doi:10.1016/B978-0-12-801238-3.66092-0.

[16] Kogan S, Sood A, Garnick MS. Zinc and wound healing: A review of zinc physiology and clinical applications. Wounds. 2017; 29(4):102–106. PMID: 28448263.

[17] Zhong W, Sun Q, Zhou Z. Chapter 12 – Role of zinc in alcoholic liver disease. In Vinood B. Patel. (ed): Molecular Aspects of Alcohol and Nutrition. Academic Press: Cambridge, MA, USA, 2016; pp. 143–156. doi:10.1016/B978-0-12-800773-0.00012-4.

[18] Garland T. Chapter 36 – Zinc. In Ramesh C. Gupta. (ed): Veterinary Toxicology, 3rd ed., Basic and Clinical Principles. Academic Press: Cambridge, MA, USA, 2018; pp. 489–492. doi:10.1016/B978-0-12-811410-0.00036-2.

[19] Offenbacher FG, Pi-Sunyer FX. Chromium in human nutrition. Ann Rev Nutr. 1988;8:543–563.

[20] Simonoff M. Chromium deficiency and cardiovascular risk. Cardiovasc Res. 1984; 18(10):591–596. doi:10.1093/cvr/18.10.591

[21] Stoecker BJ. Chromium. In Present Knowledge in Nutrition; Brown ML, Ed.; International Life Science Institute: Washington, DC, 1990; pp. 287–293.

[22] Aliasgharpour M, Farzami M. Trace elements in human nutrition: A review. Inter J Med Invest. 2013; 2:115–128.

[23] Institute of Medicine (US). Dietary reference intakes for vitamin A, vitamin K, arsenic, boron, chromium, copper, iodine, iron, manganese, molybdenum, nickel, silicon, vanadium, and zinc. In Panel on Micronutrients. National Academies Press (US): Washington, DC, 2001.7/30/2019.www.nap.edu.

[24] Aschner JL, Aschner M. Nutritional aspects of manganese homeostasis. Mol Aspects Med. 2005; 26(4–5):353–362. doi:10.1016/j.mam.2005.07.003.

[25] Li L, Yang X. The essential element manganese, oxidative stress, and metabolic diseases: Links and interactions. Oxid Med Cell Longev. 2018; Article ID 7580707, 11 pages. doi:10.1155/2018/7580707.

[26] Reilly C. The Nutritional Trace Metals. Blackwell Publishing Ltd: Brisbane, Australia, 2004.

[27] Hetzal BS, Potter BJ, Dulberg EM. The iodine deficiency disorders: Nature, pathogenesis and epidemiology. World Rev Nutr Diet. 1990; 62:59–119.

[28] Sardesai VM. Molybdenum: An essential trace element. Nutr Clin Pract. 1993; 8(6):277–281. doi:10.1177/0115426593008006277

[29] Chan S. Gerson B. Subramaniam S. The role of copper, molybdenum, selenium, and zinc in nutrition and health. Clin Lab Med. 1998; Dec18(4):673–685.

4 Drug-Nutrient Interactions

Oluwafisayo Modupe Gbadeyan,
Johnson Olaleye Oladele, and
Adenike Temidayo Oladiji

4.1 INTRODUCTION

Nutrition is the study of food and how it is used by our body as an energy source for growth, reproduction, and wellbeing (Ekesa *et al.*, 2018). It is the process of supplying the nutrients required for healthy growth, development, and life. Food is required for the body's basic metabolism, which processes energy and nutrients to support life (Smolin, 2019). It is essential for the body's fundamental metabolism, which involves the breakdown of nutrients to their absorbable form and releases of energy. It helps to sustain life, strengthen the immune system, aid in recovery from illness and disease, and aid in growth and development (Smolin, 2019).

Extrinsic and intrinsic variables impact nutrition metabolism and the function of both nutrients and non-nutrient components of food, both individually and in concert (Chen *et al.*, 2018). Examples of extrinsic variables that affect nutrient absorption and bioavailability include food, xenobiotics, interactions with prescription medicines, smoking, and alcohol usage (Moran *et al.*, 2018), while intrinsic factors include sex, age, and gene variants (Chen *et al.*, 2018).

Drugs are chemicals known to have biological effects on humans and other animals and are used to treat, cure, alleviate, prevent, diagnose, or improve physical or mental health (Hejaz and Rafik, 2015). Drugs can be taken to either prevent an ailment or to cure and/or relieve individuals of its symptoms.

Drugs are administered in a variety of ways, including oral, sublingual, rectal, intravenous, intramuscular, vaginal, and intranasal routes (Kim and De Jesus, 2022). Some medications, particularly botanicals, are inhaled. The severity of illness or sickness, the location of infection, and the status of the patients all influence the drug-delivery method.

Because of its ease and convenience, oral administration is the most often-utilized method of administration, which improves patient compliance (Bardal *et al.*, 2011). However, when certain foods and certain nutrients in foods are consumed simultaneously with certain pharmaceuticals, the total bioavailability of the food and/or the medication – as well as the pharmacokinetics, pharmacodynamics, and therapeutic effectiveness of the medications – may be affected (Mohammad and Mohammad, 2009; Van-Zyl, 2011).

4.2 DRUG ABSORPTION AND METABOLISM

Drug metabolism refers to the chemical events that occur in the body that allow medications to be readily eliminated. Drug metabolism is the biological conversion of drugs from one chemical form to another, which is generally accomplished by specialized enzyme systems (Taxak and Bharatam, 2014).

Drugs can be metabolized by hydrolysis, oxidation, conjugation, reduction, hydration, condensation, or isomerization. Pharmacological metabolism rates are altered by hereditary variables, concomitant illnesses (especially chronic liver disorders and severe heart failure), and drug interactions (particularly those involving induction or inhibition of metabolism) (Le, 2020).

Drug and xenobiotic metabolism is frequently biphasic (Testa and Bernd, 2015). The first step involves oxidation, reduction, or hydrolysis and is known as the functionalization process. CYP450, a microsomal superfamily of isoenzymes that catalyzes the oxidation of numerous medications, is

DOI: 10.1201/9781003361497-5

the most significant enzyme system in phase I metabolism (Le, 2020), while the subsequent stage includes glucuronidation. Glucuronidation is a conjugation process in which glucuronic acid, produced the cofactor UDP-glucuronic acid, is covalently bonded to a substrate bearing a nucleophilic functional group, and the resulting product, known as a glucuronide, is normally expelled in bile and urine (Hodgson, 2012). Most medications become more soluble and readily excreted by the kidneys as a result of this conjugation process, which happens mostly in the liver.

4.3   DRUG INTERACTIONS

A drug interaction is the interaction of a drug with another substance, such as another drug or a certain type of food that inhibits the drug from working properly (Debnath *et al.*, 2017). The presence of one or more interacting agents alters the pharmacokinetics or pharmacodynamics of medications in the body (Gallicano and Drusano, 2022). An interaction can change a drug's metabolism, reducing its efficacy and causing a variety of negative effects. CYP450 enzymes, which catalyze the oxidation of many medicines (Guengerich, 2018), for example, can be stimulated or inhibited by these pharmaceuticals and other related compounds, resulting in drug interactions.

Drug interactions can take different forms. It can occur when a drug interacts with another drug, with co-ingested food or nutrients, or with an ailment, herbal medicine, or other extrinsic chemicals.

4.3.1   DRUG-DRUG INTERACTION

Drug-drug interactions (DDIs) result when at least two medications react with one another. DDIs can be classified into pharmacokinetic (PK) and pharmacodynamic (PD) DDIs. Pharmacokinetic associations result from modifications in a medication's ingestion, circulation, digestion, or discharge attributes. They are collaborations that happen when one medication (the perpetrator) changes the centralization of another medication (the object), with clinical outcomes (Snyder *et al.*, 2012). Such clinical outcomes might result from changed bioavailability, digestion, and discharge of medication. Conversely, pharmacodynamic drug-drug interactions occur when interacting drugs either increase or decrease the overall effect of a drug.

4.3.2   FOOD-DRUG INTERACTION

A broader term that describes the effects of a drug on nutritional status is food-drug interactions. Food-drug interaction is defined as the alteration of pharmacodynamics or pharmacokinetics of a drug or nutritional element or a compromise in nutritional status as a result of the addition of the drug (Venkateswarulu, 2014).

Food-drug interaction is a more comprehensive word that describes the effects of medicine on nutrient status. It is characterized by a change of pharmacodynamics or pharmacokinetics of a medicine or nutrient component or a split in dietary status as a result of the medication's expansion (Venkateswarulu, 2014).

Food varieties can upset drug action at different stages in various ways. They can lessen a medication's viability by hampering it from arriving at the circulation system and respective site of activity. Food varieties may, likewise, contain supplements or different mixtures that influence how a medication is utilized in the body and discharged from the body. High fat, high protein, and fibre have been reported to significantly affect drug assimilation (Ayo *et al.*, 2005). It's fundamental to take note that taking specific medications with food diminishes the adequacy of medications, while others show stimulatory impact (Bushra *et al.*, 2011).

Chelation of dietary components is a common source of food-drug interactions. When such interaction or chelation occurs between a drug and nutrients in food, it is specifically referred to as a drug-nutrient interaction.

4.4   DRUG/NUTRIENT INTERACTION

Drug-nutrient interactions are defined as physical, physiologic, pathophysiologic, or chemical relationships between a drug and a nutrient (Chan, 2013) that results in changes in the medication's impact because of the nutrient's interaction or changes in the nutrient as a result of the drug. In other words, it refers to the change in the nutritional status of an individual or the effectiveness of a medication when drugs and diets are taken concurrently. Drug–nutrient interactions can be broadly categorized into two. The first category involves drugs that adversely influence dietary status by incapacitating the intake of food, and additionally, the assimilation, digestion, and evacuation of nutrients. The second, on the other hand, involves the impact of dietary status on drug metabolism by altering their assimilation, and in some cases, their efficacy (Van-Zyl, 2011).

Drugs may also wreak havoc on a person's nutritional status. While some drugs block the absorption of nutrients, others affect how the body utilizes and excretes them, especially vitamins and minerals (Bobroff *et al.*, 2009). These interactions can cause a lot of problems, but having enough knowledge about the drugs and when they should be taken will go a long way in limiting drug-nutrient interactions.

4.4.1   Effects of Drug Interaction

Drug-nutrient interactions occur through a variety of mechanisms. This mechanism, as illustrated in Figure 4.1, can involve a direct or indirect medication-related side-effect.

4.4.1.1   Direct Drug-Nutrient Interactions

Changes in nutrient absorption, metabolism, and excretion are all direct effects of drugs on nutrient bioavailability. Diffusion, convective transport, active transport, facilitated transport, ion-pair transport, and endocytosis are among gastrointestinal absorption mechanisms that might be hampered by drug interactions. The obstruction of absorption processes occurs majorly by chelation of compounds, adsorption of compounds, altered gastric pH, altered gastric emptying, altered intestinal motility, and altered active and passive intestinal transport (Debnath *et al.*, 2017; Kashuba and Bertino, 2022). Furthermore, medicines can enhance or reduce the urine excretion of nutrients, resulting in greater dietary needs for that nutrient (Bellows and Moore, 2022).

Direct medication side effects may be severe enough to cause nutritional insufficiency and/or toxicity, affecting body functions like bone formation, immune system function, and energy metabolism (Pronsky *et al.*, 2015).

4.4.1.2   Indirect Drug-Nutrient Interactions

Medication, on the other hand, has an indirect effect on the volume and range of foods ingested by an individual, which can result in weight gain and/or the development of nutritional deficiency illnesses.

Changes in appetite, taste and smell, a dry or sore mouth, epigastric pain, nausea, vomiting, diarrhea, and constipation are some of the indirect effects of drugs on nutritional absorption. For example, it is generally known that chemotherapy medications cause nausea and vomiting, which is linked to a higher risk of malnutrition (Genser, 2008).

4.5   CELLULAR AND MOLECULAR MECHANISMS IN DRUG-NUTRIENT INTERACTIONS

According to recent studies, the effects of medications can be changed by foods through interference with pharmacokinetic or pharmacodynamic processes (Jensen *et al.*, 2015). The terms

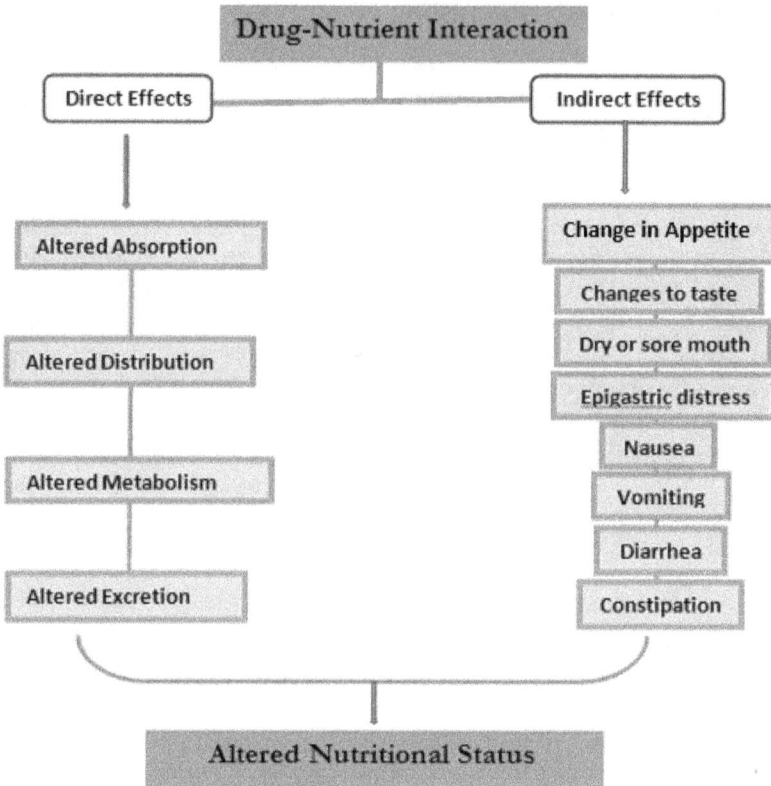

FIGURE 4.1 Mechanism of drug-nutrient interaction.

"absorption," "distribution," "metabolism," and "excretion" all refer to pharmacokinetics. On the other hand, pharmacodynamic processes are connected to the mechanisms of drug action, resulting in the therapeutic effect of pharmaceuticals; interactions between food and drugs may unintentionally lessen or improve the therapeutic effect of drugs (Bushra *et al.*, 2011).

Food-derived natural compounds (i.e., phytochemicals), which are biologically active toward a wide range of proteins involved in drug absorption, distribution, metabolism, excretion, and action, primarily exert their influence on drug pharmacokinetic or pharmacodynamic processes at the molecular level. Various mechanisms of food drug interactions are described in the following sections.

4.5.1 PHYSIOLOGIC AND PHYSICOCHEMICAL MECHANISMS

The consumption of food causes physiological reactions that modify the physicochemical characteristics of the luminal contents of the gastrointestinal system. Often, the binding of medications by food components are what produce meal-induced alterations in the physicochemical properties of intraluminal contents. Physiologic/mechanical mechanisms that alter drug absorption, distribution, metabolism, and/or excretion include delayed gastric emptying, increased bile secretion or splanchnic blood flow, and gastrointestinal pH or flora changes (Won *et al.*, 2012). Alterations of such processes can lead to reduced absorption of drugs such as penicillins and angiotensin-converting enzyme inhibitors (Singh, 1999).

4.5.1.1 Luminal Fluid Solubility

For more than 30 years, it has been understood that diet can impact how medications are metabolized (Koziolek *et al.*, 2019). Solubility as well as the availability and composition of luminal fluids is of major importance in oral drug absorption as reduced solubility limits oral drug absorption. Therefore, changes in the luminal conditions caused by food in the human GI system can cause variations in the bioavailability of medications (Koziolek *et al.*, 2019).

4.5.1.2 Concentration Gradient

Absorption can occur passively (through concentration gradients) or actively (by transporters). Passive drug absorption is fueled by the existence of a concentration gradient between the blood and the intestinal lumen (Koziolek *et al.*, 2019; Van Den Abeele *et al.*, 2017; Grimm *et al.*, 2018).

Additionally, due to non-linear pharmacokinetics, in the case of medications with poor water solubility, many transporters and drug-metabolizing enzymes in the enterocytes may be saturable, which causes even minor changes in luminal concentration to have significant consequences. It is anticipated that fluid quantities will considerably contribute to the occurrence of food effects on oral medication bioavailability, since fluid volumes have a variety of effects on luminal drug concentration (Koziolek *et al.*, 2019).

4.5.1.3 Luminal pH Value

One of the factors that determine the degree of ionization of a drug in its solution is the pH of the solution (Gaohua *et al.*, 2021). Many drugs are ionizable above or below a certain pH value; hence, luminal pH is one of the most important determinants of drug solubility and absorption (Koziolek *et al.*, 2019). Usually, a drug's ability to dissolve more quickly is aided by its increased ionization. As a result, changes in luminal pH values may have a direct impact on variations in drug solubility and even alter oral bioavailability.

4.5.1.4 Interaction with Intestinal Monolayer: Membrane Fluidity

Theoretically, since an increase in fluidity can speed up the diffusion of some medications, molecules that improve intestinal monolayer fluidity have the potential to affect drug absorption. It has been demonstrated that flavonoids, cholesterol, and tocopherol all partition into cellular membranes, enhancing the fluidity of those membranes (Arora *et al.*, 2000). These in vitro discoveries, however, have not yet been proven to have clinical relevance.

4.5.2 Biochemical Mechanisms

The food ingredient modifies the activity of drug-metabolizing enzymes and transporters through biochemical processes (Chan, 2002), some of which are detailed in the following sections.

4.5.2.1 Interaction with Uptake and Efflux Transporters

Food-drug interactions often originate when drug and nutrient molecules compete for the same transport pathway. In order to absorb, eliminate, and metabolize a wide range of nutrients, enterocytes have a large array of enzymes and transporters. Food-drug interactions at the level of the intestinal monolayer are unavoidable, since drug molecules can travel along the same pathways to enter the systemic circulation. The modulation of intestinal enzymes and transporters by a number of plant-derived drinks may have adverse pharmacokinetic (PK) and pharmacodynamic (PD) effects. Some examples of food-drug interactions involving transporters are described in the following sections.

4.5.2.1.1 Uptake Transporter-Oligopeptide Transporter (PEPT1)

Organic anion-transporting polypeptides (OATP) are multi-specific transporters located in numerous epithelia throughout the body that mediate the cellular uptake of a broad range of substrates (Roth et al., 2012). Bile acids, thyroid hormones, prostaglandins, and bilirubin glucuronides are just a few of the endogenous substrates that OATP transports (Shitara et al., 2013). Statins, protease inhibitors, fexofenadine, midazolam, montelukast, aliskiren, and talinolol are examples of common drugs that can be metabolized by them (Nakanishi and Tamai, 2015; Shitara et al., 2013; Tamai, 2012). Numerous studies in humans have proven a clinically substantial decrease in the intestinal absorption of these medications when taken with grapefruit, orange, and apple juice (Imanaga et al., 2011; Mougey et al., 2009; Shirasaka et al., 2013), which contain a variety of flavonoids that are thought to be responsible for the reduced drug absorption (Koziolek et al., 2019). OATP1A2 has been discovered to be inhibited in vitro by flavonol glycosides and catechins found in herbal extracts and green tea as well (Roth et al., 2011).

4.5.2.1.2 Efflux Transporter P-Glycoprotein

The most extensively researched efflux transporter and a recognized modulator of clinically significant interactions between food and drugs is P-glycoprotein (P-gp). This transporter is present in a variety of organs, but its prominent intestine presence is particularly important when discussing interactions between food and drugs (Marchetti et al., 2007). Medications such as antiarrhythmics, antihypertensive, cyclosporine, tacrolimus, and morphine are just a few of the many substrates of P-glycoprotein (P-gp) that have been discovered (Nakanishi and Tamai, 2015).

The primary dietary inhibitors of P-gp are believed to be furanocoumarins and flavonoids, which can be found in a wide variety of fruits and vegetables. Other efflux transporters, such as multidrug resistance associated proteins (MRPs), are frequently inhibited by flavonoids (Koziolek et al., 2019). It has been shown that sodium taurocholate (bile salt) and common lipid breakdown products limit P-gp activity in vitro (Ingels et al., 2004). In addition, when grapefruit juice is consumed along with recognized P-gp substrates, a number of clinically significant interactions have been noted.

Drug concentrations can change locally and systemically as a result of inhibiting efflux transporters. These transporters, being located on the apical (luminal) membrane of enterocytes, extrude substrates back into the intestinal lumen, which reduces systemic drug concentrations (Huang et al., 2010). Consequently, intestinal P-gp inhibition may result in increased systemic drug exposure (Won et al., 2012).

4.5.2.2 Inhibition of Drug Metabolizing Enzymes

Major enzymes in drug metabolism, such as cytochrome P450 and phase II conjugation enzymes, can be altered. There are compounds in some drinks that can modify the transporters and enzymes in the intestine that metabolize drugs. Tea, alcoholic beverages, and common fruit juices all contain phytochemicals that block phase II conjugation enzymes and intestine cytochrome P450 (Won et al., 2012; Rodríguez-Fragoso et al., 2011) as explained in the following sections.

4.5.2.2.1 Phase I of Drug Metabolism

4.5.2.2.1.1 Cytochromes P450 The majority of clinically significant adverse medication interactions are caused by the activation or inhibition of the cytochrome P450 (CYP) enzymes, which catalyze the initial Phase I metabolism of most medicines to produce more water-soluble metabolites (Lin and Lu, 2001). The CYP3A subfamily is the most prevalent among the CYPs expressed in the intestine and has been shown to affect how drugs are disposed of in vivo (Lin and Lu, 2001; Paine et al., 2006). Although substrate specificity for CYP3A is low (Wienkers, 2001), CYP3A is in charge of the oxidative metabolism of more than half of the medications now on the market (Guengerich,

1999). Increased blood levels of the parent drug and potential drug toxicity result from CYP3A, and this occurs more often than CYP3A induction (Tanaka, 1998).

Numerous studies have been conducted in vitro and on human subjects to examine the effects of various fruit juices on CYP3A expression and activity and specific inhibitory components in have also been identified and characterized.

One of the most well-investigated dietary ingredients, grapefruit juice, has been demonstrated to block the enteric metabolism of many CYP3A substrates (Hanley *et al.*, 2011). According to Paine et al., 2005, grapefruit can increase the amount of a medicine that is absorbed into the body by preventing the CYP3A-mediated pre-systemic (first-pass) metabolism in the intestine. The following oral drugs have been shown to be adversely affected by grapefruit: felodipine, nifedipine, verapamil, terfenadine, ethinyl estradiol, midazolam, saquinavir, simvastatin, and ciclosporin (Sagira *et al.*, 2003).

Furanocoumarins have been identified as key mediators of the Grape Fruit Juice (GFJ) effect in people. Examples of these compounds are bergamottin, epoxy bergamottin, and 6',7'-dihydroxybergamottin (Paine *et al.*, 2006). Flavonoids such as naringenin, naringin, quercetin, kaempferol have also been identified to be implemental in CYP3A4 inhibition. All block CYP3A4 in vitro; however, investigations with a few components in vivo have only detected minor or conflicting modulatory effect (Basheer and Kerem, 2015). Modes of intestinal CYP3A inhibition include protein degradation, reversible and mechanism-based inhibition (Paine *et al.*, 2004, 2005).

Juice prepared from Seville orange, botanically classified as *Citrus aurantium*, has been reported to contain furanocoumarins at concentrations comparable to GFJ (Guo *et al.*, 2000; Malhotra *et al.*, 2001). Seville orange juice has been shown to inhibit enteric CYP3A4 in vitro and in healthy subjects (Guo *et al.*, 2000; Malhotra *et al.*, 2001;). Trans-resveratrol (Piver *et al.*, 2001) and gallic acid (Stupans *et al.*, 2002) are also examples of substances that have been demonstrated to inhibit hepatic CYP3A in vitro in a mechanism-based and non-competitive and reversible manner.

4.5.2.2.2 Phase II of Drug Metabolism

4.5.2.2.2.1 Human Glucuronosyl Transferases (UGTs)
Human glucuronosyl transferases (UGTs) increase hydrophilicity by creating glucuronide conjugates, which aids in the removal of endogenous substrates and xenobiotics (Burchell *et al.*, 1995). In human liver microsomes, the inhibitory effects of commonly used herbal extracts on UGT1A4, 1A6, and 1A9 activities were assessed (Mohamed and Frye, 2011). Epigallocatechin gallate (EGCG), a component of green tea, reduced UGT1A4 activity (IC50 = 33.83.1 g/mL), while tea catechin supplementation increased UGT activity.

4.5.2.2.2.2 Sulfotransferases (SULTs)
A complicated, long-lived organism's growth and development must be strictly controlled, and chemical pollutants must be removed before cause serious harm the organism. The cytosolic sulfotransferases (SULTs) are a class of enzymes that perform both of these tasks in humans and are also involved in the metabolism of xenobiotics like phenol-based steroids, thyroid hormones, dopamine, and pharmaceuticals (Figure 4.2).

Sulfotransferases (SULTs) are Phase II biotransformation enzymes that catalyze the sulfate conjugation of numerous xenobiotic molecules (Suiko *et al.*, 2017). Through the reaction, they catalyze, the co-factor PAPS (3-phosphoadenosine-5-phosphosulfate) transfers a sulfonate group onto the hydroxyl (−OH) or amino (−NH$_2$) group of the substrate compound, creating a more water-soluble derivative that typically differs from the parent drug in terms of its pharmacological characteristics.

The liver, brain, colon, lung, kidney, and other tissues have all been found to have three different human SULT subfamilies (Gamage *et al.*, 2006). SULT1As are vital xenobiotic and ingested catecholamine precursor defense mechanisms (Harris and Waring, 2008).

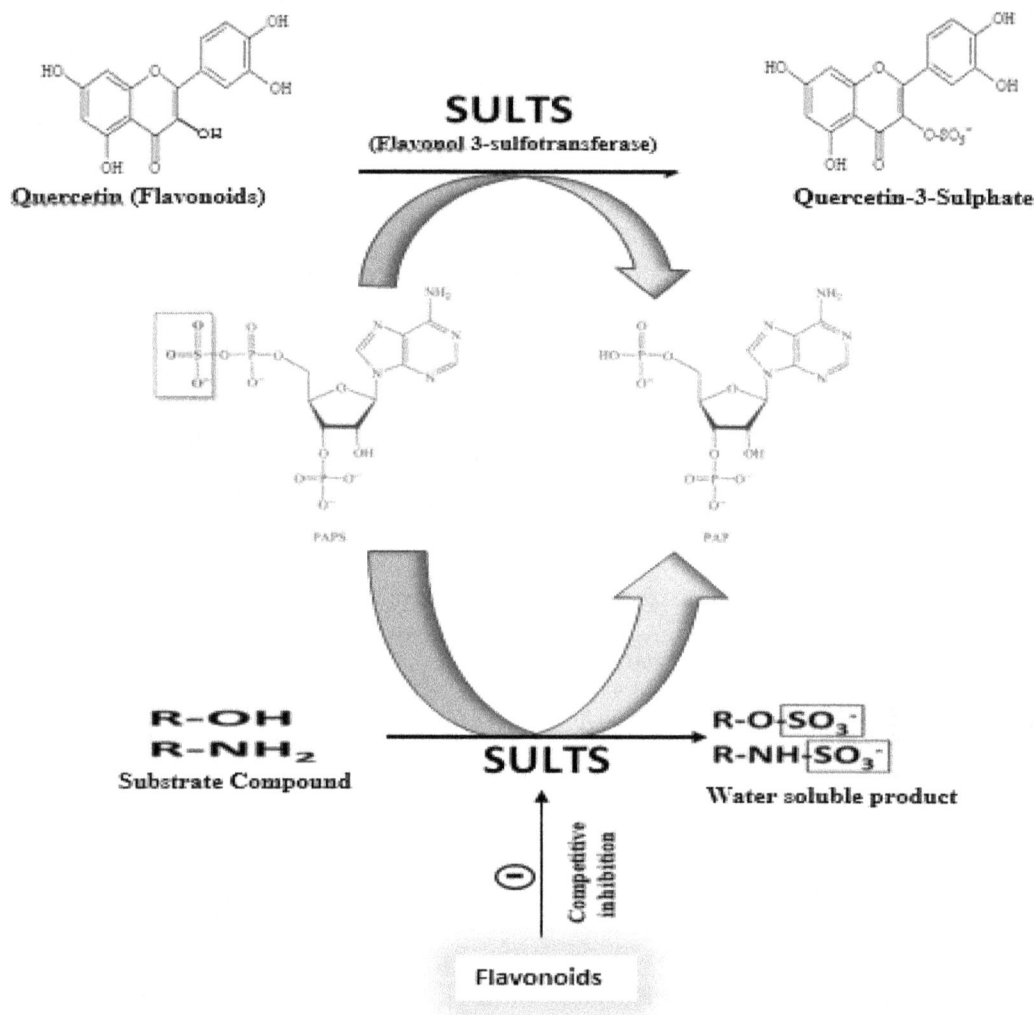

FIGURE 4.2 A diagrammatic representation of sulfation of flavonoids. PAP, 3′-phosphoadenosine 5′-phosphate; PAPS, 3′-phosphoadenosine 5′-phosphosulfate; SULTS, Sulfotransferase.

Flavonoids and isoflavonoids, classes of polyphenolic chemicals that are widely present throughout the plant kingdom, have been shown to significantly inhibit SULT 1A1. This could have a considerable impact on how pharmaceuticals are sulfated in the digestive tract, which is a crucial metabolic process for the metabolism of numerous xenobiotics, medications, and endogenous compounds (Harris and Waring, 2008). The amounts of free neurotransmitters can also rise as a result of food components inhibiting the SULT isoforms, which might increase the likelihood of a migraine attack.

The presence of two neighboring groups on a benzene ring is one motif that appears to be crucial in raising the inhibitory effectiveness of compounds for SULT 1A1. Flavonoids also possibly acts as competitive inhibitor of SULT 1A1 due to its 3, 4-hydroxyl group that can be sulfated.

4.6   TYPES OF DRUG-NUTRIENT INTERACTIONS

Based on their nature and the established mode of occurrence, drug-nutrient interactions can be categorized into four types (Type I, II, III, and IV).

4.6.1 Type I Drug-Nutrient Interaction

Type 1 reactions are ex vivo bio-inactivation events that occur before medicines or food enter an organism. They are biochemical or physical events that occur between a medicine and a dietary ingredient or formulation, such as hydrolysis, oxidation, neutralization, precipitation, or the formation of complexes (Genser, 2008).

4.6.2 Type II Drug-Nutrient Interaction

These are in vivo interactions that impact absorption and, as a result, cause bioavailability to increase or decrease (Genser, 2008). Conceivable components by which they impact assimilation in the gastrointestinal tract include alteration of the capacity/activity of enzymes, complexation, restriction or deactivation of cycles, and change of transport mechanisms.

4.6.3 Type III Drug-Nutrient Interaction

Type III drug-nutrient interactions include changes in cell or tissue circulation, systemic transport, and infiltration of medications, or supplements to specific organs or tissues can happen (Genser, 2008). These interactions occur after the medicine or nutrient has passed through the gastrointestinal tract and entered the systemic circulation.

4.6.4 Type IV Drug-Nutrient Interaction

Type IV interactions obstruct drug or nutrient removal or clearance from the body, possibly by antagonizing, impairing, or modulating renal and/or enterohepatic elimination (Chan, 2006; Genser, 2008).

4.7 DRUG INTERACTION RISK FACTORS

The likelihood of adverse interactions between foods and drugs is affected by various factors, as illustrated in Figure 4.3. These factors include age, reduced hepatic and renal function, poor nutritional and gastrointestinal status, multiple and prolonged medication therapy, intake of exclusionary diets, time of drug administration, and addiction to substances such as alcohol (Van-Zyl, 2011; Debnath *et al.*, 2017; Utermohlen, 2022).

4.7.1 Age as a Predisposing Factor of Drug-Nutrient Interaction

Different age groups have their peculiarity and response to drugs. Discoveries support the perception that basal metabolic rate decreases almost linearly with age (Shimokata and Kuzuya, 1993;

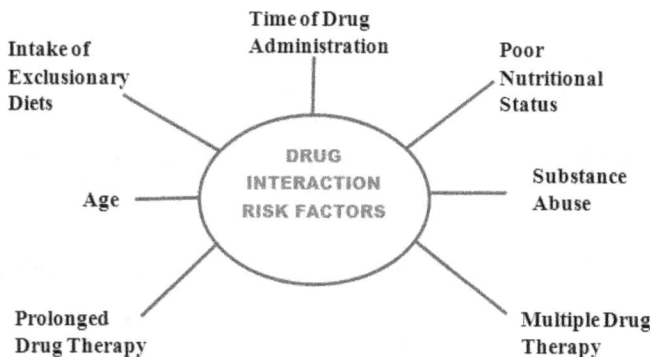

FIGURE 4.3 Major drug-interaction risk factors.

Krems *et al.*, 2005). Older patients are often treated with medications on a daily basis, and they tend to have reduced metabolic reserves, which predisposes them to drug-nutrient interactions. Drug intake, distribution, metabolism, and excretion are affected to varying degrees by the aging process itself and by diseases often associated with aging (Kirkwood, 2008).

Physiological changes associated with aging, such as decreased intestinal blood flow, altered gastrointestinal motility and absorption, decreased blood flow to the liver and kidneys, and increased gastric pH, may make it difficult for many medicines to be metabolized (Russell *et al.*, 1993; Ortolani *et al.*, 2013). Although aging has been found to inhibit processes in the first phase of drug metabolism, which includes oxidation, reduction, and hydrolysis, phase II (conjugation) does not appear to be significantly affected by age (Chapron, 2001; Ortolani *et al.*, 2013).

Age-related impact on drug or nutrient metabolism is not limited to the elderly, but it also affects children, especially those below the age of five, who find it difficult to swallow medications and tend to be selective with regard to the taste of substances. Consequently, crushing tablets, opening capsules, and mixing medications with food to enhance palatability can lead to drug-nutrient interactions (Kotzer *et al.*, 2010). Type I drug-nutrient interaction, which occurs between a medicine and a dietary ingredient or formulation before they are taken into the body, seems to be prevalent amongst this age group.

4.7.2   Nutritional Status as a Predisposing Factor of Drug-Nutrient Interaction

Malnutrition is defined as nutritional intake deficits or excesses, essential nutrient imbalances, or inadequate nutrient utilization that results in undernutrition, being overweight, or obesity (WHO, 2022)

4.7.2.1   Drug Absorption in Undernourished State

Undernutrition refers to a person's inability to achieve his or her daily energy and nutrient requirements in order to be healthy. It is characterized by exhaustion, stunting, being underweight, and vitamin and mineral deficiency (WHO, 2022). Protein Energy Malnutrition (PEM) has a deleterious impact on medication absorption, distribution, and clearance. The degree of altered body composition and function associated with PEM may affect drug disposal in different ways. Drug absorption may be reduced, protein carriers limited, and metabolism slowed in severe cases of PEM, leading to increased drug concentrations and risk of toxicity, particularly with medications with a narrow safety margin (Compher and Boullata, 2010).

4.7.2.2   Drug Absorption in Obese State

Obesity is a chronic disorder with a complex pathophysiology involving genetic and environmental factors, which ultimately impact the balance between energy intake and expenditure and manifest as excess body fat (Boullata, 2010).

The subcutaneous and transdermal routes of drug delivery were found to have lower absorption rates in obesity when compared to the oral method, most likely due to diminished blood flow locally (Cho *et al.*, 2013).

Lipophilic drugs such as steroids, benzodiazepines, and tricyclic antidepressants have been reported to have a large volume of distribution in obese people because the physicochemical properties of the drug affect their distribution in the body. Polar molecules, however, do not appear to show significant differences in the volume of distribution when obese subjects are compared with non-obese subjects (EMA, 2018).

4.7.3   Exclusionary Feeding as a Predisposing Factor of Drug-Nutrient Interaction

Many people eliminate certain foods from their diet for diagnostic, preventive, and therapeutic purposes. This can be detrimental in terms of its effects on drug metabolism. It can also result in nutrient deficiencies, especially when a physician or dietitian/nutritionist is not consulted (Johnston *et al.*, 2004).

The exclusion of all animal products from diets (intake of vegan diets) by substituting with plant products results in nutrient-drug interactions. For example, soya products have a high isoflavone content and vegetarian and vegan diets – as well as Asian foods – are mainly based on soya (Niederberger and Parnham, 2021). Cytochrome P450 (CYP) enzymes and other cellular proteins involved in drug metabolism may be altered by isoflavones (Ronis, 2016). Clinical investigations have demonstrated that genistein, one of the main isoflavones in soya, reduces CYP1A2 and CYP2A6 activity, while causing a slight induction of CYP3A4 (Xiao *et al.*, 2012). A large increase in CYP3A4 content is often a problem because, when induced, they cause decreased bioavailability of their substrates, which include drugs such as calcium channel blockers, benzodiazepines, and lipid-lowering, resulting in reduced efficacy of the drugs (Horn and Hansten, 2008; Niederberger and Parnham, 2021).

Furthermore, some drugs, such as griseofulvin, require fat for optimal absorption (Btaiche *et al.*, 2010); therefore, significant elimination of this nutrient from diets may reduce the absorption and efficacy of such drugs.

4.7.4 ABUSE OF SUBSTANCE AS A PREDISPOSING FACTOR OF DRUG-NUTRIENT INTERACTION

Enzyme induction reactions can shorten the duration of a medication's action by boosting metabolic elimination. They occur as a result of smoking and long-term alcohol or drug usage (Bibi, 2008). Smoking increases the activity of medication metabolizing enzymes like CYP1A2, which is a molecular specie of P450, making therapeutic effects more difficult to achieve (Bibi, 2008).

Excessive alcohol intake can cause malnutrition or micronutrient deficiencies, such as zinc deficiency (Barve *et al.*, 2017). A calcium, magnesium, or zinc shortage in the diet can cause drug metabolism problems. The activity of drug-metabolizing enzymes is reduced by vitamin C deficiency, especially in the elderly. Macronutrients, vitamins, and minerals, as well as other nutritional elements, influence the effectiveness of the detoxification process and, as a result, the clearance of pharmaceuticals and other xenobiotics from the body (Bidlack *et al.*, 1986). Therefore, deficiencies in certain vitamins like riboflavin, ascorbic acid, and vitamins A and E, as well as minerals like iron, copper, zinc, and magnesium, may cause alterations in drug metabolism and clearance.

4.7.5 PROLONGED OR MULTIPLE DRUG THERAPY AS A PREDISPOSING FACTOR OF DRUG-NUTRIENT INTERACTION

Prolonged use of prescription and non-prescription medications as a result of chronic conditions like hypertension, diabetes, and cardiovascular disease can be extremely harmful to one's health. For example, prolonged use of Metformin medication lowers cobalamine (Vitamin B12) levels in the blood, which can contribute to megaloblastic anemia (Owhin *et al.*, 2019; Socha *et al.*, 2020).

Drug-nutrient interactions can also occur as a result of multiple drug therapy. For example, an overdose of sorbitol, a "sugar-free" sweetener that prevents crystallization of sucrose by serving as a solubilizing agent (Rollins, 2010), can be taken when patients are administered multiple drugs that contain the substance at the same time or in short intervals. This purgative medicine can cause gastrointestinal symptoms such as severe bloating, cramps, diarrhea, and flatulence (Hyams, 1983; Rollins, 2010). Hence, excessive consumption of sorbitol as a result of multiple drug intake can alter the gastrointestinal system, leading to reduced nutrient bioavailability. Therefore, caution must be taken to avoid prolonged or multiple usage of drugs, especially without prescription.

4.8 EFFECTS OF DRUG-NUTRIENT INTERACTION

Because medications and nutrients use comparable sites for absorption and are metabolized and eliminated through the same organs, drug-nutrient interactions influence the bioavailability of nutrients in many situations. Drugs with a restricted therapeutic window or side effects that affect appetite and stomach function are the most likely to have nutritional consequences. Also, drugs that must be taken for lengthy periods of time, those that require dietary restrictions or regulation, and those that compete directly with nutrients can also have an impact on nutritional status (Van-Zyl, 2011).

Common side effects include alteration in taste sensation, appetite, and smell, which can cause a change in food intake, irritation of gastrointestinal tract, stomach upset, nausea, vomiting, diarrhea, constipation, ulcers, gastric bleeding, and change in gastric pH (Bellows and Moore, 2022). Nephrotoxicity or hepatotoxicity sometimes occurs as a result of drug-nutrient interaction, since many drugs must pass through the liver and kidney upon excretion (Bellows and Moore, 2022).

4.8.1 DRUG CLASSES AND THEIR EFFECTS ON FOOD NUTRIENTS

Drugs are categorized based on their mechanism of action, the condition they treat, and their chemical structure (Karaman, 2015). Although some classes of drugs do not have any direct effect on nutrients, others can hamper nutrient availability and invariably cause nutritional deficiencies. Potential drug/nutrient interactions associated with specific classes of drugs are illustrated in the following sections.

4.8.1.1 Antacid and Gastric Acid Suppressants

Acid blockers inhibit stomach acid production, whereas antacids neutralize stomach acid. Long-term usage of these medications may cause nutritional deficits. One class of gastric acid suppressants – proton pump inhibitors – has been linked to an increased risk of vitamin and mineral deficiencies affecting vitamin B12, vitamin C, calcium, iron, and magnesium metabolism (Heidelbaugh, 2013; Presse and Perreault, 2015). Antacids like Maalox also bind to phosphate, causing weariness, weakness, and osteomalacia (Van-Zyl, 2011).

4.8.1.2 Antibiotics

Antibiotics have a twofold influence on nutritional bioavailability. While some antibiotics reduce nutrient absorption, others exhibit stimulatory effects. Antibiotics like tetracycline bind calcium and limit its absorption, resulting in bone and tooth lesions in young people (Van-Zyl, 2011). Erythromycin also inhibits calcium, folate, vitamin B6, and vitamin B12 absorption and action, which can lead to deficiency problems if taken for a long time (Shobha, 2019). On the contrary, some antibiotics stimulate growth, possibly by suppressing intestinal gram-positive microorganisms, which interfere with the absorption of nutrients (Eyssen and Somer, 1963; Chattopadhyay, 2014).

4.8.1.3 Laxatives

By speeding up the passage of materials through the digestive tract, laxatives lessens the time available for nutrients to be absorbed. Excessive use of this medicine can lead to a shortage in vitamins like A, D, E, and K, as well as minerals required for regular human function (Debnath et al., 2017; Bobroff et al., 2009).

4.8.1.4 Anticoagulant

Anticoagulants are medications that are used to treat thromboembolic illness, which is a condition in which blood clot forms in the vein and subsequently dislodges and travels through the bloodstream. They exert their effect by hindering the use of vitamin K (Schurgers et al., 2004). These drugs, like Warfarin, slow down blood clotting by decreasing the amount of vitamin K required for the activation of clotting factors (Ardahanli et al., 2018).

4.8.1.5 Anticonvulsant

Anticonvulsant medications, though effective in controlling seizures, can cause diarrhea and a loss of appetite (Bobroff et al., 2009). Consequently, many nutrients may become less available. These medicines also reduce the availability of vitamin D for crucial activities like calcium absorption and balance (Bobroff *et al.*, 2009; Soltani *et al.*, 2016). Anticonvulsant medication can cause macrocytic anemia, rickets, osteomalacia, delirium, depression, and lowered B vitamin concentrations, particularly vitamin B1, B2, B6, B8, and B9 in epileptic patients (Van-Zyl, 2011; Brodie *et al.*, 2013).

4.8.1.6 Blood Pressure Lowering Drugs

High blood pressure is managed using antihypertensives. Mineral levels such as potassium, calcium, and zinc can be influenced by these drugs (Bobroff *et al.*, 2009).

4.8.1.7 Immunosuppressants

Immunosuppressants such as Methotrexate, which is used to treat certain types of cancer or to control severe psoriasis or rheumatoid arthritis, reduces availability of the B vitamin (folic acid) (Ortiz *et al.*, 1998; Bobroff *et al.*, 2009).

4.8.1.8 Diuretic

Diuretics may be associated with increased urinary losses of both micro and macro nutrients (Berné *et al.*, 2005). While some diuretics limit mineral loss (especially potassium loss) (Bobroff *et al.*, 2009), others increase the urinary loss of nutrients such as phosphorous, nitrogen, sodium, zinc, potassium, magnesium, chloride, bicarbonate, fat-soluble vitamin retinol, vitamin C, calcium, vitamin B6, and thiamin (Mydlik *et al.*, 1999; Greenberg, 2000; Suter *et al.*, 2000; Berné *et al.*, 2005). This increased nutrient loss indicates that individuals using diuretics may be at risk of developing nutritional deficiencies.

4.8.2 EFFECT OF NUTRIENTS ON DRUG METABOLISM

Agents affecting drug-metabolizing enzymes have been found in food. Grapefruit, for instance, inhibits the most essential enzyme in drug metabolism, cytochrome P450 3A4 (CYP3A4) (Kirby and Unadkat, 2007).

Concurrent meal and medication intake can alter the pace of medication absorption, the magnitude of absorption, or both (Genser, 2008). This alteration in the absorption and bioavailability of drugs can be either stimulatory or inhibitory. Meal consumption can promote stomach and intestinal secretions, which can help with medicine breakdown and absorption. More particularly, higher-fat meals boost the intestinal absorption of highly lipophilic medicines by stimulating the release of bile salts. They also cause the release of cholecystokinin, which reduces gastrointestinal motility and lengthens the time the drug is in touch with the intestine, potentially increasing absorption. Other medications, on the other hand, are less well absorbed when taken with food. For example, bioavailability of Azithromycin is decreased by 43% reduction when taken with food (Størmer *et al.*, 1993).

In Table 4.1 are specific examples of nutrient-induced alterations in drug absorption.

4.8.3 HOW TO LOWER THE RISK OF DRUG-NUTRIENT INTERACTIONS

It is impossible to totally avoid ingesting both nutrients and pharmaceuticals, and this predisposes people to drug-nutrient interaction. To reduce the likelihood of these interactions patients must take the following steps:

- Read the warning labels on drugs and follow the recommendations on how to take them. Medications should not be taken without a prescription.
- When a new drug is prescribed, patients must provide detailed information about the drugs they are taking as well as any dietary restrictions or other substances they are taking.
- To avoid unfavorable drug-nutrient interactions, drug prescriptions should be confined to required treatments for as short a time as feasible, with a frequent re-evaluation of the treatment choice (Schmidt and Dalhoff, 2002).

TABLE 4.1

Drug-Nutrient Interaction Affecting Drug Bioavailability

Nutrient	Drug	Drug Interaction Effects	Effects
Fibre	Statins	High-fibre diets may reduce the efficacy of statin medications like Fluvastatin.	Paeng et al., 2007
Protein	Warfarin	Increased warfarin binding to serum albumin as a result of high-protein meals could reduce warfarin's anticoagulant action.	Beatty et al., 2005
Carbohydrate	Acetaminophen	Co-administration of acetaminophen with pectin, (the starch found in fruits and vegetables) delays its absorption.	Miller and Carthan, 2003
Fat	Cycloserine	High-fat diets lower cycloserine levels in the blood.	Zhu et al., 2001
	Hydrophilic drugs	Dietary fats obstruct the absorption of hydrophilic drugs.	Van-Zyl, 2011
	Theophyll	High-fat meals may increase the amount of theophylline in the body.	Bushra et al., 2011
	Albendazole	Increased solubility and absorption of drug.	Btaiche et al., 2010
	Griseofulvin	Increased disintegration and absorption of drug.	Btaiche et al., 2010
Minerals	Tetracycline	Calcium and iron form insoluble chelates with Tetracycline, and influences its bioavailability.	Gurley and Hagan, 2003
	Antibiotics	Divalent ions, such as calcium and magnesium, form complex with some antibiotics and prevent their absorption.	Bushra et al., 2011
	Antihypertensives	Excess sodium intake impairs beneficial effects of different antihypertensive drugs.	Heerspink et al., 2012
Vitamins	Anticoagulant medications	Vitamin K interferes with effectiveness and safety of warfarin therapy.	Holt, 1998
	Salicyclates	Vitamin C increases urinary acidity, decreases elimination of salicylates – e.g., aspirin.	Van-Zyl, 2011
	Iron	Ascorbic acid inhibition of iron chelation to phytates increases iron absorption and aids reduction of iron to the ferrous form.	Btaiche et al., 2010
Casein and calcium	Ciprofloxacin	Ciprofloxacin absorption is hampered by casein and calcium in milk.	Pápai et al., 2010

4.9   CONCLUSION

Because food and pharmaceuticals are absorbed through the same organs, drug-nutrient interaction can cause a drug's absorption to be affected by the presence of food in the digestive tract and vice versa. This is a major public health concern, with symptoms and effects ranging from mild to moderate and, in extreme cases, deadly. Flavonoids and furanocoumarins have been identified as major dietary constituents that interfere with drug metabolism. Interactions between drugs and nutrients aren't always harmful. Rather, they can be utilized to increase drug absorption or reduce side effects. To prevent the risks of drug-nutrient interactions, patients should always read the directions and warning labels that come with their medications and make sure to tell their doctor about any dietary restrictions, supplements, or medications they're taking before a new prescription is made.

REFERENCES

Ardahanli, I., Cengizhan, M. S., Celik, M. (2018). Nutrition Recommendations While Taking Warfarin. www. researchgate.net/publication/327883392_Nutrition_Recommendations_While_Taking_Warfarin

Arora, A., Byrem, T. M., Nair, M. G., Strasburg, G. M. (2000). Modulation of liposomal membrane fluidity by flavonoids and isoflavonoids. *Arch Biochem Biophys.* 373:102–109. https://doi.org/10.1006/abbi.1999.1525

Ayo, J. A., Agu, H., Madaki, I. (2005). Food and drug interactions: Its side effects. *Nutr Food Sci.* 35(4):243–252. doi:10.1108/00346650510605630

Bardal, S. K., Waechter, J. E., Martin, D. S. (2011). Pharmacokinectis. In Applied Pharmacology. St. Louis, MO, Elsevier/Saunders, Chapter 2, pp. 17–34. ISBN 978-1-4377-0310-8.

Barve, S., Chen, S. Y., Kirpich, I., Watson, W. H., Mcclain, C. (2017). Development, prevention, and treatment of alcohol-induced organ injury: The role of nutrition. *Alcohol Res: Curr Rev.* 38(2):289–302.

Basheer, L., Kerem, Z. (2015). Interactions between CYP3A4 and dietary polyphenols. *Oxid Med Cell Longev.* 2015:854015. doi:10.1155/2015/854015.

Beatty, S. J., Mehta, B. H., Rodis, J. L. (2005). Decreased warfarin effect after initiation of high-protein, low-carbohydrate diets. *Ann Pharmacother.* 39(4):744–747.

Bellows, L., Moore, R. (2022). Nutrient-Drug Interactions and Food. Colorado State University Extension, Fort Collins, CL. Fact Sheet No. 9.361 Food and Nutrition Series| Health.

Berné, Y., Carías, D., Cioccia, A. M., González, E., Hevia, P. (2005). Effect of the diuretic furosemide on urinary essential nutrient loss and on body stores in growing rats. *ALAN.* 55(2).

Bibi, Z. (2008). Role of cytochrome P450 in drug interactions. *Nutr Metab (Lond).* 5:27. doi:10.1186/1743-7075-5-27

Bidlack, W. R., Brown R. C., Mohan C. (1986). Nutritional parameters that alter hepatic drug metabolism, conjugation, and toxicity. *Fed Proc.* 45(2):142–148.

Bobroff, L. B., Lentz, A., Turner, R. E. (2009). Food/drug and drug/nutrient interactions: What you should know about your medications. *EDIS.* 2009(5). doi:10.32473/edis-he776-2009

Boullata, J. I. (2010). Influence of overweight and obesity on medication. In Handbook of Drug-Nutrient Interactions. 2nd Ed. New York, NY, Humana Press, Part II, Chapter 7, pp. 167–194.

Brodie, M. J., Mintzer, S., Pack, A. M., Gidal, B. E., Vecht, C. J., Schmidt, D. (2013). Enzyme induction with antiepileptic drugs: Cause for concern? *Epilepsia.* 54:11–27.

Btaiche, I. F., Sweet, B. V., Kraft, M. D. (2010). Positive drug–nutrient interactions. In Handbook of Drug-Nutrient Interactions, 2nd ed. New York, Humana Press, Part IV, Chapter 11, pp. 303–333.

Burchell, B., Brierley, C. H., Rance, D. (1995). Specificity of human UDP-glucuronosyltransferases and xenobiotic glucuronidation. *Life Sci.* 57:1819–1831.

Bushra, R., Aslam, N., Khan, A. Y. (2011). Food-drug interactions. *Oman Med J.* 26(2):77–83. doi:10.5001/omj.2011.21.

Chan, L. N. (2002). Drug-nutrient interaction in clinical nutrition. *Curr Opin Clin Nutr Metab Care.* 5:327–332.

Chan, L. N. (2006). Drug-nutrient interactions. In Shils, M. E., Shike, M., Ross, A. C., Caballero, B., Cousins, R. J. (eds): Modern Nutrition in Health and Disease. Baltimore, Lippincott Williams & Wilkins, pp. 1540–1553.

Chan, L. N. (2013). Drug-nutrient interactions. *J Parenter Enteral Nutr.* 37(4):450–459. doi:10.1177/0148607113488799.

Chapron, D. J. (2001). Drug disposition and response. In Delafuente, J. C., Stewart, R. B. (eds): Therapeutics in the Elderly, 3rd ed. Cincinnati, Harvey Whitney Books, pp. 257–288.

Chattopadhyay, M. K. (2014). Use of antibiotics as feed additives: A burning question. *Front Microbiol.* 5:334–337. https://doi.org/10.3389/fmicb.2014.00334

Chen, Y., Michalak, M., Agellon, L. B. (2018). Importance of nutrients and nutrient metabolism on human health. *Yale J Biol Med.* 91(2):95–103.

Cho, S. J., Yoon, I. S., Kim, D. D. (2013). Obesity-related physiological changes and their pharmacokinetic 272 consequences. *J Pharm Investig.* 43(3):161–169.

Compher, C. W., Boullata, J. I. (2010). Influence of protein-calorie malnutrition on medication. In Handbook of Drug-Nutrient Interactions, 2nd ed. New York, NY, Humana Press. Part II, Chapter 6, pp. 137–160.

Debnath, S., Tejovathi, R., Babu, I., Kumar, T. H. (2017). An overview on food & drug interactions. *India Pharma Times.* 49(4).

Ekesa, B., Nabuuma, D., Namukose, S., Upenytho, G. (2018). Basic nutrition concepts & nutrition indicators: Training manual for project management unit members. 1:1–45.

European Medicines Agency (2018). Reflection paper on investigations of pharmacokinetics and pharmacodynamics in the obese population. EMA/CHMP/535116/2016. *Committee for Human Medicinal Products (CHMP)*, p. 4.

Eyssen, H., De Somer, P. (1963). Effect of antibiotics on growth and nutrient absorption of chicks. *Poult Sci.* 42(6):1373–1379.

Gallicano, K., Drusano, G. (2022). Introduction to drug interactions. In Infectious Disease: Drug Interactions in Infectious Diseases, 2nd ed. Totowa, NJ, Humana Press. http://eknygos.lsmuni.lt/springer/622/1-11. pdf extracted March, 2022

Gamage, N., Barnett, A., Hempel, N., Duggleby, R. G., Windmill, K. F., Martin, J. L., et al. (2006). Human sulfotransferases and their role in chemical metabolism. *Toxicol Sci.* 90:5–22.

Gaohua, L., Xiusheng, M., Dou, Liu (2021). Crosstalk of physiological pH and chemical pKa under the umbrella of physiologically based pharmacokinetic modeling of drug absorption, distribution, metabolism, excretion, and toxicity. *Expert Opin Drug Metab Toxicol.* 17(9):1103–1124. doi:10.1080/1742525 5.2021.1951223

Genser, D. (2008). Food and drug interaction: Consequences for the nutrition/health status. *Ann Nutr Metab.* 52(suppl 1):29–32.

Greenberg, A. (2000). Diuretic complications. *Am J Med Sci.* 319:10–24.

Grimm, M., Koziolek, M., Saleh, M., Schneider, F., Garbacz, G., Kühn, J.-P., Weitschies, W. (2018). Gastric emptying and small bowel water content after administration of grapefruit juice compared to water and isocaloric solutions of glucose and fructose: A four-way crossover MRI pilot study in healthy subjects. *Mol Pharm.* 15:548–559. https://doi.org/10.1021/acs.molpharmaceut.7b00919

Guengerich, F. P. (1999). Cytochrome P-450 3A4: Regulation and role in drug metabolism. *Annu Rev Pharmacol Toxicol.* 39:1–17.

Guengerich, F. P. (2018). Mechanisms of cytochrome P450-catalyzed oxidations. *ACS Catal.* 8(12):10964–10976. doi:10.1021/acscatal.8b03401

Guo, L. Q., Fukuda, K., Ohta, T., Yamazoe, Y. (2000). Role of furanocoumarin derivatives on grapefruit juice-mediated inhibition of human CYP3A activity. *Drug Metab Dispos.* 28:766–771.

Gurley, B. J., Hagan, D. W. (2003). Herbal and dietary supplement interactions with drugs. In McCabe, B. J., Frankel, E. H., Wolfe, J. J. (eds): Hand Book of Food-drug Interactions. Boca Raton, CRC Press, pp. 259–293.

Hanley, M. J., Cancalon, P., Widmer, W. W., Greenblatt, D. J. (2011). The effect of grapefruit juice on drug disposition. *Expert Opin Drug Metab Toxicol.* 7:267–286.

Harris, R. M., Waring, R. H. (2008). Sulfotransferase inhibition: Potential impact of diet and environmental chemicals on steroid metabolism and drug detoxification. *Curr Drug Metab.* 9(4):269–275.

Heerspink, H. J. L., Holtkamp, F. A., Parving, H. H., Navis, G. J., Lewis, J. B., Ritz, E., de Graeff, P. A., de Zeeuw. D. (2012). Moderation of dietary sodium potentiates the renal and cardiovascular protective effects of angiotensin receptor blockers *Kidney Int.* 82(3):330–337.

Heidelbaugh, J. J. (2013). Proton pump inhibitors and risk of vitamin and mineral deficiency: Evidence and clinical implications. *Ther Adv Drug Saf.* 4(3):125–133. doi:10.1177/2042098613482484.

Hejaz, H. A., Karaman, R. (2015). Drug overview. In Commonly Used Drugs. New York, Nova Science Publishers, Inc., Chapter 1. Jan. ISBN: 978-1-63463-828-9. doi:10.13140/RG.2.1.4065.9049

Hodgson, E. (2012). Introduction to Biotransformation (Metabolism) in Pesticide Biotransformation and Disposition. Boston, Academic Press, Chapter 4, pp. 53–72.

Holt, G. A. (1998). Food & Drug Interactions. Chicago, Precept Press, p. 293.

Horn, J. R., Hansten, P. D. (2008). Get to know an enzyme: CYP3A4. *Pharm Times.* 0:0.

Huang, S. M., Zhao, H., Lee, J. I., Reynolds, K., Zhang, L., Temple, R., et al. (2010). Therapeutic protein-drug interactions and implications for drug development. *Clin Pharmacol Ther.* 87:497–503.

Hyams, J. S. (1983). Sorbitol intolerance. An unappreciated cause of functional gastrointestinal complaints. *Gastroenterol.* 84:30–33.

Imanaga, J., Kotegawa, T., Imai, H., Tsutsumi, K., Yoshizato, T., Ohyama, T., Shirasaka, Y., Tamai, I., Tateishi, T., Ohashi, K. (2011). The effects of the SLCO2B1 c.1457C > T polymorphism and apple juice on the pharmacokinetics of fexofenadine and midazolam in humans. *Pharmacogenet Genomics* 21:84–93. https://doi.org/10.1097/FPC.0b013e32834300cc

Ingels, F., Beck, B., Oth, M., Augustijns, P. (2004). Effect of simulated intestinal fluid on drug permeability estimation across Caco-2 monolayers. *Int J Pharm.* 274:221–232. https://doi.org/10.1016/j. ijpharm.2004.01.014

Jensen, K., Ni, Y., Panagiotou, G., Kouskoumvekaki, I. (2015). Developing a molecular roadmap of drug-food interactions. *PLoS Comput Biol.* 10;11(2):e1004048. doi: 10.1371/journal.pcbi.1004048. PMID: 25668218; PMCID: PMC4323218.

Johnston, G. A., Bilbao, R. M., Graham-Brown, R. A. (2004). The use of dietary manipulation by parents of children with atopic dermatitis. *Br J Dermatol.* 150:1186–1189.

Karaman, R. (2015). Commonly Used Drugs – Uses, Side Effects, Bioavailability & Approaches to Improve It. New York, Nova Science Publishers, Inc. ISBN: 9781634638289. doi:10.13140/RG.2.1.1444.4640

Kashuba, A., Bertino, J. S. (2022). Mechanisms of drug interactions I absorption, metabolism, and excretion. In Piscitelli, S. C., Rodvold, K. A. (eds): Infectious Disease: Drug Interactions in Infectious Diseases, 2nd ed. Totowa, NJ, Humana Press. http://eknygos.lsmuni.lt/springer/622/13-39.pdf

Kim, J., De Jesus, O. (2022). Medication routes of administration. In StatPearls [Internet]. Treasure Island, FL, StatPearls Publishing. www.ncbi.nlm.nih.gov/books/NBK568677/

Kirby, B. J., Unadkat, J. D. (2007). Grapefruit juice, a glass full of drug interactions? *Clin Pharmacol Ther.* 81(5):631–633. doi:10.1038/sj.clpt.6100185.

Kirkwood, T. B. (2008). A systematic look at an old problem. *Nature.* 451(7179):644–647.

Kotzer, L. M., Mascarenhas, M. R., Wallac, E. (2010). Drug–nutrient interactions in infancy and childhood. In Handbook of Drug-Nutrient Interactions, 2nd ed. New York, NY, Humana Press. Part V, p. 576.

Koziolek, M., Alcaro, S., Augustijns, P., Basit, A. W., Grimm, M., Hens, B., Hoad, C. L., Jedamzik, P., Madla, C. M., Maliepaard, M., Marciani, L., Maruca, A., Parrott, N., Pávek, P., Porter, C. J. H., Reppas, C., van Riet-Nales, D., Rubbens, J., Statelova, M., Trevaskis, N. L., Valentová, K., Vertzoni, M., Čepo, D. V., Corsetti, M. (2019). The mechanisms of pharmacokinetic food-drug interactions – A perspective from the UNGAP group. *Eur J Pharm Sci.* Jun;15(134):31–59. doi:10.1016/j.ejps.2019.04.003. Epub 2019 Apr 8. PMID: 30974173.

Krems, C., Lührmann, P., Straßburg, A. (2005). Lower resting metabolic rate in the elderly may not be entirely due to changes in body composition. *Eur J Clin Nutr.* 59:255–262. doi:10.1038/sj.ejcn.1602066

Le, J. (2020). Drug Metabolism. Kenilworth, NJ, USA, Merck Sharp & Dohme Corp., a subsidiary of Merck & Co., Inc.

Lin, J. H., Lu, A. Y. (2001). Interindividual variability in inhibition and induction of cytochrome P450 enzymes. *Annu Rev Pharmacol Toxicol.* 41:535–567.

Malhotra, S., Bailey, D. G., Paine, M. F., Watkins, P. B. (2001). Seville orange juice-felodipine interaction: Comparison with dilute grapefruit juice and involvement of furocoumarins. *Clin Pharmacol Ther.* 69:14–23.

Marchetti, S., Mazzanti, R., Beijnen, J. H., Schellens, J. H. M. (2007). Concise review: Clinical relevance of drug and herb drug interactions mediated by the ABC transporter ABCB1 (MDR1, P-glycoprotein). *Oncologist.* 12:927–941. https://doi.org/10.1634/theoncologist.12-8-927

Miller, B., Carthan, N. (2003). Non-prescription drug and nutrient interaction. In McCabe, B. J., Frankel, E. H., Wolfe, J. J. (eds): Handbook of Food-drug Interactions. Boca Raton, CRC Press, pp. 251–258.

Mohamed, M. E., Frye, R. F. (2011). Inhibitory effects of commonly used herbal extracts on UDP-glucuronosyltransferase 1A4, 1A6, and 1A9 enzyme activities. *Drug Metab Dispos.* 39:1522–1528.

Mohammad, Y., Mohammad, I. (2009). Drug-food interactions and role of pharmacist. *Asian J Pharm Clin Res.* 2(4).

Moran, N. E., Mohn, E. S., Hason, N., Erdman, J. W., Johnson, E. J. (2018). Intrinsic and extrinsic factors impacting absorption, metabolism, and health effects of dietary carotenoids. *Advan Nutr (Bethesda, Md.).* 9(4):465–492. doi:10.1093/advances/nmy025

Mougey, E. B., Feng, H., Castro, M., Irvin, C. G., Lima, J. J. (2009). Absorption of montelukast is transporter mediated: A common variant of OATP2B1 is associated with reduced plasma concentrations and poor response. *Pharmacogenet Genomics* 19:129–138. https://doi.org/10.1097/FPC.0b013e32831bd98c

Mydlik, M., Derzsiova, K., Zemberova, E. (1999). Influence of water and sodium diuresis on furosemide on urinary excretion of vitamin B6, oxalic acid and vitamin C in chronic renal failure. *Miner Electrolyte Metab.* 25:352–356.

Nakanishi, T., Tamai, I. (2015). Interaction of drug or food with drug transporters in intestine and liver. *Curr Drug Metab.* 16:753–764. https://doi.org/10.2174/1389200216091512011135357

Niederberger, E., Parnham, M. J. (2021). The impact of diet and exercise on drug responses. *Int J Mol Sci.* 22:7692. doi:10.3390/ijms22147692

Ortiz, Z., Shea, B., Suarez-Almazor, M. E., Moher, D., Wells, G. A., Tugwell, P. (1998). The efficacy of folic acid and folinic acid in reducing methotrexate gastrointestinal toxicity in rheumatoid arthritis. A meta-analysis of randomized controlled trials. *J Rheumatol.* 25:36–43.

Ortolani, E., Landi, F., Martone, A. M., Onder, G., Bernabei, R. (2013). Nutritional status and drug therapy in older adults. *J Gerontol Geriat Res.* 2:123.

Owhin, O., Kalejaiye, O. O., Fasipe, O. J., Adaja, T. M., Akhideno, P. E., Kehinde, M. O. (2019). Assessment of serum vitamin B12 levels and chronic haemato-toxicologic adverse profile induced by metformin pharmacotherapy among type 2 diabetic patients: A prospective analytical study. *Toxicol Res Appl.* 3:1–13.

Paeng, C. H., Sprague, M., Jackevicius, C. A. (2007). Interaction between warfarin and cranberry juice. *Clin Ther.* 29(8):1730–1735.

Paine, M. F., Criss, A. B., Watkins, P. B. (2004). Two major grapefruit juice components differ in intestinal CYP3A4 inhibition kinetic and binding properties. *Drug Metab Dispos.* 32:1146–1153.

Paine, M. F., Criss, A. B., Watkins, P. B. (2005). Two major grapefruit juice components differ in time to onset of intestinal CYP3A4 inhibition. *J Pharmacol Exp Ther.* 312:1151–1160.

Paine, M. F., Hart, H. L., Ludington, S. S., Haining, R. L, Rettie, A. E., Zeldin, D. C. (2006). The human intestinal cytochrome P450 "pie". *Drug Metab Dispos.* 34:880–886.

Pápai, K., Budai, M., Ludányi, K., Antal, I., Klebovich, I. (2010). In vitro food-drug interaction study: Which milk component has a decreasing effect on the bioavailability of ciprofloxacin? *J Pharm Biomed Anal.* 52(1):37–42.

Piver, B., Berthou, F., Dreano, Y., Lucas, D. (2001). Inhibition of CYP3A, CYP1A and CYP2E1 activities by resveratrol and other non volatile red wine components. *Toxicol Lett.* 125:83–91.

Presse, N., Perreault, S. (2015). Vitamin B12 deficiency induced by the use of gastric acid inhibitors: Calcium supplements as a potential effect modifier. *J Nutr Health Aging.* 20(5). doi:10.1007/s12603-015-0605-x

Pronsky, Z. M., Elbe, D., Ayoob, K. (2015). Food Medication Interactions, 18th ed. Birchrunville, PA, FMI, p. 444.

Rodríguez-Fragoso, L., Martínez-Arismendi, J. L., Orozco-Bustos, D., Reyes-Esparza, J., Torres, E., Burchiel, S. W. (2011). Potential risks resulting from fruit/vegetable-drug interactions: Effects on drug-metabolizing enzymes and drug transporters. *J Food Sci.* 76:R112–R124.

Rollins, C. J. (2010). Drug–nutrient interactions in patients receiving enteral nutrition. In Handbook of Drug-Nutrient Interactions, 2nd ed. New York, NY, Humana Press. Part IV, Chapter 13, pp. 367–406.

Ronis, M. J. (2016). Effects of soy containing diet and isoflavones on cytochrome P450 enzyme expression and activity. *Drug Metab Rev.* 48:331–341.

Roth, M., Obaidat, A., Hagenbuch, B. (2012). OATPs, OATs and OCTs: The organic anion and cation transporters of the SLCO and SLC22A gene superfamilies. *Br J Pharmacol.* 165(5):1260–1287. doi:10.1111/j.1476-5381.2011.01724.x

Roth, M., Timmermann, B. N., Hagenbuch, B. (2011). Interactions of green tea catechins with organic anion-transporting polypeptides. *Drug Metab Dispos.* 39:920–926. https://doi.org/10.1124/dmd.110.036640

Russell, T. L., Berardi, R. R., Barnett, J. L., Dermentzoglou, L. C., Jarvenpaa, K. M., Schmaltz, S. P., Dressman, J. B. (1993). Upper gastrointestinal pH in seventy-nine healthy, elderly, North American men and women. *Pharm Res.* 10(2):187–196.

Sagira, A., Schmitt, M., Dilger, K., Häussinger, D. (2003). Inhibition of cytochrome P450 3A: Relevant drug interactions in gastroenterology. *Digestion.* 68:41–48.

Schmidt, L. E., Dalhoff, K. (2002). Food-drug interactions. *Drugs.* 62:1481–1502.

Schurgers, L. J., Shearer, M. J., Hamulyák, K., Stöcklin, E., Vermeer, C. (2004). Effect of vitamin K intake on the stability of oral anticoagulant treatment: Dose-response relationships in healthy subjects. *Blood.* 104(9).

Shimokata, H., Kuzuya, F. (1993). Aging, basal metabolic rate, and nutrition. *Nihon Ronen Igakkai Zasshi.* 30(7):572–576.

Shirasaka, Y., Shichiri, M., Mori, T., Nakanishi, T., Tamai, I. (2013). Major active components in grapefruit, orange, and apple juices responsible for OATP2B1-mediated drug interactions. *J Pharm Sci.* 102:3418–3426. https://doi.org/10.1002/jps. 23653

Shitara, Y., Maeda, K., Ikejiri, K., Yoshida, K., Horie, T., Sugiyama, Y. (2013). Clinical significance of organic anion transporting polypeptides (OATPs) in drug disposition: Their roles in hepatic clearance and intestinal absorption. *Biopharm. Drug Dispos.* 34:45–78. https://doi.org/10.1002/bdd.1823

Shobha. (2019). Antibiotics and nutritional implications- the drugs-nutrients interactions. *Acta Sci Nutr Health.* 51–54.

Singh, B. N. (1999). Effects of food on clinical pharmacokinetics. *Clin Pharmacokinet.* 37:213–255.

Smolin, L. A., Grosvenor, M. B. (2019). Nutrition: Science and Applications, 4th ed. Mississauga, ON, Canada, John Wiley & Sons.

Snyder B. D., Polasek, T. M., Doogue, M. P. (2012). Drug interactions: Principles and practice. *Aust Prescr.* 35:85–88.

Socha, D. S., DeSouza, S. I., Flagg, A., Sekeres, M., Rogers, H. J. (2020). Severe megaloblastic anemia: Vitamin deficiency and other causes. *Cleveland Cli J Med.* 87(3).

Soltani, D., Ghaffar, P. M., Tafakhori, A., Sarraf, P., Bitarafan, S. (2016). Nutritional aspects of treatment in epileptic patients. *Iranian J Child Neurol.* 10(3):1–12.

Størmer, F. C., Reistad, R., Alexander, J. (1993). Glycyrrhizic acid in liquor ice–evaluation of health hazard. *Food Chem Toxicol.* 31(4):303–312. doi:10.1016/0278-6915(93)90080-I.

Stupans, L., Tan, H. W., Kirlich, A., Tuck, K., Hayball, P., Murray, M. (2002). Inhibition of CYP3A-mediated oxidation in human hepatic microsomes by the dietary derived complex phenol, gallic acid. *J Pharm Pharmacol.* 54:269–275.

Suiko, M., Kurogi, K., Hashiguchi, T., Sakakibara, Y., Liu, M. C. (2017). Updated perspectives on the cytosolic sulfotransferases (SULTs) and SULT-mediated sulfation. *Biosci Biotechnol Biochem.* 81(1):63–72.

Suter, P. M., Haller, J., Hany, A., Vetter, W. (2000). Diuretic use: A risk for subclinical thiamine deficiency in elderly patients. *J Nutr Health Aging.* 4:69–71.

Tamai, I. (2012). Oral drug delivery utilizing intestinal OATP transporters. *Adv Drug Deliv Rev.* 64:508–514. https://doi.org/10.1016/j.addr.2011.07.007

Tanaka, E. (1998). Clinically important pharmacokinetic drug-drug interactions: Role of cytochrome P450 enzymes. *J Clin Pharm Ther.* 23:403–416.

Taxak, N., Bharatam, P. V. (2014). Drug metabolism A fascinating link between chemistry and biology. *Resonance.* 19:259–282.

Testa, B., Bernd, C. (2015). Biotransformation reactions and their enzymes. In Camille Georges Wermuth, David Aldous, Pierre Raboisson, Didier Rognan. (eds): The Practice of Medicinal Chemistry, 4th ed. San Diego, Academic Press. Chapter 24.

Utermohlen, V. (2022). Nutrient–drug interactions. In Encyclopedia of Food and Culture. Retrieved March 28, 2022 from Encyclopedia.com: www.encyclopedia.com/food/encyclopedias-almanacs-transcripts-and-maps/nutrient-drug-interactions

Van Den Abeele, J., Rubbens, J., Brouwers, J., Augustijns, P. (2017). The dynamic gastric environment and its impact on drug and formulation behaviour. *Eur J Pharm Sci.* 96:207–231. https://doi.org/10.1016/j.ejps.2016.08.060.

Van-Zyl, M. S. (2011). The effects of drugs on nutrition. *Afr J Clin Nutr.* 24(3):S38–S41.

Venkateswarulu, V. (2014). Biopharamaceutics & Pharmacokinetics, 2nd ed. Hyderabad, India, Pharma Med Press, pp. 72–73.

Wienkers, L. C. (2001). Problems associated with in vitro assessment of drug inhibition of CYP3A4 and other P-450 enzymes and its impact on drug discovery. *J Pharmacol Toxicol Methods* 45:79–84.

Won, C. S., Oberlies, N. H., Paine, M. F. (2012). Mechanisms underlying food-drug interactions: Inhibition of intestinal metabolism and transport. *Pharmacol Ther.* Nov;136(2):186–201. doi:10.1016/j.pharmthera.2012.08.001. Epub 2012 Aug 4. PMID: 22884524; PMCID: PMC3466398.

World Health Organisation (Extracted 2022). www.who.int/health-topics/malnutrition#tab=tab_2

Xiao, C. Q., Chen, R., Lin, J., Wang, G., Chen, Y., Tan, Z. R., Zhou, H. H. (2012). Effect of genistein on the activities of cytochrome P450 3A and P-glycoprotein in Chinese healthy participants. *Xenobiotica.* 42:173–178.

Zhu, M., Nix, D. E., Adam, R. D., Childs, J. M., Peloquin, C. A. (2001). Pharmacokinetics of cycloserine under fasting conditions and with high-fat meal, orange juice, and antacids. *Pharmacotherapy.* 21(8):891–897.

5 Food Preservation, Spoilage and Food Adulteration

Ebenezer I. O. Ajayi

5.1 INTRODUCTION

Food spoilage and adulteration have continually been the major threat to achieving global food security, as about one-third of the total world foods do not get to the consumers, but rather, become spoilt, unsafe and non-redundant, as stated by the FAO some decades ago (Gustavsson *et al.*, 2011; Saini *et al.*, 2021). Meanwhile, food is much prone to contamination from different activities during processing, packaging and storage, leading to spoilage of the food as it goes in the line from producer through retailer to final consumer. Although some of these spoilt foods are discovered and discarded as waste by the producer, the majority get to consumers directly through retail shops and/or restaurants (Barth *et al.*, 2009). More alarming is the recent global food fraud, which involves deliberate misrepresentation, alteration or change of food products and/or constituents in either raw or finished form or presenting false information about the food product in order to increase economic gain. Food adulteration embodies both deliberate alterations that deteriorate food quality or substance and incidental contaminations during food processing, including harvest, production, storage, transportation and distribution. Apparently, the act of adulteration, which includes elimination or substitution of genuine components of food for counterfeit, artificial and fraudulent ones, which could be poisonous or hazardous, is done without the consumers' consent and knowledge, thus putting them at risk of health issues and death, in the worst cases (Banti, 2020).

However, some alterations during food processing are intentionally for preservation, to improve the appearance, texture and biochemical properties of the food, including shelf life, without the ulterior motive of economic gain. This makes adulteration easy to be confounded with preservation and *vice versa*. Preservation has, since time immemorial, been the redeeming factor that minimizes loss of essential foodstuffs to spoilage resulting from physical, chemical or biological activities, such as unintended atmospheric microbial contamination. Food preservation is the process of subjecting food to physical, chemical or biological processes, including applying substances obtained either from plants or microorganisms (natural) or synthesized from chemical compounds (synthetic), capable of controlling the biotic and abiotic component that could cause the spoilage of food (Seetaramaiah *et al.*, 2011; Amit *et al.*, 2017; Sherawat *et al.*, 2021).

The main purpose behind adding any substance (in the form of additives) to food or subjecting it to any process determines the additive as either adulterant or preservative, thereby creating a clear-cut difference between adulteration and preservation. Food spoilage and adulteration therefore deteriorate the safety of food, especially processed food, and expose the consumer to life-threatening risks as well as create economical and statutory problems to the food industry, resulting in significant global economic loss throughout the chain (Saini *et al.*, 2021). On the contrary, preservation will not only increase the longevity of shelf-life, improve the quality and characteristics and stabilize the nutritional content of the food to impede spoilage; it maintains the desirable properties, assures consumers of improving health benefits at no cost or lost to either the food industry or the global economy (Amit *et al.*, 2017; Mukhopadhyay *et al.*, 2018).

 DOI: 10.1201/9781003361497-6

5.2 FOOD SPOILAGE

Spoilage of food is implicated by any alteration in the nutritional properties, biochemical quality and organoleptic properties of food due to any form of contamination at any stage (from grow raw material to final product) of food processing, such that the food becomes unacceptable for human consumption (WHO, 2020). To put it simply, food spoilage is the resultant effect of either direct or indirect contamination of food by biological and/or non-biological agents at any point prior to the consumption of the food. Generally, contamination is the root of most spoilage, some intrinsic properties of food (such as light and oxygen sensitivity, presence of catabolic compounds and metabolites) could also mediate spoilage. Lipid oxidation, which results in the release of toxic substances and microbial proliferation, is indicative of food spoilage implicated by foul odour, change in pH and taste, making it unacceptable for consumption, through sensory evaluation (Saini *et al.*, 2021). Technically, the direct correlation between some inherent feature such as origin, water activity, pH, content and storage condition of food and possible microflora of food during and after production can be exploited to impede or delay proliferation of microorganisms. Furthermore, good hygiene and manufacturing practices with adequate and traceable approaches could be relatively employed to minimize occurrence of contamination and monitor exposure of populaces to spoilt food.

Some of these organisms are not only capable of deteriorating the food quality; they are potential pathogens to humans, which is the most deleterious consequent of food spoilage (Lorenzo *et al.*, 2018). The presence of any form of contaminant in food subjects it to spoilage, which is a major economic loss to the food industry which threatens food sufficiency (security). Perhaps, such spoilt foods become ingested by consumers and it leads to different health-related issues, ranging from mild food-borne infections like diarrhoea, vomiting, nausea, intestinal cramps and fever, to a life-threatening disease such as chronic ulcers (Raposo *et al.*, 2017; Saini *et al.*, 2021).

5.2.1 CAUSES OF FOOD SPOILAGE

Basically, the colour, texture, nutrient content and edibility of food are subject of deterioration, indicating food spoilage. Causes of food spoilage could be naturally mediated through intrinsic properties of the food or artificially mediated by extrinsic properties, including environmental factors. Biological action through microbial (including their metabolic product) contamination and non-biological actions through exogenous chemicals and alteration of normal physicochemical properties of the food are the two major categorical causes of food spoilage. However, the mechanism by which each of these factors causes food spoilage does not require emphasis, since spoilage caused by one can stimulate another (Amit *et al.*, 2017).

5.2.1.1 Non-Biological Causes of Food Spoilage

Non-biological food spoilage can be categorized into physical and chemical kinds of spoilage which are respectively mediated by several factors that cause change in either stability or sensory properties of food. Unstable moisture content and difference by temperature in the ingredients, moisture value and component of food, compared to the standard, is indicative of physical spoilage (Steele, 2004), while oxidation of lipids, which often results in unpleasant colour and odour, indicates chemical spoilage (Van Boekel, 2008).

5.2.1.1.1 *Factors Affecting Physical Spoilage of Food*

Moisture content, also known as water content (in the form of gain, loss or migration) of a food, is a major contributor to deterioration of food quality. The thermodynamic property of water, also known as water activity (a_w), changes as temperature changes, causing instability in the physical attribute of the food – a suitable situation for the occurrence of other factors that lead to food spoilage (Roudaut and Debeaufort, 2010).

Temperature is the most essential factor that causes spoilage of food because it enhances several, if not all, intrinsic and extrinsic metabolic activities in food, and consequently, causes instability in food constituents. There is an optimum temperature range required by all foods at different conditions to maintain their physical quality; any shift in the required temperature leads to alteration and/or deterioration in the food. For instance, a very low temperature, such as freezing temperature, causes cell breakage, which lowers the food quality, while a high temperature will induce a proteolysis in a protein-filled food (Steele, 2004; Amit *et al.*, 2017).

Crystallization occurs through crystal growth, which is formed as small and large extracellular ice within food cells during slow and quick or multiple freezing respectively. Such ice-filled cells undergo crystallization due to either temperature rise or accumulation of water, thereby mediating food spoilage by disrupting the cell and initiating metabolism (Steele, 2004). However, water binding agents like emulsifiers can be added to prevent the development of large crystal ice growth and crystallization (Amit *et al.*, 2017).

Glass transition temperature (T_g) is a temperature-specific transition of the amorphous matrix of a food from a viscous glass state to a liquid-like rubber state (Karmas *et al.*, 1992; Amit *et al.*, 2017). This transition process depends on specific temperature, relative humidity, moisture and solid content of the food, to determine the stability of physical constituent of food, which has a negative effect on the shelf life of foodstuffs (Amit *et al.*, 2017).

5.2.1.1.2 Factors Affecting Chemical Spoilage of Food

Chemical factors, such as oxidation, proteolysis, putrefaction and pectic hydrolysis, that affect food spoilage are directly related to causes of microbial spoilage, in that the mechanisms involved are synonymous with or require enzymatic reaction traceable to microorganisms and their metabolites.

Oxidation is the conversion of essential components of food to organic compounds and ammonia in the presence of oxygen. A typical example is rancidification, which involves oxidation of unsaturated fats that liberates carbonyl compound that causes the rancid taste and ammonia with its foul flavour, discoloration and formation of toxic substance (Steele, 2004; Enfors, 2008). Oxidation of amino acids in fresh meat and fish, which liberated organic acid and ammonia, is another example of such a spoilage reaction (Jay, 2000).

Proteolysis is a post-translational modification with high ubiquity, which specifically breaks the peptide and iso-peptide bond of protein components of foods in the presence of enzyme protease (Igarashi *et al.*, 2006). This irreversible process leaves with the food several amino acids gotten from the peptide component, which may be bitter or sweet in taste, depending on the amino acids (Enfors, 2008). Change in the taste depletes the sensory status of the food, and thus, the acceptability.

Putrefaction is an anaerobic reaction that serially leads from a change of amino acids to a mixture of organic acids, amines and stiff-smelling sulfur compounds in the presence of mediating bacteria. Furthermore, the phenomenon also liberates several chemicals with unpleasant odour, such ammonia, phenols and indole. High temperatures above 15°C also facilitate the process which leads to food spoilage (Panda, 2003; Enfors, 2008).

Mailland reaction is a non-enzymatic browning which occurs due to presence of proteins or amino acids in food like dry milk and eggs, with a significant, dark colouration. The colour change is an indication of reduced protein stability and nutritional content of some amino acids, creating a foul flavour that indicates food spoilage (Singh and Desrosier, 2014).

Chemical contaminant: heavy metals of industrial origin such as cadmium, polychlorinated biphenyl (PCB) and lead; organic pollutants such as DDT and chlordane; and industrial pollutants such as dibenzofurans and dibenzodioxins, which could be introduced into food during packaging, storage and transportation, are also agents of food spoilage. Ingestion of foods contaminated with these chemicals has been associated with several chronic disease such as cancer, including impairment of different biological systems (Ritter *et al.*, 1995; Saini *et al.*, 2021).

5.2.1.2 Biological Causes of Food Spoilage

The major biological cause of food spoilage is by microbial contamination, the proliferation of adventitious microorganisms and/or their metabolic products such as spores and enzymes, in food. Foods are highly nutritious with enhancing properties such as slight acid and moisture content, which makes them prone to contamination from these ubiquitous and microscopic agents, microorganisms (Saini *et al.*, 2021).

5.2.1.2.1 Microbial Contamination

Microbial contamination is the most common cause of food spoilage, causing significant health issues, with increasing records of associated food-borne outbreaks and diseases (Raposo *et al.*, 2017). Technically, depending on type and the biotic/abiotic condition of food, any microorganism whose multiplication is enhanced by a food is capable of causing spoilage in the food. Although multiple microbes could be responsible for food spoilage, there are some of these microbes that are food-specific, while many others are ubiquitous (Saini *et al.*, 2021). Spoilage microorganisms can broadly be categorized into different classes of bacteria such as Gram-positive, Gram-positive spore former, Gram-negative rod-shaped and lactic acids bacteria, yeasts, moulds, parasites and viruses (Figure 5.1) (Lorenzo *et al.*, 2018; Saini *et al.*, 2021).

5.2.2 HEALTH-RELATED EFFECT OF FOOD SPOILAGE

As earlier explained, the height of the injurious effect of food spoilage lies in the fact that some of the contaminants do not only cause off-odour, off-colour and other indications of spoilage; ingestion of such contaminants are deleterious to human health in one form or the other (Raposo *et al.*, 2017; Saini *et al.*, 2021). Ingestion of these agents of spoilage in food is directly linked with several health-related issues, majorly known as food-borne diseases and food poisoning, including some life-threatening conditions such as heart disorder and neuromuscular disorder (Saini *et al.*, 2021). Records on the frequency and prevalence of these conditions are on the increase in recent times, serving as a great burden on world health.

Another major consequence of food spoilage is the economic loss of the food industry, country and entire world, which serves as a hindrance to accomplishment of world food security (Gustavsson *et al.*, 2011; Saini *et al.*, 2021).

5.2.3 DETECTION OF FOOD SPOILAGE AND ITS CAUSES

Apparently, even before altered sensory status like off-odour, off-colour and softening, among others, indicative of spoilage of foods, are observed, the physical, chemical or biological deterioration

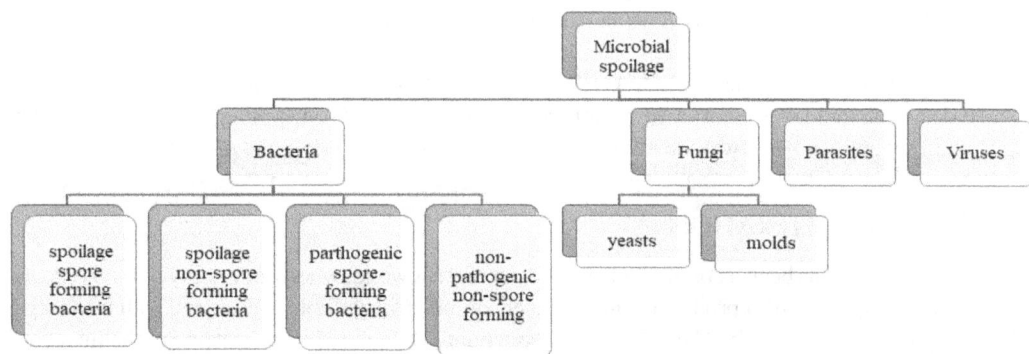

FIGURE 5.1 Category of major microorganisms involved in food spoilage (Lorenzo *et al.*, 2018).

has begun. Hence, early detection of spoilage agents will lead to possible impediment of food spoilage, leading to reduction of food loss and also to minimization of the health-related hazard (Lorenzo *et al.*, 2018). Conventionally, several methods involving determination of concentration of spoilage agents has been used to detect food spoilage, but inconsistent/unreliable results, tediousness and required time and labour remained as disadvantages of these methods. With the latest scientific and technological developments, several methods that employ advanced techniques with sensitive capacity for sensory detection and measurement of micro level of the contaminants (Saini *et al.*, 2021) have been developed, in the place of traditional methods like colorimetric, nucleic acid-based assay (Oh and Park, 2016; Srisa-Art *et al.*, 2018).

Amongst the most recent and advanced methods employed in food spoilage detection are:

Microfluidic system methods are an integrated high-throughput technique capable of detecting and studying a single cell in a biological analysis. They include:

- **Single-Cell Droplet Microfluidic System**, reportedly used to detect *Bacillus coagulans, Esherichia coli, Listeria monocytogenes, Salmonella* sp. (Jang *et al.*, 2017;Zhu *et al.*, 2018; Zhu *et al.*, 2019).
- **Microfluidic paper-based analytical devices (µPADs)**, a portable technology that utilizes paper in a microfluidic, analytical system to monitor environmental contaminants, is capable of measuring the quantity of analyte using the standard (Barbosa *et al.*, 2015).
- **Biosensor methods** are analytical devices majorly consisting of detector, signal generator, signal transducer and amplifier, used to estimate analytes. The detector and transducer of a biosensor determines the name and type of the sensor including magnetic, mass, optical, micromechanical, thermal and electrochemical biosensor (Shahzad *et al.*, 2017; Zhao *et al.*, 2017).
- **Nano-biosensor** that uses magnetic nano-particles, for instance, has been applied in the estimation of different contaminants and biological agents (Bunney *et al.*, 2017).
- **DNA-biosensor,** coupled with PCR, reportedly utilizes target oligonucleotides that are immobilized on a carbon paste electrode with primer, which quickly and simultaneously detects different bacterial pathogens (Palchetti and Mascini, 2008; Elsholz *et al.*, 2006; Alsammarraie and Lin, 2017).
- **Smartphone-based biosensor,** which reportedly employs the latest operating system, portability, sensitivity, transducer and data processor of the smartphone, supplemented with some optical or electrochemical biosensor to swiftly detect different food contaminants, including pathogens (Lin *et al.*, 2017; Ji *et al.*, 2017; Hu *et al.*, 2019; Wang *et al.*, 2019; Xu *et al.*, 2019; Zhang *et al.*, 2019).
- **Apta sensor**, a sensor that uses a class of molecule, called aptamer, has been reportedly useful in the detecting toxins, especially aflatoxin, and contaminants in foods (Liu *et al.*, 2017; Roushani *et al.*, 2018; Pourmadadi *et al.*, 2019; Krishnan *et al.*, 2021).

The potential of other methods, like Elisa-based detection, Omics tools based on PCR and LAMP detection and DNA microarray techniques in detection of food spoilage, have equally been reported in several studies (Bertone *et al.*, 2005; Zeinhom *et al.*, 2018; Hu *et al.*, 2020).

5.3 FOOD ADULTERATION

Adulteration of food has been a common menace to our current world, where the quality of food is deliberately debased by disdainful producers and/or traders of foods for gullible consumers, with the motive of accruing huge financial gain. Considering the essentiality of food to humans, who are the final consumer in food chain, posting the injurious and debilitating effect of food adulteration on humans (Banti, 2020), apparently, these food frauds are most often perpetrated in countries with poor control laws and monitoring agencies on food quality standards and usage of chemicals, undermining the real purpose of the World Health Organization (WHO) and Food Agricultural Organization (FAO) regarding food safety (Pardeshi, 2019). Although several developed countries, after significant effort, have been able to minimize the malpractice, they have not been able to achieve a total eradication, which thereby remains as a global threat to food safety and security (Banti, 2020; Saini *et al.*, 2021).

Food adulteration could be in form of partial or total replacement of essential components of food with less valuable components, the addition of unauthorized substances to maximize some other component of food and/or removal of valuable components of the food, all with the purpose of economic gain, without reflecting the misleading advertisement of the producer (Pardeshi, 2019; Banti, 2020). This malpractice has existed with the same age as buying and selling practices, in a metamorphic manner with time, which includes adding cheaper substitutes of a particular item of food to make larger quantity. The increasing occurrence of food fraud can be attributed to several factors such as the disdainful intentions of making higher profit or masking food spoilage by producer and ignorance of the gullible consumers (Manasha and Janani, 2016). Majorly, the unessential, unauthorized and invaluable substances or chemical components that are added to food or used for replacement during food fraud are termed adulterant, some of which are poisonous and injurious to human health. Several studies have established the consequential effect of food adulteration to human health and food safety worldwide (Manasha and Janani, 2016; Pardeshi, 2019; Banti, 2020; Saini *et al.*, 2021).

5.3.1 TYPES OF FOOD ADULTERATION

Generally, adulteration of foods can intentionally be perpetrated by producers with different motives, mostly of financial gain, or can occur incidentally due to natural occurrence relating to food substances, carelessness and inadequate hygiene during food processing (Faraz *et al.*, 2013; Awasthi *et al.*, 2014).

5.3.1.1 Deliberate Adulteration of Food

Deliberate types of food adulteration, which are mostly for purpose of high gains, either take the form of adding extraneous substances to increase the quantity of food or counterfeit the quality of the product or substituting essential constituent of food with inexpensive and valueless items (Pardeshi, 2019; Banti, 2020). Several studies have reported on the different deliberate forms of adulteration, which include adding white powder stone to salt, chalk to sugar, washing powder to ice-cream, water to honey or milk, argemone oil to groundnut oil, chicory to coffee, argemone seed to mustard seed, urea to milk, among others (Momtaz *et al.*, 2023; Faraz *et al.*, 2013; El-Loly *et al.*, 2013; Misgana, 2020; Bansal *et al.*, 2015). Genetically modified food (GMF) has gained increased acceptance due to some attributed advantages associated with both producers and consumers; nonetheless, it remains a form of deliberate adulteration when true information about it is inadequate (Banti, 2020; Momtaz *et al.*, 2023).

Furthermore, several activities – such as metallic lead from green colours used to give fresh colour to leafy vegetables; excessive pesticides, herbicides and chemical fertilizers used for plant growth; wax used to add shine to apples; oxytoxin and calcium carbide used respectively to fasten the growth and ripening of different fruits – are also examples of acts of adulteration in food processing, if not well communicated to the consumer (Momtaz *et al.*, 2023; Asrat and Ermias, 2015).

5.3.1.2 Incidental Adulteration of Food

This type of food adulteration happens unintentionally, partly due to the natural attributes of food, carelessness, usage of improper facilities and inadequate hygiene at any point during food processing, from the initial planting of raw materials to the final stage of finished product (Faraz *et al.*, 2013; Awasthi *et al.*, 2014). This type of adulteration occurs outside the producers' knowledge, in that adulterants may get into the food chain through the way the food was cultivated, harvested, processed, handled, stored, marketed and transported. Among such adulterants are metallic contaminations, including heavy metals such as mercury/lead from effluent or water, inorganic chemicals such as arsenic from pesticide, herbicides and fertilizers, tin from storage cans. Antinutrient substances peculiar with some foods like green vegetables and some seafoods, droppings from rodents, larva of different organisms and other exogenous substances can accidentally get into food as adulterants (Momtaz *et al.*, 2023; Banti, 2020).

5.3.2 EFFECT OF FOOD ADULTERATION

Adulteration of food, as a threat to food safety and security, not only confers a deleterious consequence on the health of the gullible victims; it also has a negative impact on the economy relating to the food industry and the country at large. Food adulteration is the top menace against food safety, as it limits the nutritional values of foods accessible to humans, which could result in an undernourished population and heighten the risk of exposure to life-threatening diseases (Pardeshi, 2019; Banti, 2020; Saini *et al.*, 2021). Economically, owing to illiteracy and ignorance of issues relating to this malpractice, adulterated food serves dual harms of depleted health status and financial cheating, as it is acquired at the rate required for unadulterated products.

5.3.3 DETECTION OF FOOD ADULTERATION

Traditionally, sensory evaluation that involves assessment of organoleptic features of foods has been applied in the detection of food adulteration. Several physical, chemical and biochemical methods that employ very sensitive analytical techniques have, however, been more promising in the detection of adulterants in foods (Banti, 2020).

Sensory method involves evaluation of taste, odour, size, colour, and other organoleptic characteristics to detect adulteration in food items. Although organoleptic assessment is often included in the routine evaluation of food samples for adulteration, sensory evaluation is not globally accepted for exclusive detection of adulterants. Some sensory methods for detecting adulteration in some foods have, however, been developed and recommended by reputable organizations like International Standard Organization (ISO), which are reportedly useful in trading for grading food items (Vesireddi, 2013).

Physical methods which involve assessment of physical parameters like texture, solubility, morphology and density of food, using microscopic and macroscopic techniques to detect adulterants in food commodities. A typical example is assessment of grains to detect adulterants like stones, weed seeds, weevil grain, rodent excreta, which could easily be achieved by physical examination in a plain plate (Banti, 2020).

Chemical and biochemical methods which employ analytical procedures with/without sensitive techniques such as spectroscopy, electrophoresis, immunology and chromatography in the detection of food adulteration (Bansal *et al.*, 2015). Among sensitive techniques that have been reported with impressive potential for adulterant detection are high performance liquid chromatography (HPLC), gas chromatography-mass spectroscopy/Fourier-transformed infrared spectroscopy (GC), near-infrared spectroscopy (NIR), nuclear magnetic-resonance (NMR), enzyme-linked immune-sorbent assay (ELISA) and atomic absorption spectrometry (AAS) (Nielsen, 2010; Xue *et al.*, 2010; Bansal *et al.*, 2015; Fiorini *et al.*, 2018).

Overall, supplement of chromatographic with spectroscopic techniques has proven more advantageous, as it not only offers a more accurate result; it accounts for the identity of adulterants and also discriminates among samples (Bansal *et al.*, 2015). Addition of about three drops of iodine to about a half-teaspoon of butter/ghee is a typical example of a simple, analytical procedure to detect starchy adulterants (Banti, 2020).

5.4   FOOD PRESERVATION

The nutritional composition and other inherent properties of food makes foods prone to biological, physical and chemical contamination that ultimately leads to spoilage of foods after a short period of time. Basically, foods are classified as perishable, which can spoil in no time if preservation is not employed, including meats, dairy products, eggs, sea foods, milk; semi-perishable, which can be preserved for a longer time of about six months when stored properly – examples are cheeses, potatoes, vegetables and fruits; or non-perishable, which are capable of not getting spoilt when stored for years or longer – examples are flour, peanuts, sugar, dry beans and others (Barth *et al.*, 2019). Food preservation becomes very essential to retain nutritional value, texture, colour and flavour, and most importantly, extends the shelf life of food (Amit *et al.*, 2017).

The basic aim of preserving food, which differentiates it from adulteration, is to avoid spoilage by extending the shelf life. Conventionally, foods are preserved following methods such as chilling, drying, freezing, pasteurization, irradiation (Chen, 2023) and application of chemical preservatives. More advanced methods, like high-pressure technology and pulse-field technology, are currently being applied, owing to recent developments in science and technology.

5.4.1 Methods of Food Preservation

There are three categories of conventional methods employed for food preservation, which include physical, chemical and biological methods.

5.4.1.1 Conventional Methods

5.4.1.1.1 Physical Methods

Drying involves the use of evaporation technique to reduce moisture in food below the threshold of 0.88 suitable for microbial survival, thereby preserving the food from microbial invasion and proliferation (Jay, 2000; Syamaladevi *et al.*, 2016). Drying, as one of the oldest and cheapest forms of preservation, has numerous advantages, such as weight and volume reduction and extended storage time, and a few limitations, such as loss of flavour and some compounds like vitamin C, lipids and proteins (Kutz, 2008).

Pasteurization is employed to kill spoilage microorganisms and enzymes by heating food to a certain temperature, thereby prolonging the shelf life of food (Cavazos-Garduño *et al.*, 2016). Pasteurization is based on temperature-time combination categorized as high-temperature short-time (HTST), ultra-high temperature (UHT) and low-temperature long-time (LTLT) (Amit *et al.*, 2017). Longer shelf life is attributed to food processed with UHT pasteurization. However, it has been reported that pasteurization reduces vitamin C, B-12 and phosphorus in food by 20%, 10% and 5% respectively, although the reductions have insignificant effect on their nutritional value (Fellows, 2009).

Freezing, particularly, slows down physiochemical and biochemical reactions, which ultimately hinders the growth of both pathogenic and spoilage organisms in food (George, 2008). Slow freezing enhances formation of large ice crystals in extracellular spaces, while rapid freezing forms small ice crystals that are distributed all around the tissue (Ramaswamy and Tung, 1984).

Chilling involves reduction of the initial temperature of food products to lower temperature, usually between -1°C and 8°C, and maintaining the final temperature over a long period of time (Saravacos and Kostaropoulous, 2016), with the aim of reducing the biochemical and microbiological activity that may pose a threat to the shelf life of both fresh and processed food products (Indira and Sudheer, 2008). The chilling method of preservation can be achieved with the use of a jacket-heat exchanger, an ice-bank cooler, a vacuum attribution system, a cryogenic chamber or a plate-heat exchanger (James, 2008). The rate of chilling depends on the size and weight of food, initial temperature, moisture content, absence and presence of a lid, packaging and thermal conductivity. Among the limitations of the chilling method are dehydration of uncovered food and reduction of crispness of some food (Saravacos and Kostaropoulous, 2016).

Irradiation, one of the most recent and common of physical methods of food preservation, uses a certain dose of ionizing radiation (IR) (kGy) (Toldrá, 2010). The irradiation process, a non-thermal technique (Figure 5.2), employs IR, which could be natural such as gamma rays, X-rays and high-energy ultraviolet (UV) radiation or artificial IR, including an induced secondary radiation

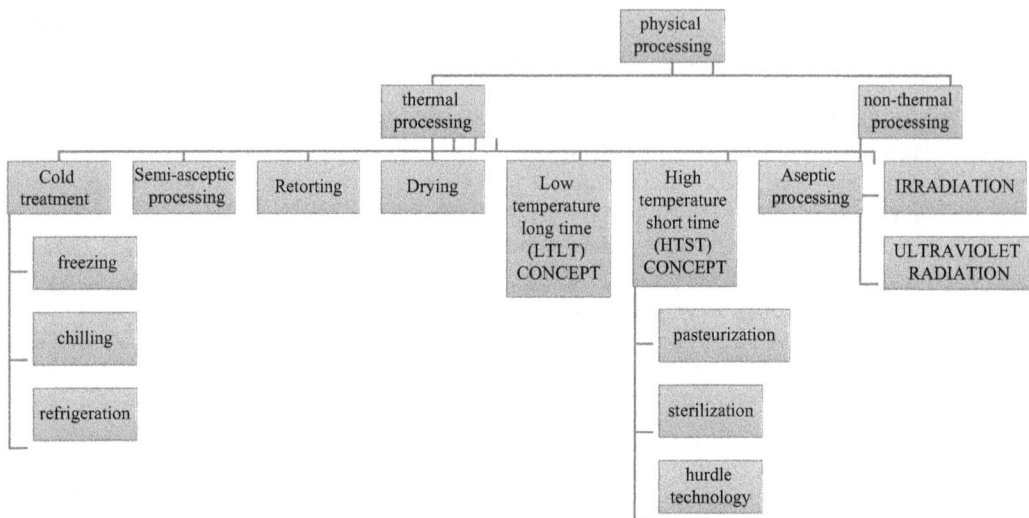

FIGURE 5.2 Classification of physical methods of food preservation (Amit *et al.*, 2017).

and accelerated electrons (Moniruzzaman *et al.*, 2016). IR preserves and improves shelf life of grains, fruits and vegetables by stopping sprouting and killing deteriorating organisms (Amit *et al.*, 2017). Irradiation, just like other conventional methods, has been reported to cause loss of some nutritional value, especially that a high dose of IR causes loss of vitamins A, C, B1 and E (Smith and Pillai, 2004).

Other physical methods applicable in food preservation are depicted in Figure 5.2.

5.4.1.1.2   Chemical Methods

The use of chemical substances to preserve food, which is ideally monitored by regulatory bodies in different countries, depends on the concentration and selectivity of the chemical agents, physico-chemical characteristics of the food and spoilage organisms (Islam *et al.*, 2016). Chemical preservations are either natural, such as salt, sugar, vinegar and rosemary extract, or artificial, synthesized industrially and classified as anti-enzymatic, antioxidant and antimicrobial (Sati and Sati, 2013). Most chemical preservatives are regarded as safe, except for a few that have reportedly been associated with life-threatening effects such as causing migraines, triggering asthmatic syndromes and causing carcinogenic effects (Nogrady, 2013).

5.4.1.1.3   Biological Processes

Fermentation is among the oldest methods of preservation, which uses microorganisms such as bacteria, mould, yeast, and/or microbial enzymes to preserve food by decomposing carbohydrate in food to alcohol and carbon-dioxide (alcohol fermentation), lactic acid and water (lactic acid fermentation) and acetic acid and water (vinegar fermentation) (Koutchma *et al.*, 2016). As oppose to the chemical method of preservation, fermentation improves the nutritional values and digestibility of foods (Lewin, 2012).

5.4.1.2   Modern Methods of Food Preservation

A few advanced methods of food preservation have so far been reported with promising potentials; they include:

> **High-pressure (HP) processing technology**, also known as ultra-high-pressure processing, employs hydrostatic pressures of about 900 MPa for few minutes to eliminate

microorganisms present in food (Amit *et al.*, 2017). HPP kills vegetative microorganism by inducing structural changes at the cell membrane and deactivating microbial enzymes (Heinz and Buckow, 2010). Foods like salad, fruit juice and vegetables are better processed using HPP. Although some microorganisms like *Lactobacillus* sp., Enterohemorrhagic *Escherichia coli* and *Listeria monocytogens* have tolerance for high pressure (Casadei, 2002), high pressure above 300 MPa at ambient temperature is capable of inactivating vegetative bacteria, viruses and yeast (Buckow and Bull, 2013). HPP has the advantages of being environmentally friendly, capable of ensuring food safety by extending shelf life and improving nutritional value and taste of food, without affecting the colour, flavour and vitamins (Buckow and Bull, 2013). This technology is, however, limited by high cost and availability of limited information regarding the technology (Amit *et al.*, 2017).

High-pressure thermal processing (HPT) combines the effect of pressure of about 600MPa and temperature above 60°C, which has proven synergistic potential in eradicating spores and spore-forming microorganisms (Olivier, 2011; Scepankova *et al.*, 2022). Since pressure is involved in the use of HPT, the need for excessive, long heating is reduced. The quality of food's flavour, texture, colour and nutritional content is enhanced, as the heat received by them is less (Oey, 2008). HPT conditions required for inactivating non-proteolytic *Clostridium botulinum* are moderate, compared to what is needed against proteolytic *C. botulinum* (Margosch, 2004).

Pulse Electric-Field processing (PEF) involves placing food in between two electrodes, or pumping it through electrodes, before exposing it to pulsed, high-voltage pulses of about 40 KV/cm for 20–1000ms in order to inactivate microorganisms in the food (Buckow and Bull, 2013). Extrinsic factors of food, such as water activity, pH, electric conductivity and soluble solids, and cell characteristics, such as structure and size, determine how susceptible the spoilage microorganisms will be to the effect of PEF. The mechanism of action of PEF on microorganisms is simply that it perforates the cell membrane and forces open the protein channels (Gášková, 1996). PEF has advantages in processing liquid food, especially that contains heat labile bioactive components, as it does not change the flavour or nutrient content of such food (Amit *et al.*, 2017).

Cool plasma is mostly applicable for total eradication of bacterial spores on the surface of foods, glass, steel and plastic. Cool plasma uses an ionized gas state generated from gas or liquid treated with a power source. It consists of few components, such as free radicals, atoms and molecules (at excited states), charged particles and ultraviolet (UV) photons that affect biological systems (Kong, 2012). Cool plasma processing can be used to preserve thermo-sensitive food materials without leaving any residues on food, as the process does not require water or chemicals (Kong, 2012).

5.5 CONCLUSIONS

Apparently, food spoilage and adulteration has been a drawback to the global effort towards food safety and security, as they deteriorate food and expose consumers to risks as well as create economic problems for food industries. Preservation of food is often associated erroneously with food fraud, also known as adulteration, which is a menace to the food industry worldwide. Meanwhile, a clear-cut difference that depends on the main purpose exists between adulteration and preservation, in that the former creates problems, while the latter is a problem-solving practice. Modern methods, including HP, HPT, PEF processing technology, are more promising for food preservation, with the ability to expand shelf life without devaluing the nutritional content of food. However, government intervention with legal control and standard surveillance policy is urgently needed to avert the threat of adulteration spoilage on food security and safety.

REFERENCES

Alsammarraie, F. K. and Lin, M. (2017). Using standing gold nanorod arrays as surface-enhanced Raman spectroscopy (SERS) substrates for detection of carbaryl residues in fruit juice and milk. *J. Agric. Food Chem.*, **65**: 666–674. [CrossRef] [PubMed]

Amit, S. K., Uddin, M. M., Rahman, R. A., Islam, S. M. R. and Khan, M. S. (2017). Review on mechanisms and commercial aspects of food preservation and processing. *Agric. Food Secur.*, **6**: 51. doi:10.1186/s40066-017-0130-8.

Asrat, A. and Ermias, B. E. (2015). Food adulteration: Its challenges and impact. *Food Sci. Qual. Manag.*, 50–56.

Awasthi, S., Jain, K., Das, A., Alam, R., Surti, G. and Kishan, N. (2014). Analysis of food quality and food adulterants from different departmental & local grocery stores by qualitative analysis for food safety. *J. Env. Sci. Toxicol. Food Technol.*, **8**(2): 22–26.

Bansal, S., Apoorva, S., Manisha, M., Anupam, K. M. and Sanjiv, K. (2015). Food adulteration: Sources, health risks and detection methods. *Crit. Rev. Food Sci. Nutr.* **57**(6): 1174–1189. doi:10.1080/10408398.2014.967834

Banti, M. (2020). Food adulteration and some methods of detection, review. *Int. J Nutr. Food Sci.*, **9**(3): 86–94. doi:10.11648/j.ijnfs.20200903.13

Barbosa, A. I., Gehlot, P., Sidapra, K., Edwards, A. D. and Reis, N. M. (2015). Portable smartphone quantitation of prostate specific antigen (PSA) in a fluoropolymer microfluidic device. *Biosens. Bioelectron.*, **70**: 5–14. [CrossRef]

Barth, M., Hankinson, T. R., Zhuang, H. and Breidt, F. (2009). Microbiological spoilage of fruits and vegetables. In: Compendium of the microbiological spoilage of foods and beverages. Sperber, W. H. and Doyle M. P., editors. Food Microbiology and Food Safety. Springer, New York: Dordrecht Heidelberg, London. doi:10.1007/978-1-4419-0826-1_6

Bertone, P., Gerstein, M. and Snyder, M. (2005). Applications of DNA tiling arrays to experimental genome annotation and regulatory pathway discovery. *Chromosome Res.*, **13**: 259–274. [CrossRef] [PubMed]

Buckow, R. and Bull, M. K. (2013). Advanced food preservation technologies. *Microbiol Australia.*, **34**(2): 108–111. doi:10.1071/MA13037

Bunney, J., Williamson, S., Atkin, D., Jeanneret, M., Cozzolino, D., Chapman, J., Power, A. and Chandra, S. (2017). The use of electrochemical biosensors in food analysis. *Curr. Res. Nutr. Food Sci. J.*, **5**: 183–195. doi.org/10.12944/CRNFSJ.5.3.02

Casadei, M. A. (2002). Role of membrane fluidity in pressure resistance of Escherichia coli NCTC 8164. *Appl. Environ. Microbiol.*, **68**: 5965–5972. doi:10.1128/AEM.68.12.5965-5972.2002

Cavazos-Garduño, A., Serrano-Niño, J. C., Solís-Pacheco, J. R., Gutierrez Padilla, J. A., González-Reynoso, O., García, H. S. and Aguilar-Uscanga, B. R. (2016). Effect of pasteurization, freeze-drying and spray drying on the fat globule and lipid profile of human milk. *J. Food Nutr. Res.*, **4**(5): 296–302.

Chen, Z. (2023). Food adulteration: Understanding the risks and safeguarding our health. *J. Food Microbiol. Saf. Hyg.*, **8**: 197. doi:10.35248/2476-2059.23.8.197

El-Loly, M., Mansour, A. I. A. and Ahmed, R. O. (2013). Evaluation of raw milk for common commercial additives and heat treatments. *Int. J Food Saf.*, **15**: 7–10. https://api.semanticscholar.org/CorpusID:534 94940

Elsholz, B., Wörl, R., Blohm, L., Albers, J., Feucht, H., Grunwald, T., Jurgen, T., Schweder, T. and Hintsche, R. (2006). Automated detection and quantitation of bacterial RNA by using electrical microarrays. *Anal. Chem.*, **78**(14): 4794–4802. https://doi.org/10.1021/ac0600914

Enfors, S. O. (2008). Food Microbiology. Stockholm: KTH-Biotechnology. http://www.biotech.kth.se/bio process/enfors/Downloads/FoodMicrobioloy.pdf

Faraz, A., Lateef, M., Mustafa, M. I., Akhtar, P., Yaqoob, M. and Rehman, S. (2013). Detection of adulteration, chemical composition and hygienic status of milk supplied to various canteens of educational institutes and public places in Faisalabad. *J. Animal Plant. Sci.*, **23**(1): 119–124. https://thejaps.org.pk/docs/Supplementary/vol-3-sup-1/24.pdf

Fellows, P. J. (2009). Food processing technology: Principles and practice. 3rd ed. Cambridge: Woodhead Publishing. https://www.webpal.org/SAFE/aaarecovery/2_food_storage/Food%20Processing%20Tech nology.pdf

Fiorini, D., Boarelli, M. C., Conti, P., Alfei, B., Caprioli, G., Ricciutelli, M., Sagratini, G., Fedeli, D., Gabbianelli, R. and Pacetti, D. (2018). Chemical and sensory differences between high price and low price extra virgin olive oils. *Food Res Int.*, **105**: 65–75. doi:10.1016/j.foodres.2017.11.005

Gášková, D. (1996). Effect of high-voltage electric pulses on yeast cells: Factors influencing the killing efficiency. *Bioelectrochem. Bioenerg.*, **39**: 195–202. doi:10.1016/0302 4598(95)01892-1

George, M. (2008). Freezing. In: Food biodeterioration and preservation. Tucker, G. S., editor. Singapore: Blackwell Publisher, pp. 117–135. http://ndl.ethernet.edu.et/bitstream/123456789/87738/24/Food%20 Biodeterioration%20and%20Preservation%20by%20Gary%20S.%20Tucker%20%28z-lib.org%29.pdf

Gustavsson, J., Cederberg, C., Sonesson, U., Van Otterdijk, R. and Meybeck, A. (2011). The methodology of the FAO study: Global food losses and food waste – Extent, causes and prevention. FAO report. Rome, Italy: Food and Agriculture Organization (FAO) of the United Nations. https://www.diva-portal.org/ smash/get/diva2:944159/FULLTEXT01.pdf

Heinz, V. and Buckow, R. (2010). Food preservation by high pressure. *J. Verbrauch. Lebensm.*, **5**: 73–81. doi:10.1007/s00003-009-0311-x

Hu, W., Feng, K., Jiang, A., Xiu, Z., Lao, Y., Li, Y. and Long, Y. (2020). An in situ-synthesized gene chip for the detection of food-borne pathogens on fresh-cut cantaloupe and lettuce. *Front. Microbiol.*, **10**: 3089. doi: 10.3389/fmicb.2019.03089

Hu, X., Shi, J., Shi, Y., Zou, X., Arslan, M., Zhang, W., Huang, X., Li, Z. and Xu, Y. (2019). Use of a smart phone for visual detection of melamine in milk based on Au@ carbon quantum dots nanocomposites. *Food Chem.*, **272**: 58–65. doi: 10.1016/j.foodchem.2018.08.021

Igarashi, Y., Eroshkin, A., Gramatikova, S., Gramatikoff, K., Zhang, Y., Smith, J. W., Osterman, A. L. and Godzik, A. (2006). CutDB: A proteolytic event database. *Oxford J.*, **35**(1): D546–9.38. doi:10.1093/nar/ gkl813

Indira, V. and Sudheer, K. P. (2008). Post-Harvest technology of horticultural crops. In: Peter, K. V., editor. Horticulture science. New Delhi: New India Publishing Agency; (2007). Product quality. *Trends Food Sci. Technol.*, **19**(8): 418–424.

Islam, M. N., Mursalat, M. and Khan, M. S. (2016). A review on the legislative aspect of artificial fruit ripening. *Agric. Food Secur.*, **5**(1): 8.

James, S. (2008). Food biodeterioration and preservation. Singapore: Blackwell.

Jang, M., Jeong, S. W., Bae, N. H., Song, Y., Lee, T. J., Lee, M. K., Lee, S. J. and Lee, K. G. (2017). Droplet-based digital PCR system for detection of single-cell level of foodborne pathogens. *BioChip. J.*, **11**: 329–337. [CrossRef]

Jay, J. M. (2000). Modern food microbiology. 6th ed. Gaithersburg: Aspen Publishers.

Ji, D., Liu, L., Li, S., Chen, C., Lu, Y., Wu, J. and Liu, Q. (2017). Bioelectronics: Smartphone-based cyclic voltammetry system with graphene modified screen printed electrodes for glucose detection. *Biosens. Bioelectron.*, **98**: 449–456. [CrossRef] [PubMed]

Karmas, R., Pilar, B. M. and Marcus, K. (1992). Effect of glass transition on rates of nonenzymic browning in food systems. *J. Agric. Food Chem.*, **40**:873–879.

Kong, M. G. (2012). Microbial decontamination of food by non-thermal plasmas. In: Microbial decontamination in the food industry. Demirci, A. and Ngadi, M. O., editors. Sawston: Woodhead Publishing, pp. 472–492. Woodhead Publishing Series in Food Science, Technology and Nutrition. doi:10.1533/9780857 095756.2.472.

Koutchma, T., Popovi, C. V., Ros-Polski, V. and Popielarz, A. (2016). Effects of ultraviolet light and high-pressure processing on quality and health-related constituents of fresh juice products. *Compr. Rev. Food Sci. Food Saf.*, **15**(5): 844–867.

Krishnan, S., Kumar Narasimhan, A., Gangodkar, D., Dhanasekaran, S., Kumar Jha, N., Dua, K., Thakur, V. K. and Kumar Gupta, P. (2021). Aptameric nanobiosensors for the diagnosis of COVID-19: An update. *Mater. Lett.*, **2021**: 131237. [CrossRef]

Kutz, M. (2008). Handbook of farm, dairy, and food machinery. 1st ed. New York: William Andrew.

Lewin, A. (2012). Real food fermentation: Preserving whole fresh food with live cultures in your home kitchen. 4th ed. Gloucester, MA: Quarry Books.

Lin, H.Y., Huang, C.H., Park, J., Pathania, D., Castro, C.M., Fasano, A., Weissleder, R. and Lee, H. (2017). Integrated magneto-chemical sensor for on-site food allergen detection. *ACS Nano.*, **11**: 10062–10069. [CrossRef]

Liu, S., Wang, Y., Xu, W., Leng, X., Wang, H., Guo, Y. and Huang, J. A. (2017). A novel sandwich-type electrochemical aptasensor based on GR-3D Au and aptamer-AuNPs-HRP for sensitive detection of oxytetracycline. *Biosens. Bioelectron.*, **88**: 181–187. [CrossRef]

Lorenzo, J. M., Munekata, P. E., Dominguez, R., Pateiro, M., Saraiva, J. A. and Franco, D. (2018). Main groups of microorganisms of relevance for food safety and stability: General aspects and overall description. In: Innovative technologies for food preservation. Barba, Francisco J., Sant'Ana, Anderson S., Orlien, Vibeke, Koubaa, Mohamed, editors. Academic Press, pp. 53–107. London EC2Y 5AS, United Kingdom.

Manasha, M. and Janani, F. (2016). Food adulteration and its problems (intentional, accidental and natural food adulteration). *Int. J Res. Fin Market.*, **6**(4): 131–140.

Margosch, D. (2004). Comparison of pressure and heat resistance of *Clostridium botulinum* and other endo-spores in mashed carrots. *J. Food Prot.*, **67**: 2530–2537.

Misgana, B. (2020). Food adulteration and some methods of detection, review. *Int. J. Nutr. Food Sci.*, **9**(3): 86–94. https://doi.org/10.11648/j.ijnfs.20200903.13

Momtaz, M., Bubli, S. Y. and Khan, M. S. (2023). Mechanisms and health aspects of food adulteration: A comprehensive review. *Foods*, **12**(1): 199. doi:10.3390/foods12010199

Moniruzzaman, M., Alam, M. K., Biswas, S. K., Pramanik, M. K., Islam, M. M. and Uddin, G. S. (2016). Irradiation to ensure safety and quality of fruit salads consumed in Bangladesh. *J. Food Nutr. Res.*, **4**(1):40–45.

Mukhopadhyay, S., Ukuku, D.O., Juneja, V.K., Nayak, B. and Olanya, O.M. (2018). Microbial control and food preservation: Theory and practice: Principles of food preservation. Book Chapter. https://doi.org/10.1016/j.cofs.2018.01.013

Nielsen, S. S. (2010). Food analysis, food science texts series. 4th edition ed. Purdue University, West Lafayette, IN: Springer. doi:10.1007/978-1-4419-1478-1_6

Nogrady, B. (2013). The hard facts of food additives. ABC Health and Wellbeing. www.abc.net.au/health/features/stories/2013/02/14/3684208.htm.

Oey, I. (2008). Effect of high-pressure processing on colour, texture and flavour of fruit- and vegetable-based food products: A review. *Trends Food Sci. Technol.*, **19**: 320–328. doi:10.1016/j.tifs.2008.04.001

Oh, J. H. and Park, M. K. (2016). Immunosensors combined with a light microscopic imaging system for rapid detection of Salmonella. *Food Control*, **59**: 780–786. [CrossRef]

Olivier, S. A. (2011). Strong and consistently synergistic inactivation of spores of spoilage associated *Bacillus* and *Geobacillus* spp. by high pressure and heat compared with inactivation by heat alone. *Appl. Environ. Microbiol.*, **77**: 2317–2324. doi:10.1128/AEM.01957-10

Palchetti, I. and Mascini, M. (2008). Electroanalytical biosensors and their potential for food pathogen and toxin detection. *Anal. Bioanal. Chem.*, **391**: 455–471. [CrossRef]

Panda, H. (2003). Herbal foods and its medicinal values. Delhi: National Institute of Industrial Research.

Pardeshi, S. (2019). Food adulteration: Injurious adulterants and contaminants in foods and their health effects and its safety measures in India. *Int. J. Sci. Dev. Res.*, **4**(6): 229–236.

Pourmadadi, M., Shayeh, J. S., Omidi, M., Yazdian, F., Alebouyeh, M. and Tayebi, L. (2019). A glassy carbon electrode modified with reduced graphene oxide and gold nanoparticles for electrochemical aptasensing of lipopolysaccharides from Escherichia coli bacteria. *Microchim. Acta.*, **186**: 1–8. [CrossRef]

Ramaswamy, H. S. and Tung, M. A. (1984). A review on predicting freezing times of foods. *J. Food Process. Eng.*, **7**(3): 169–203.

Raposo, A., Pérez, E., de Faria, C. T., Ferrús, M. A. and Carrascosa, C. (2017). Food spoilage by *Pseudomonas* spp. – An overview. In: Food borne pathogens and antibiotic resistance. Hoboken, NJ: John Wiley & Sons, Inc, pp. 41–58.

Ritter, L., Solomon, K. R., Forget, J., Stemeroff, M. and O'leary, C. (1995). A review of selected persistent organic pollutants. *The International Programme on Chemical Safety (IPCS).*; World Health Organization: Geneva, Switzerland, **65**: 66–71.

Roudaut, G. and Debeaufort, F. (2010). Moisture loss, gain and migration in foods and its impact on food quality. In: Food science, technology and nutrition, chemical deterioration and physical instability of food and beverages. Skibsted, L. H., Risbo, J., Andersen, M. L., editors. Woodhead Publishing, pp. 143–185, Cambridge CB22 3HJ, UK: Woodhead Publishing Series. ISBN 9781845694951, https://doi.org/10.1533/9781845699260.2.143.

Roushani, M., Nezhadali, A. and Jalilian, Z. (2018). An electrochemical chlorpyrifos aptasensor based on the use of a glassy carbon electrode modified with an electropolymerized aptamer-imprinted polymer and gold nanorods. *Microchim. Acta.*, **185**: 551. [CrossRef] [PubMed]

Saini, R. V., Vaid, P., Saini, N. K., Siwal, S. S., Gupta, V. K., Thakur, V. K. and Saini, A. K. (2021). Recent advancements in the technologies detecting food spoiling agents. *J. Funct. Biomater.* **12**: 67. https://doi.org/10.3390/jfb12040067

Saravacos, G. and Kostaropoulous, A. E. (2016). Handbook of food processing equipment. Food Engineering Series. New York: Kluwer Academic/Plenum Publishers. doi: 10.1007/978-3-319-25020-5

Sati, S. P. and Sati, N. (2013). Artificial preservatives and their harmful effects: Looking towards nature for safer alternatives. *Int. J. Pharm. Sci. Res.*, **4**(7): 2496–2501.

Scepankova, H., Pinto, C. A., Estevinho, L. M. and Saraiva, J. A. (2022). High-pressure-based strategies for the inactivation of *Bacillus subtilis* endospores in honey. *Molecules*, **27**(18): 5918. doi:10.3390/molecules27185918

Seetaramaiah, K., Smith, A. A., Murali, R. and Manavalan, R (2011). Preservatives in food products; *Review. Int. J. Pharm. Biol. Archiv.*, **2**(2): 583–599.

Shahzad, F., Zaidi, S. A. and Koo C. M. (2017). Highly sensitive electrochemical sensor based on environmentally friendly biomass-derived sulfur-doped graphene for cancer biomarker detection. *Sens. Actuators. B. Chem.*, **241**: 716–724. [CrossRef]

Sherawat, M., Rahi, R. K., Gupta, V., Neelam, D. and Sain, D. (2021). Prevention and control of food spoilage: An overview. *Int. J. Pharm. Biol. Sci.*, **11**(1): 124–130.

Singh, R. P. and Desrosier, N. W. (2014). Food preservation. Encyclopaedia Britannica Inc. Chicago. www.britannica.com/topic/food-preservation.

Smith, J. S. and Pillai, S. (2004). Irradiation and food safety. *Food Technol.*, **58**(11): 48–55.

Srisa-Art, M., Boehle, K. E., Geiss, B. J. and Henry, C. S. (2018). Highly sensitive detection of Salmonella typhimurium using a colorimetric paper-based analytical device coupled with immunomagnetic separation. *Anal. Chem.*, **90**: 1035–1043. [CrossRef] [PubMed]

Steele, R. (2004). Understanding and measuring the shelf-life of food. 1st ed. Sawston: Woodhead Publishing Limited.

Syamaladevi, R. M., Tang, J., Villa-Rojas, R., Sablani, S., Carter, B. and Campbell, G. (2016). Influence of water activity on thermal resistance of microorganisms in low-moisture foods: A review. *Compr. Rev. Food Sci. Food Saf.*, **15**(2): 353–370.

Toldrá, F. (2010). Irradiation of food commodities: Techniques, applications, detection, legislation, safety and consumer opinion. Ioannis S. Arvanitoyannis, editor. School of Agricultural Sciences, Department of Agriculture Ichthyology & Aquatic Resources, University of Thessaly, Hellas, Greece. Published by: Academic Press, an imprint of Elsevier, p. 710. Also published in 2010. *Trends in Food Science & Technology*, 22(1), 50. https://doi.org/10.1016/j.tifs.2010.12.003

Van Boekel, M. A. (2008). Kinetic modeling of food quality: A critical review. *Compr. Rev. Food Sci. Food. Saf.*, **7**: 144–58.

Vasireddi, O. (2013). Food adulteration & control mechanism. In: Workshop on Food defense awareness for food business operators and exporters. Hyderabad.

Wang, S., Zheng, L., Cai, G., Liu, N., Liao, M., Li, Y., Zhang, X. and Lin, J. A. (2019). Microfluidic biosensor for online and sensitive detection of *Salmonella typhimurium* using fluorescence labeling and smartphone video processing. *Biosens. Bioelectron.*, **140**: 111333. [CrossRef] [PubMed]

World Health Organization (WHO) (2020). The state of food security and nutrition in the world 2020: Transforming food systems for affordable healthy diets. Rome, Italy: Food & Agriculture Organization.

Xu, G., Cheng, C., Liu, Z., Yuan, W., Wu, X., Lu, Y., Low, S. S., Liu, J., Zhu, L. and Ji, D. (2019). Battery-free and wireless epidermal electrochemical system with all-printed stretchable electrode array for multiplexed in situ sweat analysis. *Adv. Mater. Technol.*, **4**: 1800658. [CrossRef]

Xue, H. Y., Hu, W. W., Son, H., Han, Y. and Yang, Z. Y. (2010). Indirect ELISA for detection and quantification of bovine milk in goat milk. *Food Sci.*, **31**: 370–373.

Zeinhom, M. M. A., Wang, Y., Song, Y., Zhu, M. J., Lin, Y. and Du, D. A. (2018). Portable smart-phone device for rapid and sensitive detection of *E. caoli* O157:H7 in yoghurt and egg. *Biosens. Bioelectron.*, **99**: 479–485. [CrossRef]

Zhang, H., Xue, L., Huang, F., Wang, S., Wang, L., Liu, N. and Lin, J. A. (2019). Capillary biosensor for rapid detection of Salmonella using Fe-nanocluster amplification and smart phone imaging. *Biosens. Bioelectron.*, **127**: 142–149. [CrossRef]

Zhao, C. Q., Jin, H., Gui, R. J. and Wang, Z. H. (2017). Facile fabrication of dual-ratiometric electrochemical sensors based on a bare electrode for dual-signal sensing of analytes in electrolyte solution. *Sens. Actuators B Chem.*, **409**: 71–78. [CrossRef]

Zhu, X. D., Shi, X., Chu, J., Ye, B., Zuo, P. and Wang, Y. H. (2018). Quantitative analysis of the growth of individual Bacillus coagulans cells by microdroplet technology. *Biores. Bioprocess.*, **8**(5): 1–8. [CrossRef]

Zhu, X. D., Shi, X., Wang, S. W., Chu, J., Zhu, W. H., Ye, B. C., Zuo, P. and Wang, Y. H. (2019). High-throughput screening of high lactic acid-producing Bacillus coagulans by droplet microfluidic based flow cytometry with fluorescence activated cell sorting. *RSC Adv.*, **9**: 4507–4513. [CrossRef]

6 Alcohol Nutrition

John Adeolu Falode

6.1 INTRODUCTION

The human race has been consuming fermented drinks for some centuries now, and there has been debate over the benefits and drawbacks of such drinks, particularly in terms of human health. Alcohol is best defined as a beverage to boost energy and make the drinker feel high or relaxed, and as a very toxic substance, with the dose determining the outcome. Alcohol use in moderation can be of assistance to the cardiovascular system. Nonetheless, in most nations, heavy drinking is a leading reason for premature death. Alcohol consumption is involved partly in roughly all fatal road accidents in the almost all parts of the world (NIAAA, 10). Furthermore, heavy alcohol use has been associated with harm to various key organs, including the liver, heart, stomach, brain, and kidneys, due to the active element ethanol; it also causes harm to the fetus during pregnancy, raises the possibility of breast and other cancers, leads to despair and violent behaviors, and interrupts relationships. Furthermore, it has a negative impact on blood lipids, insulin, inflammation, and coagulation. The mood, focus, and coordination of the individual are as well affected.

6.2 NUTRITION AND ALCOHOL

Human nutrition serves two purposes: energy production and bodily structure and function maintenance. Foods provide the energy and macromolecules needed to produce the biomolecules needed to repair worn out or damaged cells as well as the dietetic machineries required for physiological tasks. Alcoholics frequently feed defectively, restricting their intake of important nutrients and negatively impacting both energy production and structure repairs. Also, drinking impairs one's ability to concentrate by influencing nutrient digestion, storage, usage, and excretion (Lieber, 1988).

6.2.1 ALCOHOL AS THE BASIS OF NUTRITIONAL DEFICIENCIES IN ALCOHOLICS

The intestines are responsible for the absorption of nutrients from digested foods; the nutrients then enter the bloodstream and are transported to the liver. The liver either processes nutrients for instantaneous consumption or for long-term storage. Drinkers typically substitute alcohol for food, which eventually leads to malnutrition. Nutritional insufficiency and health crises can result from feeding poorly on any of the important nutritional elements (carbohydrates, protein, fats, vitamins, and/ or minerals). Alcohol, on the other hand, changes drinkers' body metabolism, preventing absorption, digestion, and use of certain food nutrients, resulting in nutrient insufficiency. Eventually, a slew of health issues arises. Alcohol prevents these nutrients from being broken down into useful molecules. This is carried out by lowering the amount of digestive enzymes produced from the pancreas (Korsten, 1989). Alcohol, as well, hinders nutritional absorption by harming the cells lining the stomach and intestines and stopping a large portion of nutrients from being transported into the bloodstream (Feinman, 1989). Furthermore, nutrient-deficient diets may result in additional absorption issues. Folate deficiency, for example, affects the cells lining the small intestine, causing electrolyte and folate assimilation to be disrupted (Feinman, 1989). Although nutrients are digested and absorbed, alcohol can encumber them from being used to their utmost potential by altering their transit, storage, and elimination (Thompson and Pratt, 1992). Increased excretion of nutrients

DOI: 10.1201/9781003361497-7

like fat, as well as decreased vitamin storage in the liver, indicates inadequate nutrient utilization in alcoholics (Feinman, 1989).

6.2.2 ALCOHOL AND SUPPLY OF ENERGY

Because most alcoholics get roughly half of their daily calories from alcohol, they prefer to avoid eating, which is a primary source of nutritional components like lipids, proteins, and carbohydrates that the body system needs (Feinman, 1989; Feinman and Lieber, 1992). However, even during enough food intake, the mechanisms through which the body regulates blood glucose concentration can be influenced by alcohol, resulting in either upraised or lowered blood glucose levels (Patel, 1989). Increased blood sugar, as a result of decreased insulin secretion, is usually transient and has no penalty in non-diabetic alcoholics. When a hungry or malnourished individual takes alcohol, hypoglycemia can occur. In the absence of energy supply through food, the sugar store is exhausted, and the by-products of alcohol metabolism prevent glucose from being formed from other substances like amino acids (Patel, 1989). Consequently, alcohol depletes the glucose supply to the brain and other body tissues, which is required for energy and function. Even if hypoglycemia (low blood sugar) is only present for a short time, it can cause catastrophic harm. While alcohol is a source of energy, its energy cannot be calculated using a simple calorie conversion number (USDHHS, 1988). Subjects lose weight when alcohol is swapped for carbs, calorie for calorie, demonstrating that alcohol provides less energy than carbohydrates. The mechanisms behind this low-energy alcohol conversion are complex and poorly understood (World et al., 1984), but various hypotheses have been advanced. Chronic drinking, for example, activates an inept alcohol metabolism system called the microsomal ethanol-oxidizing system (MEOS) (Lieber, 1988). The greater part of the energy formed by MEOS-driven alcohol metabolism is wasted as heat instead of being utilized to provide energy to the body.

6.3 THE EFFECTS OF ALCOHOL CONSUMPTION ON CELLULAR STRUCTURE (ORGANIZATION) AND FUNCTION

6.3.1 STRUCTURE AND FUNCTION

Because proteins constitute the majority of the cell, a high-protein diet is necessary for healthy cell upkeep. Alcohol has been shown to influence protein nutrition through impairing protein digestion to amino acids as well as the small intestine and liver's processing of amino acids, damaged protein synthesis from amino acids, as well as hepatic protein secretion (Feinman, 1989). Alcohol is well-known for affecting bodily function by blocking nutritional metabolism, resulting in vitamin shortages.

6.3.2 VITAMINS

Vitamins are essential for proper biological functioning, including development, metabolism, and function. Because of reduced intake of diets and impaired assimilation, metabolism, and use, persistent high alcohol consumption is linked to vitamin deficits in many people (Lieber, 1988, 1989). Alcohol, for example, hinders fat absorption, and hence, prevents the fat-soluble vitamins A, D, E, and K from being absorbed (Lieber, 1989; Leo and Lieber, 1989). Vitamin A insufficiency has been associated with night blindness, while vitamin D deficiency has been linked to bone deterioration (Feinman and Lieber, 1992). Vitamins A, C, D, E, F, K, and B vitamins are crucial in wound healing and cell conservation and homeostasis, and some alcoholics are low in them (Tortora and Anagnostakos, 1987). Vitamin K deficiency, in particular, can cause delayed clotting and excessive bleeding because the vitamin is required for blood clotting. Deficits in other vitamins important in brain function can potentially cause brain injury.

6.3.2.1   B1 Vitamin (Thiamine)

Several enzymes rely on thiamine for their structure and activity. Thiamine (vitamin B1) is found in a variety of foods, consisting of cereal grains, beans, nuts, yeast, and meat. Skeletal muscles, liver, brain, kidney, and heart all contain substantial levels of it. The breakdown of sugar molecules into different forms of molecules require enzymes whose actions and composition are dependent on thiamine, the production of some brain chemicals (such as neurotransmitters), as well as the manufacture of several other critical molecules and the body's capability to fight free radicals. When alcohol is combined with an uneven diet, thiamine levels drop quickly, disrupting absorption, storage, activation, and excretion. Beriberi is a thiamine-deficiency disease condition often associated with pain and the inability to move, among other symptoms. Weakness, weariness, and emotional disturbance are also early signs of thiamine insufficiency. As a result of the deficit, Beriberi develops, which can lead to heart failure, neuropathy, or peripheral edema. It's difficult to determine how much thiamine to provide to rectify a shortage as long as alcohol is consumed, since the alcohol will prevent thiamine from being effectively absorbed and converted to its active form. For men 14 years and older, the recommended dietary allowance (RDA) for thiamine is 1.2 milligrams (mg), while women over the age of 18 receive 1.1 milligrams (mg). 50 mg of oral thiamine supplement is recommended daily for people who have or are at risk of thiamine deficiency, and in severe situations, 50–100 mg of thiamine should be injected three to four times daily into the vein.

6.3.2.2   Folate

Folate aids in the formation and maintenance of fresh cells. It can be found in a range of foods, including vegetables (the largest concentrations are in spinach, asparagus, and Brussels sprouts), nuts, beans, peas, fruits and fruit juices, meat (the highest concentration is in liver), eggs, shellfish, yeast, and dairy products. Folate deficiency has been linked to cancer and birth abnormalities. Alcohol disrupts folate absorption, transport, metabolism, storage, and release via the liver. In healthy men, even moderate alcohol consumption over a short period of time (two weeks) can drastically lower serum folate concentration. An elevated level of folate in the blood has been associated with a reduced risk of breast cancer. For men and women over the age of 18, the RDA for folate is 400 micrograms (mcg). A well-balanced diet, on the other hand, is sufficient to meet the RDA.

6.3.2.3   B12 (Cobalamin)

Vitamin B12 is essential for the development and maintenance of healthy red blood cells, nerve cells, DNA, and protein metabolism. Alcohol inhibits vitamin B12 absorption, distribution, metabolism, and excretion by interfering with dietary folate intake, absorption, distribution, metabolism and excretion. Loss of balance, numbness or tingling in the arms and legs, weakness, weariness, constipation, disorientation, melancholy, poor memory, tenderness of the mouth or tongue, weight loss, and megaloblastic anemia are all symptoms of low vitamin B12 levels. Animal goods such as seafood, poultry, meat, eggs, and milk products contain vitamin B12, whereas plant products do not. According to studies, both moderate and high alcohol use has an effect on vitamin B12 levels. For men and women above the age of 14, the RDA for vitamin B12 is 2.4 micrograms. When a person's capability to absorb this vitamin is impaired, a deficit can be corrected with injections. Oral supplements are beneficial when doses are started at 2,000 mcg per day, then reduced to 1,000 mcg per day, weekly, and eventually monthly.

6.3.2.4   A Vitamin

Vitamin A is critical to our survival as humans; it is required for cell division and differentiation as well as for night vision, immune system regulation, bone formation, and reproduction. It is a fat-soluble vitamin – one of the four. Vitamin A can be sourced from fish, fortified cereals, and dairy products; it is also found in broccoli, carrots, squash, and cantaloupe. For men over the age of 18, the RDA for vitamin A is 900 mcg, and for women over the age of 18, it is 700 mcg. Alcohol has been linked to vitamin A deficiency and increasing the toxicity of the vitamin, when taken in large doses. Alcohol affects its metabolism, making it unavailable to drinkers, and supplementation is not an option because vitamin A is lethal in high doses, and taking too much in the form of supplements can be precarious. Dietary supplements of beta carotene (a precursor to vitamin A) are available. If abstinence from alcohol is not possible, moderate alcohol intake is the only smart decision.

6.3.3 MINERALS

Mineral deficiency often results in a variety of health problems, ranging from calcium-related bone ill health to zinc-related night blindness and skin diseases. Mineral deficiencies such as calcium, magnesium, iron, and zinc are common in alcoholics, despite the fact that alcohol does not appear to influence mineral absorption (Marsano and McClain, 1989). However, alcohol causes secondary issues like a drop off in calcium incorporation due to fat malabsorption; a magnesium deficit owing to reduced ingestion, enhanced urinary excretion, nausea, and diarrhea (Flink, 1986); insufficiency of iron due to bleeding from the gut (gastrointestinal track) (Marsano and McClain, 1989); and zinc malabsorption or losses due to other nutrient deficiencies (Marsano and McClain, 1989; McClain et al., 1986).

6.3.3.1 Calcium

Calcium is, moreover, important for the correct functioning of cells and the entire body structure. It is necessary for bone tissue growth, vasoconstriction and dilation, and muscle contraction and expansion, hormone and enzyme secretion, and as a second messenger in the transmission of messages through the nervous system. It is the body's most prevalent mineral. Milk, yogurt, and cheese are the best sources of calcium. Alcohol use has been linked to calcium loss in the body due to increased urine calcium excretion, resulting in calcium insufficiency. Osteoporosis can be caused by a calcium shortage. Adolescents and young adults who use large amounts of alcohol on a regular basis can have a significant impact on bone health and increase their chance of developing osteoporosis later in life. The RDA for men aged 19–70 is 1,000 mg, and for men aged 71 and above, 1,200 mg; and for women aged 19–50, the RDA is 1,000 mg, and for women aged 51 and up, 1,200 mg. Supplementing with calcium may be useful.

6.3.3.2 Protein

Alcohol changes the way amino acids and proteins are processed. Proteins and amino acids assist to preserve and sustain cell structure by transporting chemicals in and out of cells and acting as enzymes. Alcohol inhibits the absorption of amino acids in the small intestine. Alcohol abuse usually has a fatal effect on the liver, causing alcohol-induced hepatitis, cirrhosis, hepatic failure, and, in some circumstances, liver cancer and death. A number of consequences emerge as a result of abnormal protein metabolism in chronic liver failure, including reduced albumin, ascites, and an increased risk of hepatic encephalopathy. Chronic alcohol consumption also affects the pancreas, and decreased production of pancreatic enzymes leads to malabsorption of fats and proteins long before other indications of chronic pancreatic damage appear.

6.4 CONSUMPTION OF ALCOHOLIC BEVERAGES SHOULD BE KEPT TO A MINIMUM

There is no commonly agreed standard drink definition, even among alcohol academics, if the truth be told (Kloner and Rezkalla, 2007). Some experts believe that red wine makes the distinction, but another study suggests that beverage preference has minimal impact on cardiovascular health (DGA, 2018). Modest drinking is characterized as a level of alcohol consumption that is balanced. It could also be described as a state where the health benefits of alcohol clearly exceed the hazards.

6.5 CELLULAR PERSPECTIVE OF POTENTIAL HEALTH BENEFITS OF ALCOHOL

The results of various research have revealed that drinking alcohol in moderation has advantages over abstention for better health and a longer life expectancy. The impact of confounding variables and systematic flaws, which may have been accidentally ignored in the early research, have come under scrutiny, nevertheless (Nova et al., 2012).

6.5.1 MODERATE ALCOHOL USE, ILLNESS, AND MORTALITY

Numerous observational studies have revealed the nuanced connection between alcohol use, mortality, and health maintenance. The U-shaped connection between alcohol usage and mortality demonstrates that light to moderate alcohol intake is more linked to reduced mortality than high or total alcohol abstinence (Nova et al., 2012). Although numerous studies since then have constantly indicated that moderate drinkers outlive heavy and abstaining drinkers, there is debate about the significance of confounding factors and the validity of such results if they are taken into account.

6.5.2 ALCOHOL CONSUMPTION IN MODERATION, INFLAMMATION, AND CVD

Literature has thoroughly covered the advantages of moderate alcohol drinking on the cardiovascular system (Klatsky, 2010). These cardioprotective benefits have been seen in patients with myocardial infarction, stroke, and hypertension risk as well as in healthy persons (Brugger-Andersen et al., 2009; Bos et al., 2010; Ronksley et al., 2011). Studies in the fields of epidemiology, medicine, and science have shown that the pathogeneses of cardiovascular disease, particularly atherosclerosis, involve inflammatory pathways (McNeill et al., 2010; Espinola-Klein et al., 2011). Endothelial dysfunction, the first sign of atherosclerosis, is characterized by an imbalance between vasodilation and vasoconstriction. This imbalance is a result of increased production of adhesion molecules, pro-inflammatory cytokines, pro-thrombotic factors, and oxidative stress (Sitia et al., 2010). C-reactive protein (CRP) is one inflammatory marker that is used to track the progression of disease and cardiovascular risk (Mangalmurti and Davidson, 2011). Through a number of methods, moderate alcohol use can lower the risk of CVD, including elevating HDL, apoA1, and adiponectin levels and lowering LDL concentrations, blood pressure, coronary blood flow, platelet aggregation, fibrinogen levels, and other factors (Klatsky, 2010; Brien et al., 2011). Despite the fact that moderate alcohol drinking protects the cardiovascular system and other disorders linked to it, some of the effects appear to be unique to wine consumption. In addition to ethanol, wine contains additional compounds like resveratrol and hydroxytyrosol that have significant anti-inflammatory and antioxidant properties (Bertelli and Das, 2009). According to numerous studies, moderate wine drinking has some health benefits for the cardiovascular system that are not seen with other alcoholic beverages (Huang et al., 2010; Vazquez-Prieto et al., 2011).

6.5.3 ALCOHOL CONSUMPTION IN MODERATION AND THE IMMUNE SYSTEM

The quantity, frequency, and duration of alcohol administration are just a few of the variables that affect how alcohol affects immunological function. Romeo et al. discuss the dearth of studies examining the effects of moderate alcohol use on immunity at that time (Romeo et al., 2007a). Others describe anti-inflammatory effects, such as those on the adhesion properties of monocytes (Badia et al., 2004), fibrinogen (Estruch et al., 2004), and inflammatory cytokine production (Estruch et al., 2004; Winker et al., 2006; Mandrekar et al., 2006) as well as the transcription factor NF-kB. Other studies have shown a decrease in the frequency of the common pro-inflammatory mediators such as TNF-A and IL-1β (Mandrekar et al., 2006). Romeo et al. studies reveal improvements in a variety of immunological parameters, including leucocyte counts (only in women), cytokine production, and

Ig concentrations (Romeo et al., 2007b, 2007c). Although wine and beer are sources of alcohol, it is important to keep in mind that they also contain other nutrients that can affect the immune system, such as carbs, soluble fibre, minerals, and vitamins (Vinson et al., 2003; Boscolo et al., 2003; Magrone and Jirillo, 2010). Xanthohumol, the main prenylated flavonoid found in beer, and resveratrol, a polyphenolic phyto-alexin found in red wine, have both been linked to possible health and immune system advantages. In addition to its significant immunosuppressive effects on T-cell development, IL-2 activated killer cell production, cytotoxic T-lymphocyte production, and Th1 cytokine production (IL-2, interferon-g, and TNFa), xanthohumol also has anti-inflammatory and antioxidant properties (Gao et al., 2009). Numerous studies have demonstrated the vast range of biological benefits that resveratrol and its derivatives have, including anti-tumor (Mahyar-Roemer et al., 2001; Fujita et al., 2011), antioxidant (Goldberg, 1996), and anti-inflammatory activities. According to Wirleitner et al. (2005), this substance may decrease interferon-g-mediated biochemical pathways and interfere with immune activation and cytokine cascades, which could be extremely important to halt the onset and progression of several immune-related disorders.

6.6   ALCOHOL'S NEGATIVE EFFECTS

Alcohol abuse frequently develops into a difficult-to-control-or-abandon habit. Though some people find it simple to stop, the greater part of people do not. The impact of excessive alcohol use on human bodily systems cannot be underestimated. It has been reported that it can cause liver inflammation (alcohol-induced hepatitis), which can lead to liver cirrhosis; it can cause heart muscle injury (cardiomyopathy); and it has been linked to a variety of cancers, including cancers of the mouth, throat, pharynx, liver, breast among others (WCRF/AICR, 2007). The lethal effects of alcohol consumption may be connected to two molecules found in it: ethanol and acetaldehyde, a compound generated when ethanol is broken down. In large doses, both have been discovered to be carcinogenic to humans (Scoccianti et al., 2015). Drinkers who also smoke tobacco or eat a bad diet, according to reports, multiply the negative effects of alcohol. Alcohol misuse has an economic impact on alcoholics' families, friends, and communities. Alcohol use has been connected to over 30% of violent crime instances (Rand and Catalano, 2007), and hundreds, if not millions, of people have died too soon as a result of drunk drivers (CDCP, 2018). Drinking moderately still has its drawbacks. Alcohol usually causes sleep disturbances and has a detrimental impact on one's ability to make good decisions. Alcohol-drug interaction occurs with a number of drugs, including pain relievers, acetaminophen, antidepressants, anticonvulsants, and sedatives, and this interaction is frequently potentially harmful ways. It also has the potential for addiction, especially for persons with a such history in their family.

6.6.1   ALCOHOL CONSUMPTION ENHANCES THE RISK OF BREAST CANCER AND OTHER CANCERS

More than a few studies have connected chronic and continuous use of alcohol to the development of cancers, especially breast cancer (Smith-Warner et al., 1998; Scoccianti et al., 2015; Allen et al., 2009; Kim et al., 2017). A very large, 30-year prospective research of 88,084 women and 47,881 men indicated that even one drink per day increased the risk of alcohol-related cancers in women (female breast, oral cavity, pharynx, larynx, liver, and oesophagus), particularly breast cancer, in both smokers and nonsmokers. In men who did not smoke, however, one to two drinks per day were not linked to an increased risk of alcohol-related malignancies (Cao et al., 2015). The presence of folate, a micronutrient and vitamin, in people's meals lowers the risk of developing breast cancer in women. Folate is indispensable in the production of new cells as well as the prevention of DNA modifications; however, its deficit can occur as a result of excessive alcohol use, and this can lead to mutations in specific genes, which can lead to cancer. A daily folate intake of 400 micrograms has been recommended (Baglietto et al., 2005; Zhang et al., 1999).

6.7   THE MOLECULAR UNDERPINNINGS OF ALCOHOL'S ADVERSE EFFECTS AND THE RESULTANT PATHOLOGICAL STATES (MEDICAL CONSEQUENCES)

6.7.1   LIVER DISEASE CAUSED BY ALCOHOL (ALD)

Chronic alcohol consumption has serious consequences for the liver, heart, and brain, among other organs. While moderate alcohol consumption may benefit some pathological diseases, such as cardiovascular disease (heart ischemia), long-term alcohol intake intensifies the risk of alcoholic-related liver disease (ALD) (Lim et al., 2010). Excessive and ongoing alcohol consumption can cause alcohol-induced hepatitis (AH), which typically results in severe clinical symptoms such as indicators of liver decompensation (such as jaundice, ascites, infection, and bleeding from esophageal varices, among others) (Thursz et al., 2015). Several alcohol-induced vicious pathways have been linked to liver damage, including the following.

6.7.1.1   Oxidative Stress in (ALD)

The main kind of cells responsible for ethanol metabolism are hepatocytes. Alcohol dehydrogenase is principally responsible for converting ethanol to acetaldehyde. Cytosolic aldehyde dehydrogenase (ALDH1) and mitochondrial ALDH2 then convert acetaldehyde into the non-toxic compound acetate. Another alcohol-metabolizing enzyme, CYP2E1, converts ethanol to acetaldehyde at high ethanol concentrations, producing reactive oxygen species (ROS) (Nagy et al., 2016). Although acetaldehyde and ethanol are direct liver poisons, increased ROS generation and the subsequent release of inflammatory cytokines might facilitate alcohol-induced liver inflammation and injury. Chronic alcohol use increases hepatic CYP2E1 levels, which boosts the production of ROS (Nagy et al., 2016). Furthermore, ethanol and acetaldehyde directly damage the mitochondria of hepatocytes, increasing mitochondrial ROS production and worsening liver inflammation and injury. Neutrophils are another source of ROS and play an important role in the progression of alcoholic hepatitis (AH). Neutrophils have an impact on the severity of AH illness (Altamirano et al., 2014). Ethanol increases the expression of E-selectin on sinusoidal endothelial cells and intercellular adhesion molecule-1 (ICAM-1) on neutrophil surfaces, allowing circulating neutrophils to move to the liver. Kupffer cells and hepatic stellate cells also secrete chemokines (CXCL1, C-C motif chemokine ligand (CCL2), and CXCL8) that promote neutrophil migration and infiltration into injured liver regions (Bertola et al., 2013). The IL-1b and TNFa produced by Kupffer cells as well as the ROS produced by neutrophils promote hepatocyte death and local inflammation (Xu et al., 2014). As a result, excess ROS production by alcohol breakdown, impaired mitochondria, and neutrophils cause liver inflammation and eventual liver injury by the ethanol so produced.

6.7.1.2   ALD Has Altered Lipid Metabolism

Because ethanol alters hepatic lipid metabolism, lipid precipitates are formed as a result of steatosis caused by alcohol in the cytoplasm of hepatocytes containing triglyceride and esterified cholesterol. Ethanol inhibits adenosine monophosphate-activated kinase (AMPK), peroxisome proliferator activated receptor (PPAR), and sirtuin 1 (SIRT1), lowering FA b-oxidation (Nakajima et al., 2004). Decreased b-oxidation promotes steatosis. Furthermore, ethanol reduces hepatic SIRT1 activity, which increases SREBP-1c transcriptional activity (You et al., 2008; Crabb and Liangpunsakul, 2006). Ethanol causes a decrease in SIRT1 activity, which is linked to a decrease in DEP domain-containing mTOR-interacting protein (DEPTOR), a negative watchdog of mTORC1 that promotes the transcription of SREBP-1c and lipin-1 movement to the cytoplasm while inhibiting PPAR transcription. Alcohol promotes lipogenesis by increasing the manifestation and activity of SREBP-1c, ACC1, and PPARg while decreasing the activity of AMPK, SIRT1, and PPAR (You et al., 2008; Chen et al., 2018; Zhang et al., 2016). Lipin-1's critical function has been linked to ALD. Alcohol induces fatty liver by increasing hepatic lipin-1 expression while inhibiting lipin-1 nuclear translocation, which prevents FA bioxidation (You et al., 2017). Alcohol-induced steatosis is also connected with lower levels of very-low-density lipoprotein (VLDL). The microsomal triglyceride transfer protein (MTP) amasses VLDL for the production of lipids. Ethanol reduced MTP levels in hepatocytes and the PPAR agonist can upturn VLDL secretion by upregulating MTP. Lipin-1 overexpression in ALD also plays a role in lowering VLDL secretion (Bi et al., 2015). Furthermore, ethanol raises the level of the fatty acids (FAs) in circulation in the liver, which encourages alcoholic steatosis by increasing lipids breakdown in peripheral and visceral fat tissues (Ramirez et al., 2013). Furthermore, by activating TLR4 signaling, circulating FAs can cause liver inflammation (Ohashi et al., 2018). Alcohol abuse also impairs hepatocytes' ability to lipolyze and degrade lipid droplets. Lipid breakdown is controlled by neutral lipases in the cytosol such as adipose triglyceride lipase (ATGL) and lipophagy, a type of autophagy linked to destruction of lipid droplets in the lysosomes. Alcohol inhibits adrenergic-mediated lipid droplet disintegration in hepatocytes by preventing phosphorylation of hormone-sensitive lipase by protein kinase A and ATGL recruitment to lipid droplets (Schott et al., 2017).

6.7.1.3   ALD Patients' Impaired Liver Regeneration

Although hepatocytes have a remarkable ability to repair following liver damage or the loss of liver tissues, this ability is severely compromised in ALD. This was seen in AH patients and rat models exposed to prolonged ethanol (Dubuquoy et al., 2015). Chronic ethanol use in rodent models reduces the ability of the liver to regenerate following partial hepatectomy by preventing the induction of cell cycle genes and changing the liver's miRNA profile (Dippold et al., 2013).

6.7.2   ALCOHOL-INDUCED NEUROPATHOLOGICAL CONDITIONS

A combination of ethanol toxicity and malnutrition may have long-term consequences and exacerbate clinical signs of neurological damage (Crews and Nixon, 2009). In general, chronic alcohol use may result in erratic notches of cerebral injury, comprising serious dementia, as well as a steady decline in psychological status (Kwok, 2016). Alcohol is the second major cause of dementia in adults in the United States (10%), after Alzheimer's disease (40–60%) (Crews, 1999). Nutrition, alcohol consumption, and its frequency and duration are lifestyle factors that have a relationship with the severity of neurological consequences. Chronic alcoholics typically get 50% of their calories from alcohol, which puts them at risk for severe malnutrition (Diamond and Francisco, 1993). Alcohol intake may raise the likelihood of epileptic seizures, brain infections, cerebrovascular lesions, and change the balance of the neurotransmitters in the body (Freedland and McMicken, 1993). High order executive function may be impacted by cognitive impairment, and this may result in secondary disabilities that last the remainder of one's life.

6.7.2.1   Alcohol Metabolism's Pathophysiology and How it Affects BBB Malfunction

The molecular basis of cell death caused by alcohol is unknown, despite thousands of studies investigating the impact of alcohol on the nervous system. Many long-term AUD patients have neurocognitive and neurovascular impairment due to ethanol metabolites, which is linked to BBB failure (Haorah et al., 2005a). The BBB is an extremely selective semipermeable membrane formed by brain microvascular endothelial cells (BMVEC). Pericytes and astrocytes connect to the BMVEC via a tight junction, ensuring the structural integrity of the BBB. This close connection acts as a natural defender and is critical for maintaining normal brain homeostasis (Daneman and Prat, 2015). The brain's cytoskeletal structure may interact with ethanol metabolites or neurotoxic chemicals to increase BBB permeability and trigger neuroinflammation (Haorah et al., 2005b; Liu et al., 2017). Because ALDH (aldehyde dehydrogenase) is found in brain cell mitochondria, it is known that acetaldehyde is oxidized in brain cells. ALDH then changes acetaldehyde to acetate, which has additional effects on the brain by increasing lipid peroxidation and free radical formation. In addition to cumulative ROS production, EtOH causes oxidative metabolizing enzymes to express catalytically. As a result, ethanol increases the oxidative stress response while decreasing antioxidant function indirectly. Alcohol consumption is thought to produce ROS, specifically in the cytochrome P450–2E1 (CYP2E1)-metabolized EtOH, which produces H_2O_2, superoxide, and other free radicals. The Rho kinase (ROCK/JNK) signaling cascade is then activated by the free radicals, resulting in the production of inflammatory cytokines and vascular endothelial growth factor (VEGF) in the brain endothelial cells (for instance, ICAM-1 and E-selectin upregulation and IL-6 release) (Zehendner et al., 2013; Haorah et al., 2008). Excessive ROS effects activate transcription-modulated lipid peroxidation in neurons, raising the levels of 4-HNE (lipid peroxidation products) while decreasing the levels of neuronal cytoskeletal proteins (Maffi et al., 2008). The primary cause of alcohol-related neurodegeneration is interruption of neuron-specific neurofilaments or neuronal death (Haorah et al., 2008). Both short-term and long-term alcohol consumption can alter the structure of phospholipid-containing cell membranes, increasing ROS formation, enhancing peroxidation of lipids, proteins, and mitochondria, and decreasing ATP production (Amano et al., 2010). Astrocytes protect the blood-brain barrier (BBB) by coordinating the flow of blood in the CNS and neural activity between pericytes and CNS vasculature (Sweeney et al., 2016). Alcohol typically causes tight junction disassembly by activating protein kinase C (PKC), allowing harmful chemicals into the brain and impairing CNS homeostasis. Furthermore, empirical studies show that the primary cause of brain damage by alcohol is an oxidative stress reaction induced by proinflammatory cytokines activated in the course of alcohol intemperance. Pro-inflammatory cytokines induce anti-inflammatory and immune response signals, contributing to tissue atrophy and neuronal deterioration. NF-kB (transcription factor) mediates and participates in these processes (Thameem Dheen et al., 2007; Collins and Neafsey, 2012). In reaction to alcohol-induced oxidative stress-related inflammation, large families of released proteins known as cytokines are moved from blood serum to neural tissue (Collins and Neafsey, 2012). Increased cytokine production, particularly of macrophage chemotactic protein 1 (CCL 2), tumor necrotic factor (TNF), and interleukin IL-1 and IL-1, causes neuroinflammation and nerve axon damage in nociceptive synaptic terminals, leading to intracortical network dysfunction and neuropathy (Noor et al., 2020).

6.7.2.2 Neurodegeneration is Caused by the Glucose Transport System Being Compromised

Previous research has found a link between impaired glucose metabolism and neuronal death at the boundary of alcohol-induced BBB failure, which leads to CNS neurodegeneration (Shah et al., 2012; Niccoli et al., 2016). As a result of a BBB rupture, protein channels for glucose transport (GLUT 1 and GLUT 3) may be expressed less and glucose uptake within brain tissue may be reduced (Muneer et al., 2011). Almost 90% of brain part relies on a steady source of glucose to sustain its energetic task. The GLUT 1 glucose transporter transports glucose from capillary endothelium to astrocytes, where it is metabolized and transported to neurons as energy for tissue plasticity and anti-oxidation via the GLUT 3 transporter to regenerate (Niccoli et al., 2016; Barros et al., 2017). Glucose intake decreases steadily in nerve cells in the hippocampus, corpus callosum, and cerebral cortex during the preclinical stage of dementia. In an animal model, this results in lactate production, aerobic glycolysis, among other cellular events (Hagen et al., 2002; Shah et al., 2012). Clinical symptoms appear eventually with connection to dementia, ataxia, spasticity, and mild to severe cognitive impairments. As a result, maintaining the standard glucose homeostasis is critical for optimum utility of the brain; if this balance is altered or disrupted, it causes neuronal toxicity, which leads to cell death and has a negative impact on cognitive performance.

6.7.2.3 Neurotoxicity Induced by NMDA Receptors

The primary excitatory brain neurotransmitter N-methyl-D-aspartate (NMDA) interacts with the glutamate binding site located in cells in the brain. The influx of various ions (Na+ and Ca2+) into the cell via the NMDA receptors maintains cell depolarization and nerve action potential activation.

NMDA receptors are required for synaptic plasticity and signal transmission throughout the cellular processes of learning, the development of working memory through neural synchronization via intra-cortical communication, and visuospatial memory (Zhou and Baudry, 2006). Alcohol is thought to act as an NMDA receptor antagonist, so in the case of AUD, it causes NMDA receptor hypofunction, which may result in neural network dysfunction with loss of synaptic plasticity (Chandrasekar, 2013). The physiological functions of the NMDA receptor are required to maintain homeostasis and appropriate neural function. Numerous controversial studies suggested that NMDA receptors play an important role in excitotoxicity, which reduces cell life and causes cell death (Collins and Neafsey, 2016). The latest proof supports the notion that NMDA receptor excitotoxicity affects both healthy brain function and neurodegenerative diseases such as Alzheimer's and Huntington's disease (Crews and Nixon, 2009). Nevertheless, there is no entrenched theory that distinguishes the use of alcohol as an NMDA receptor antagonist or as a neuroprotective drug. This is due to the fact that effective use of NMDA antagonists would necessitate preventing excessive activation while not interfering with normal physiological processes (Collins and Neafsey, 2016). Earlier research, however, suggested that chronic alcohol use could reduce the production of brain-derived neurotrophic factor (BDNF) due to ethanol-induced blocking of the NMDA receptor, potentially worsening neurotoxicity (Bhave et al., 1999). More research is needed to determine the role of the NMDA receptor in the mechanism of neurodegeneration or neuro-regeneration in patients with AUD.

6.8   OTHER LIFE-THREATENING FALLOUTS FROM ALCOHOLISM

Anyone who has ever had a hangover can relate to the fact that drinking alcohol is bad for your health. Reduced inhibitions, indistinct and inaudible speech, damage to motor coordination, confusion, memory-loss issues, problems with attention, loss of consciousness, respiratory problems, and even mortality are among risks associated with alcohol consumption. The vital body organs like brain, liver, heart, pancreas, and the immune system can all be affected by chronic and incessant alcohol consumption. It can also cause malignancies of the mouth, throat, breast, and liver, among others. When taken by expectant women, it can induce fetal alcohol syndrome in the baby. In pregnant and nursing women, there is no known safe level of alcohol consumption.

6.8.1   LIVER DISEASE

Because it is the seat of biotransformation and metabolism of medicines and xenobiotics, the liver is the internal organ most vulnerable to injury. The primary cause of alcoholic liver damage is alcohol; however, undernourishment is also a hazardous for alcohol-related liver damage. Alcohol use has been shown to impact liver-bound nutrients such as carotenoids, which are the primary sources of vitamin A, and vitamin E compounds (Leo et al., 1992; Leo et al., 1993). Considerable reduction of these nutrients may have a role in the liver damage caused by alcohol.

6.8.2   PANCREATITIS

Malnutrition and protein-deficient diet have been associated with an enhanced risk of developing alcoholic pancreatitis (Korsten et al., 1992), while overeating has also been connected to pancreatitis (Korsten et al., 1990).

6.8.3   BRAIN

Thiamine deficiency in the brain, which is common in alcoholics, can cause serious neurological issues, including Wernicke/Korsakoff syndrome, which comprises poor mobility and memory loss (Victor, 1992). The impact of nutritional deficits on brain function can be severe and long-lasting.

6.8.4 Pregnancy

Alcohol has a direct, harmful effect on embryonic development, resulting in birth abnormalities such as fetal alcohol syndrome. Alcohol can influence fetal development when it is combined with a nutritional shortage (Phillips et al., 1989). Food intake could rise up to about 140% to fulfill the demands of both mother and fetus during pregnancy, which is 10 to 30% higher than normal (Phillips et al., 1989). Although an alcoholic mother's poor nutrition has a direct negative impact on the fetus' nutrition, alcohol can also impede nourishment flow to the fetus (Phillips et al., 1989).

6.8.5 The Dicey Impact of Alcohol on Blood Sugar Concentration

The major metabolic fuel in our body system is blood glucose. Excess glucose is stored as glycogen in the muscle and liver and is normally obtained from the meals we eat. Insulin and glucagon are hormones that regulate blood glucose levels by sensing blood glucose levels and either storing surplus glucose or delivering signals to release glucose from its stores when blood glucose levels are low. The body considers alcohol to be a xenobiotic or toxicant. Alcohol interacts with all the sources of glucose as well as the hormones required to maintain good and healthy blood glucose levels, according to some studies. The most significant effect is noticed in heavy drinkers who consume large amounts of alcohol on a regular basis. When a heavy drinker's diet lacks sufficient carbohydrates, their glycogen stores are depleted within a few hours. Excessive alcohol consumption might reduce the efficacy of insulin over time, resulting in elevated blood sugar levels. Heavy drinkers are more likely to develop alcohol-induced liver disease, glucose intolerance, or diabetes. Alcohol has a negative effect on blood glucose levels, regardless of how often it is consumed. Drinking on an empty stomach could trigger hypoglycemia. Acute alcohol consumption has been shown to enhance insulin secretion, resulting in low blood sugar (hypoglycemia), which affects the hormonal response. Alcohol changes hypoglycemic medications, making it a difficult problem for anyone with diabetes. Anyone with diabetes should exercise extreme caution while ingesting alcohol.

6.8.6 The Effects of Alcohol on Weight Gain

Although moderate alcohol use contains about 100–150 calories on average, according to a study, higher alcohol use increases the likelihood of slight weight gain (Downer et al., 2017). Additionally, drinkers' higher calorie consumption from non-alcoholic sources tends to contribute to greater calorie intake from alcoholic ones.

6.9 ALCOHOL'S POTENTIAL HEALTH BENEFITS

6.9.1 Protection against Cardiovascular Disease

Several studies have revealed that reasonable alcohol consumption does not increase the risk of cardiac arrest, ischemic stroke, sudden cardiac fatality, or mortality from any cause (Goldberg et al., 2001). Increased alcohol consumption, on the other hand, has been linked to hypertension, irregular cardiac rhythms, stroke, cardiac arrest, and death (Scoccianti et al., 2015; O'Keefe et al., 2014; Zhang et al., 2014; Bell et al., 2017). The scientific basis for showing the benefits of moderate alcohol use is that moderate alcohol usage raises levels of high-density lipoprotein (HDL) (Booyse et al., 2007), and higher HDL levels are linked to a lower risk of heart disease. Reasonable alcohol use has also been associated with a number of constructive effects, including increased insulin sensitivity and improvements in blood clotting factors such tissue type plasminogen activator, fibrinogen, clotting factor VII, and von Willebrand factor (Booyse et al., 2007). This usually avoids the production of small blood clots in the heart, neck, and the brain, which is the leading cause of heart attacks and strokes.

6.9.2 ADDITIONAL ADVANTAGES

Moderate alcohol use has health benefits not only for the heart, but also for other essential organs.

Moderate alcohol consumption has been shown to reduce the possibility of gallstones (Leitzmann et al., 1999) and type 2 diabetes (Leitzmann et al., 1999; Koppes et al., 2005; Diousse et al., 2007).

6.10 ALCOHOLICS' NUTRITIONAL STATE

Both heavy and mild alcohol consumption leads to poor eating habits, with drinkers frequently consuming less food than is required to provide adequate food nutrients such as carbohydrates, proteins, fats, vitamins A, C, B, and minerals – for example, calcium and iron (Feinman, 1989; Hillers and Massey, 1985). Another issue is that alcohol causes mild malnutrition to progress to severe malnutrition by interfering with meal digestion and nutrient use. According to studies, even the heaviest drinkers have few nutritional deficits, yet many alcoholics who are hospitalized for medical repercussions of alcoholism suffer from ruthless undernourishment (Lieber, 1988, 1989).

Body parameters such as weight, height, mass, and skin fold thickness can be used to estimate fat reserves, as well as the calculation of some blood biomarkers that can offer measurements of circulating proteins, vitamins, and minerals. However, these methods are frequently erroneous, and for many nutrients, there is no obvious "cut-off" point that would allow a precise characterization of insufficiency (Thompson and Pratt, 1992). As a result, the limitations of the methodologies make assessing the nutritional condition of alcoholics difficult. Dietary habits can yield inferences regarding the likelihood of developing nutritional deficiencies.

6.11 THE ROLE OF GENETICS IN ALCOHOLISM

Individuals react to medications or xenobiotics in different ways, and genetic polymorphism revealed this. Genetics has been shown to play a significant effect in defining an individual's alcohol preferences and likelihood of developing alcoholism in studies. In most cases, Gregor Mendel's inheritance rule does not apply to alcoholism. Then again, alcoholism is controlled by a number of genes that form a network with one another over and above external circumstances (NIAAA, 2017). According to research, the effect of alcohol on the cardiovascular system is influenced by some genes. Alcohol dehydrogenase is a metabolizing enzyme that comes in two forms. Alcohol dehydrogenase type 1C (ADH1C) is one form of this enzyme that comes in two "types". The first breaks down alcohol fast, while the second takes longer. Moderate consumers with two copies of the slow-acting enzyme gene have a significantly reduced risk of cardiovascular disease than moderate drinkers with two copies of the fast-acting enzyme gene (Hines et al., 2001). Those who have both the slow-acting and fast-acting enzyme genes are in the middle. It's possible that the fast-acting enzyme degrades alcohol before it has a positive impact on HDL and clotting factors. However, changes in the ADH1C gene have no effect on the risk of heart disease in those who do not consume alcohol. This lends credence to the notion that alcohol lessens the risk of heart disease.

6.12 WRAPPING UP

The pros and cons of sensible alcohol consumption cannot be really defined as years pass. Until middle age, when cardiovascular disease begins to account for an increasingly considerable share of the burden of disease and death, moderate alcohol consumption tends to have more harmful effects than beneficial effects.

REFERENCES

Allen NE, Beral V, Casabonne D, Kan SW, Reeves GK, Brown A, Green J. Moderate alcohol intake and cancer incidence in women. J Nat Cancer Inst. 2009 Mar 4;101(5):296–305.

Altamirano J, Miquel R, Katoonizadeh A. A histologic scoring system for prognosis of patients with alcoholic hepatitis. Gastroenterology. 2014;146:1231e1239 (e1–e6)

Amano M, Nakayama M, Kaibuchi K. Rho-kinase/ROCK: A key regulator of the cytoskeleton and cell polarity. Cytoskeleton (Hoboken). 2010;67:545–554.

Badía E, Sacanella E, Fernàndez-Solà J et al. Decreased tumor necrosis factor-induced adhesion of human monocytes to endothelial cells after moderate alcohol consumption. Am J Clin Nutr. 2004;80:225–230.

Baglietto L, English DR, Gertig DM, Hopper JL, Giles GG. Does dietary folate intake modify effect of alcohol consumption on breast cancer risk? Prospective Cohort Study. BMJ. 2005 Oct 6;331(7520):807.

Barros LF, San Martín A, Ruminot I, et al. Near-critical GLUT1 and Neurodegeneration. J Neurosci Res. 2017;95:2267–2274.408

Bell S, Daskalopoulou M, Rapsomaniki E, George J, Britton A, Bobak M, Casas JP, Dale CE, Denaxas S, Shah AD, Hemingway H. Association between clinically recorded alcohol consumption and initial presentation of 12 cardiovascular diseases: Population based cohort study using linked health records. BMJ. 2017 Mar 22;356:j909.

Bertelli AA, Das DK. Grapes, wines, resveratrol, and heart health. J Cardiovasc Pharmacol. 2009;54:468–476.

Bertola A, Park O, Gao B. Chronic plus binge ethanol feeding synergistically induces neutrophil infiltration and liver injury in mice: A critical role for Eselectin. Hepatology. 2013;58:1814e1823

Bhave SV, Ghoda L, Hoffman PL. Brain-derived neurotrophic factor mediates the antiapoptotic effect of NMDA in cerebellar granule neurons: Signal transduction cascades and site of ethanol action. J Neurosci. 1999;19:3277–3286.

Bi L, Jiang Z, Zhou J. The role of lipin-1 in the pathogenesis of alcoholic fatty liver. Alcohol Alcohol. 2015;50:146e151.

Booyse FM, Pan W, Grenett HE, Parks DA, Darley-Usmar VM, Bradley KM, Tabengwa EM. Mechanism by which alcohol and wine polyphenols affect coronary heart disease risk. Ann Epidemiol. 2007 May 1;17(5):S24–31.

Bos S, Grobbee DE, Boer JM et al. Alcohol consumption and risk of cardiovascular disease among hypertensive women. Eur J Cardiovasc Prev Rehabil. 2010;17:119–126.

Boscolo P, del Signore A, Sabbioni E et al. Effects of resveratrol on lymphocyte proliferation and cytokine release. Ann Clin Lab Sci. 2003;33:226–231.

Brien SE, Ronksley PE, Turner BJ et al. Effect of alcohol consumption on biological markers associated with risk of coronary heart disease: Systematic review and metaanalysis of interventional studies. BMJ. 2011;22:342–357.

Brügger-Andersen T, Pönitz V, Snapinn S et al. OPTIMAAL study group. Moderate alcohol consumption is associated with reduced long-term cardiovascular risk in patients following a complicated acute myocardial infarction. Int J Cardiol. 2009;133:229–232.

Cao Y, Willett WC, Rimm EB, Stampfer MJ, Giovannucci EL. Light to moderate intake of alcohol, drinking patterns, and risk of cancer: Results from two prospective US cohort studies. BMJ. 2015 Aug 18;351:h4238.

Centers for Disease Control and Prevention. Impaired driving: Get the facts. 2018. https://www.cdc.gov/transportationsafety/impaired_driving/impaired-drv_factsheet.html. Accessed 4/23/2018.

Chandrasekar R. Alcohol and NMDA receptor: Current research and future direction. Front Mol Neurosci. 2013;6:14.

Chen H, Shen F, Sherban A et al. DEP domain-containing mTOR-interacting protein suppresses lipogenesis and ameliorates hepatic steatosis and acute-on-chronic liver injury in alcoholic liver disease. Hepatology. 2018;68:496e514.

Collins MA, Neafsey EJ. Alcohol, excitotoxicity and adult brain damage: An experimentally unproven chain-of-events. Front Mol Neurosci. 2016;9:8.

Collins MA, Neafsey EJ. Neuroinflammatory pathways in binge alcohol-induced neuronal degeneration: Oxidative stress cascade involving aquaporin, brain edema, and phospholipase A2 activation. Neurotox Res. 2012;21:70–78.

Crabb DW, Liangpunsakul S. Alcohol and lipid metabolism. J Gastroenterol Hepatol. 2006;3:S56eS60.

Crews FT. Alcohol and neurodegeneration. CNS Drug Rev. 1999;5:379–394.

Crews FT, Nixon K. Mechanisms of neurodegeneration and regeneration in alcoholism. Alcohol Alcohol. 2009;44:115–127.

Daneman R, Prat A. The blood-brain barrier. Cold Spring Harb Perspect Biol. 2015;7:a020412.

Diamond I, Francisco S. Neurologic effects of alcoholism. West J Med. 1993;161:279–287.

Dietary guidelines for Americans 2015–2020. U.S. Department of Agriculture. https://health.gov/dietaryguidelines/2015/guidelines/appendix-9/. Accessed 7/23/2018.

Dippold RP, Vadigepalli R, Gonye GE, Patra B, Hoek JB. Chronic ethanol feeding alters miRNA expression dynamics during liver regeneration. Alcohol Clin Exp Res. 2013;37:E59eE69.

Downer MK, Bertoia ML, Mukamal KJ, Rimm EB, Stampfer MJ. Change in alcohol intake in relation to weight change in a cohort of US men with 24 years of follow-up. Obesity. 2017 Nov;25(11):1988–1996.

Dubuquoy L, Louvet A, Lassailly G et al. Progenitor cell expansion and impaired hepatocyte regeneration in explanted livers from alcoholic hepatitis. Gut. 2015;64:1949e1960.

Espinola-Klein C, Gori T, Blankenberg S et al. Inflammatory markers and cardiovascular risk in the metabolic syndrome. Front Biosci. 2011;16:1663–1674.

Estruch R, Sacanella E, Badia E et al. Different effects of red wine and gin consumption on inflammatory bio-markers of atherosclerosis: A prospective randomized crossover trial: Effects of wine on inflammatory markers. Atherosclerosis. 2004;175:117–1123.

Feinman L. Absorption and utilization of nutrients in alcoholism. Alcohol Res. Health World. 1989;13(3):207–210.

Feinman L, Lieber CS. Nutrition: Medical problems of alcoholism. In: Lieber CS, ed. Medical and Nutritional Complications of Alcoholism: Mechanisms in Management. New York: Plenum Publishing Corp., 1992. pp. 515–530. https://doi.org/10.1007/978-1-4615-3320-7_17

Flink EB. Magnesium deficiency in alcoholism. Alcohol Clin Exp Res. 1986;10(6):590–594.

Freedland ES, McMicken DB. Alcohol-related seizures, part I: Pathophysiology, differential diagnosis, and evaluation. J Emerg Med. 1993;11:463–473.

Fujita Y, Islam R, Sakai K et al. Aza-derivatives of resveratrol are potent macrophage migration inhibitory factor inhibitors. Invest New Drugs. 2011 (In the Press).

Gao X, Deeb D, Liu Y et al. Immunomodulatory activity of xanthohumol: Inhibition of T cell proliferation, cell-mediated cytotoxicity and Th1 cytokine production through suppression of NF-kappaB. Immunopharmacol Immunotoxicol. 2009;31:477–484.

Goldberg DM. More on antioxidant activity of resveratrol in red wine. Clin Chem. 1996;42:113–114.

Goldberg IJ, Mosca L, Piano MR, Fisher EA. Wine and your heart: A science advisory for healthcare professionals from the Nutrition Committee, Council on Epidemiology and Prevention, and Council on Cardiovascular Nursing of the American Heart Association. Circulation. 2001 Jan 23;103(3):472–475.

Hagen TM, Liu J, Lykkesfeldt J et al. Feeding acetyl-L-carnitine and lipoic acid to old rats significantly improves metabolic function while decreasing oxidative stress. Proc Natl Acad Sci U S A. 2002;99:1870–1875.

Haorah J, Heilman D, Knipe B et al. Ethanol-induced activation of myosin light chain kinase leads to dysfunction of tight junctions and blood-brain barrier compromise. Alcohol Clin Exp Res. 2005a;29:999–1009.

Haorah J, Knipe B, Leibhart J et al. Alcohol-induced oxidative stress in brain endothelial cells causes blood-brain barrier dysfunction. J Leukoc Biol. 2005b;78:1223–1232.

Haorah J, Ramirez SH, Floreani N et al. Mechanism of alcohol-induced oxidative stress and neuronal injury. Free Radic Biol Med. 2008;45:1542–1550.

Hillers VN, Massey LK. Interrelationships of moderate and high alcohol consumption with diet and health status. Am J Clin Nutr. 1985;41(2):356–362.

Hines LM, Stampfer MJ, Ma J, Gaziano JM, Ridker PM, Hankinson SE, Sacks F, Rimm EB, Hunter DJ. Genetic variation in alcohol dehydrogenase and the beneficial effect of moderate alcohol consumption on myocardial infarction. N Engl J Med. 2001 Feb 22;344(8):549–555.

Huang PH, Chen YH, Tsai HY et al. Intake of red wine increases the number and functional capacity of circulating endothelial progenitor cells by enhancing nitric oxide bioavailability. Arterioscler Thromb Vasc Biol. 2010;30:869–877.

Kim HJ, Jung S, Eliassen AH, Chen WY, Willett WC, Cho E. Alcohol consumption and breast cancer risk in younger women according to family history of breast cancer and folate intake. Am J Epidemiol. 2017 Aug 10;186(5):524–531.

Klatsky AL. Alcohol and cardiovascular health. Physiol Behav. 2010;100:76–81.

Kloner RA, Rezkalla SH. To drink or not to drink? That is the question. Circulation. 2007 Sep 11;116(11):1306–1317.

Koppes LL, Dekker JM, Hendriks HF, Bouter LM, Heine RJ. Moderate alcohol consumption lowers the risk of type 2 diabetes: A meta-analysis of prospective observational studies. Diabetes Care. 2005 Mar 1;28(3):719–725.

Korsten MA. Alcoholism and pancreatitis: Does nutrition play a role? Alcohol Res. Health. 1989;13(3):232–237.

Korsten MA, Pirola RC, Lieber CS. Alcohol and the pancreas. In: Lieber CS, ed. Medical and Nutritional Complications of Alcoholism: Mechanisms in Management. New York: Plenum Publishing Corp., 1992. pp. 341–358.

Korsten MA, Wilson JS, Lieber CS. Interactive effects of dietary protein and ethanol on rat pancreas: Protein synthesis and enzyme secretion. Gastroenterology. 1990;99(1):229–236.

Kwok CL. Central nervous system neurotoxicity of chronic alcohol abuse. Asia Pac J Med Toxicol. 2016;2:70–71.

Leitzmann MF, Giovannucci EL, Stampfer MJ, Spiegelman D, Colditz GA, Willett WC, Rimm EB. Prospective study of alcohol consumption patterns in relation to symptomatic gallstone disease in men. Alcohol Clin Exp Res. 1999 May;23(5):835–841.

Leo MA, Kim C-I, Lowe N, Lieber CS. Interaction of ethanol with *-carotene: Delayed blood clearance and enhanced hepatotoxicity. Hepatology. 1992;15(5):883–891.

Leo MA, Lieber CS. Alcohol and vitamin A. Alcohol Health Res World. 1989;13(3):250–254.

Leo MA, Rosman AS, Lieber CS. Differential depletion of carotenoids and tocopherol in liver disease. Hepatology. 1993;17(6):977–986.

Lieber CS. Alcohol and nutrition: An overview. Alcohol Health Res World. 1989;13(3):197–205.

Lieber CS. The influence of alcohol on nutritional status. Nutr Rev. 1988;46(7):241–254.

Lim SS, Vos T, Flaxman AD et al. A comparative risk assessment of burden of disease and injury attributable to 67 risk factors and risk factor clusters in 21 regions, 1990–2010: A systematic analysis for the Global Burden of Disease Study 2010. Lancet. 2012;380:2224e2260.

Liu X, Sui B, Sun J. Blood-brain barrier dysfunction induced by silica NPs in vitro and in vivo: Involvement of oxidative stress and Rho-kinase/JNK signaling pathways. Biomaterials. 2017;121:64–82.

Maffi SK, Rathinam ML, Cherian PP et al. Glutathione content as a potential mediator of the vulnerability of cultured fetal cortical neurons to ethanol-induced apoptosis. J Neurosci Res. 2008;86:1064–1076.407

Magrone T, Jirillo E. Polyphenols from red wine are potent modulators of innate and adaptive immune responsiveness. Proc Nutr Soc. 2010;69:279–285.

Mahyar-Roemer M, Katsen A, Mestres P et al. Resveratrol induces colon tumor cell apoptosis independently of p53 and precede by epithelial differentiation, mitochondrial proliferation and membrane potential collapse. Int J Cancer. 2001;94:615–622.

Mandrekar P, Catalano D, White B et al. Moderate alcohol intake in humans attenuates monocyte inflammatory responses: Inhibition of nuclear regulatory factor kappa B and induction of interleukin 10. Alcohol Clin Exp Res. 2006;30:135–139.

Mangalmurti SS, Davidson MH. The incremental value of lipids and inflammatory biomarkers in determining residual cardiovascular risk. Curr Atheroscler Rep. 2011;13:373–380.

Marsano L, McClain CJ. Effects of alcohol on electrolytes and minerals. Alcohol Health Res World. 1989;13(3):255–260.

McClain CJ, Antonow DR, Cohen DA, Shedlofsky SI. Zinc metabolism in alcoholic liver disease. Alcohol Clin Exp Res. 1986;10(6):582–589.

McNeill E, Channon KM, Greaves DR. Inflammatory cell recruitment in cardiovascular disease: Murine models and potential clinical applications. Clin Sci (Lond). 2010;118:641–655.

Muneer PMA, Alikunju S, Szlachetka AM et al. Inhibitory effects of alcohol on glucose transport across the blood-brain barrier leads to neurodegeneration: Preventive role of acetyl-L carnitine. Psychopharmacology (Berl). 2011;214:707–718.

Nagy LE, Ding WX, Cresci G, Saikia P, Shah VH. Linking pathogenic mechanisms of alcoholic liver disease with clinical phenotypes. Gastroenterology. 2016;150:1756e1768.

Nakajima T, Kamijo Y, Tanaka N et al. Peroxisome proliferator-activated receptor alpha protects against alcohol-induced liver damage. Hepatology. 2004;40:972e980

National Institute on Alcohol Abuse and Alcoholism. 10th Special Report to the U.S. Congress on Alcohol and Health.

National Institute on Alcohol Abuse and Alcoholism. Alcohol Facts and Statistics. June 2017. www.niaaa.nih.gov/alcohol-health/overview-alcohol-consumption/alcohol-facts-and-statistics. Accessed 4/23/2018.

Niccoli T, Cabecinha M, Tillmann A et al. Increased glucose transport into neurons rescues Ab toxicity in drosophila highlights d overexpression of glucose transporter glut1 rescues a drosophila Ab toxicity model d glut1 overexpression reduces Grp78 protein levels and induces the UPR d A Grp78 dominant-negative mutant also rescues Ab toxicity in drosophila d metformin rescues Ab toxicity and leads to reduced Grp78 expression. Curr Biol. 2016;26:2291–2300.

Noor S, Sanchez JJ, Sun MS et al. The LFA-1 antagonist BIRT377 reverses neuropathic pain in prenatal alcohol-exposed female rats via actions on peripheral and central neuroimmune function in discrete pain-relevant tissue regions. Brain Behav Immun. 2020;87:339–358.

Nova E, Baccan GC, Veses A, Zapatera B, Marcos A. Potential health benefits of moderate alcohol consumption: Current perspectives in research, Proc Nutr Soc. 2012;71:307–315. doi:10.1017/S0029665112000171

Ohashi K, Pimienta M, Seki E. Alcoholic liver disease: A current molecular and clinical perspective. Liver Res. 2018;2:161e172.

O'Keefe JH, Bhatti SK, Bajwa A, DiNicolantonio JJ, Lavie CJ. Alcohol and cardiovascular health: The dose makes the poison . . . or the remedy. Mayo Clin Proc. 2014 Mar 1;89(3):382–393. Elsevier.

Patel DG. Effects of ethanol on carbohydrate metabolism and implications for the aging alcoholic. Alcohol Health Res World. 1989;13(3):240–246.

Phillips DK, Henderson GI, Schenker S. Pathogenesis of fetal alcohol syndrome: Overview with emphasis on the possible role of nutrition. Alcohol Health Res World. 1989;13(3):219–227.

Ramirez T, Longato L, Dostalek M, Tong M, Wands JR, de la Monte SM. Insulin resistance, ceramide accumulation and endoplasmic reticulum stress in experimental chronic alcohol-induced steatohepatitis. Alcohol Alcohol. 2013;48:39e52.

Rand, Michael, Catalano, Shannan. Criminal victimization, 2006. Bureau of Justice Statistics Bulletin. U.S. Department of Justice. December 2007. https://bjs.ojp.gov/content/pub/pdf/cv06.pdf

Romeo J, Wärnberg J, Díaz LE et al. Effects of moderate beer consumption on first-line immunity of healthy adults. J Physiol Biochem. 2007a;63:153–159. doi: 10.1007/BF03168226

Romeo J, Wärnberg J, Nova E et al. Changes in the immune system after moderate beer consumption. Ann Nutr Metab. 2007b;51:359–366. doi: 10.1159/000107679

Romeo J, Wärnberg J, Nova E et al. Moderate alcohol consumption and the immune system: A review. Br J Nutr. 2007c;98(Suppl. 1):S111–S115. https://doi.org/10.1017/S0007114507838049

Ronksley PE, Brien SE, Turner BJ et al. Association of alcohol consumption with selected cardiovascular disease outcomes: A systematic review and meta-analysis. BMJ. 2011;342:d671.

Schott MB, Rasineni K, Weller SG et al. beta-Adrenergic induction of lipolysis in hepatocytes is inhibited by ethanol exposure. J Biol Chem. 2017;292:11815e11828.

Scoccianti C, Cecchini M, Anderson AS, Berrino F, Boutron-Ruault MC, Espina C, Key TJ, Leitzmann M, Norat T, Powers H, Wiseman M. European code against cancer 4th edition: Alcohol drinking and cancer. Cancer Epidemiol. 2015 Dec 1;39:S67–74.

Shah K, DeSilva S, Abbruscato T. The role of glucose transporters in brain disease: Diabetes and Alzheimer's disease. Int J Mol Sci. 2012;13:12629–12655.

Sitia S, Tomasoni L, Atzeni F et al. From endothelial dysfunction to atherosclerosis. Autoimmun Rev. 2010;9:830–834.

Smith-Warner SA, Spiegelman D, Yaun SS, Van Den Brandt PA, Folsom AR, Goldbohm RA, Graham S, Holmberg L, Howe GR, Marshall JR, Miller AB. Alcohol and breast cancer in women: A pooled analysis of cohort studies. JAMA. 1998 Feb 18;279(7):535–540.

Sweeney MD, Ayyadurai S, Zlokovic BV. Pericytes of the neurovascular unit: Key functions and signaling pathways. Nat Neurosci. 2016;19:771–783.

Thameem Dheen S, Kaur C, Ling EA. Microglial activation and its implications in the brain diseases. Curr Med Chem. 2007;14:1189–1197.

Thomson AD, Pratt OE. Interaction of nutrients and alcohol: Absorption, transport, utilization, and metabolism. In: Watson RR, Watzl B, eds. Nutrition and Alcohol. Boca Raton, FL: CRC Press, 1992. pp. 75–99.

Thursz MR, Richardson P, Allison M et al. Prednisolone or pentoxifylline for alcoholic hepatitis. N Engl J Med. 2015;372:1619e1628.

Tortora GJ, Anagnostakos NP, eds. Principles of Anatomy and Physiology. 5th ed. New York: Harper & Row Publishers, 1987.

U.S. Department of Health and Human Services. The Surgeon General's Report on Nutrition and Health. DHHS Pub. No. (PHS)88–50210. Washington, DC: Supt. of Docs., U.S. Govt. Print. Off., 1988.

Vazquez-Prieto MA, Renna NF, Diez ER et al. Effect of red wine on adipocytokine expression and vascular alterations in fructose-fed rats. Am J Hypertens. 2011;24:234–240.

Victor M. The effects of alcohol on the nervous system: Clinical features, pathogenesis, and treatment. In: Lieber CS, ed. Medical and Nutritional Complications of Alcoholism: Mechanisms in Management. New York: Plenum Publishing Corp., 1992. pp. 413–457.

Vinson JA, Mandarano M, Hirst M et al. Phenol antioxidant quantity and quality in foods: Beers and the effect of two types of beer on an animal model of atherosclerosis. J Agric Food Chem. 2003;51:5528–5533.

Winkler C, Wirleitner B, Schroecksnadel K et al. Beer down-regulates activated peripheral blood mononuclear cells in vitro. Int Immunopharmacol. 2006;6:390–395.

Wirleitner B, Schroecksnadel K, Winkler C et al. Resveratrol suppresses interferon-gamma-induced biochemical pathways in human peripheral blood mononuclear cells in vitro. Immunol Lett. 2005;100:159–163.

World Cancer Research Fund/American Institute for Cancer Research. Diet, Nutrition, Physical Activity and Cancer: A Global Perspective. Continuous Update Project Expert Report. Washington (DC): American Institute for Cancer Research, 2007.

World MJ, Ryle PR, Pratt OE, Thomson AD. Alcohol and body weight. Alcohol and Alcoholism. 1984;19(1):1–6.

Xu R, Huang H, Zhang Z, Wang FS. The role of neutrophils in the development of liver diseases. Cell Mol Immunol. 2014;11:224e231

You M, Jogasuria A, Lee K, et al. Signal transduction mechanisms of alcoholic fatty liver disease: Merging role of lipin-1. Curr Mol Pharmacol. 2017;10:226e236.

You M, Liang X, Ajmo JM, Ness GC. Involvement of mammalian sirtuin 1 in the action of ethanol in the liver. Am J Physiol Gastrointest Liver Physiol. 2008;294:G892eG898.

Zehendner CM, Librizzi L, Hedrich J, et al. Moderate hypoxia followed by reoxygenation results in blood-brain barrier breakdown via oxidative stress-dependent tight-junction protein disruption. PLoS One. 2013;8:e82823.

Zhang C, Qin YY, Chen Q, Jiang H, Chen XZ, Xu CL, Mao PJ, He J, Zhou YH. Alcohol intake and risk of stroke: A dose–response meta-analysis of prospective studies. Int J Cardiol. 2014 Jul 1;174(3):669–77.

Zhang S, Hunter DJ, Hankinson SE, Giovannucci EL, Rosner BA, Colditz GA, Speizer FE, Willett WC. A prospective study of folate intake and the risk of breast cancer. JAMA. 1999 May 5;281(17):1632–1637.

Zhang W, Sun Q, Zhong W, Sun X, Zhou Z. Hepatic peroxisome proliferator activated receptor gamma signaling contributes to alcohol-induced hepatic steatosis and inflammation in mice. Alcohol Clin Exp Res. 2016;40:988e999.

Zhou M, Baudry M. Developmental changes in NMDA neurotoxicity reflect developmental changes in subunit composition of NMDA receptors. J Neurosci. 2006;26:2956–2963.

7 Functional Foods and Nutraceuticals in Health Maintenance

Monica Butnariu

7.1 INTRODUCTION

Those foods that contain a nutritious bioactive component (vitamins, minerals, proteins, etc.) or non-nutritive (prebiotic fibres, polyphenols, etc.) are considered "functional", which positively influences the functioning of the body, protects against the occurrence of diseases, prevents nutritional deficits and can help the normal growth and development of the human body. The concept of "functional food" was introduced around 1980 in Japan, when the government began to approve and promote foods with proven benefits in order to improve the health of the population as well as to try to observe their benefits. The wide range of food products introduces a diversity of essential bio-compounds, both nutritious and non-nutritive. They have the possibility to ameliorate people's well-being and may even decrease the possibility or delay the onset and development of substantial conditions such as cardiovascular sickness, malignant diseases, and systemic skeletal disorder (osteoporosis) by acting on oxidative stress. Progress in food knowledge and technology provides food manufacturing with elaborated procedures for controlling and modifying the physical conformation and chemical configuration of food bio-compounds.

7.2 FUNCTIONAL FOODS: CURRENT ATTESTATIONS AND APPROACHES

The use of functional foods (FFs) decreases the risk of disease (Rkd), but they are not preplanned to act as a support for fortifiers that express deficiencies in the body. FFs are not created with the intention of treating sickness or being consumed in palliative/calmative care. Attestations by Well-being Canada and other agencies consider FFs to have a content of essential bioactive compounds (EBCs) added into a product. Thus, tomatoes with a high content of lycopene or other plants (vegetables) with a content of natural substances that are similar to cholesterol (sterols). These bio-compounds can be relatively readily added into the individual's daily diet. Unlike FFs, nutraceutical (NTs) bio-compounds contain BCs, which are extracted from their matrix (the food product [EBcs]) and added in the form of pills, capsules, ampoules (capsules of bioflavonoids, γ-linoleic acid).

Natural bio-compounds are determined as substances that can be consumed for an extended period of time and fall under the category of curative bio-compounds (echinacea, herbal teas, St. John's wort). Curing some sicknesses can be accomplished with natural bio-compounds, while, according to the attestation given by Well-being Canada, FFs are consumed only to decrease the Rkd. So, FFs and NTs can be foods in which the nature or bioavailability of one or more constituent has been adjusted or a integration of these opportunities (Puttasiddaiah et al. 2022).

FFs and NTs can be practical for all members of a community or for specific categories of a community, which can be determined by standards of age or genetic organization. European experts put forward the following attestation: an EBcs can be considered practical if it has been acceptably proven to favorably influence one or more goal qualities in the body, beyond the appropriate nutritional consequences, in a significant way, to improve well-being and/or decrease the possibility of sickness.

DOI: 10.1201/9781003361497-8

Specific attestations:

- The FFs is/or may be almost identical in essential quality to a formalistic food, is consumed as part of a regular diet, and is shown to have beneficial physiological consequences in reducing the possibility of chronic sickness in addition to its basic nutritional qualities.
- FFs is a EBcs or drink that confers a physiological benefit that ameliorates general well-being, helps prevent or treat a sickness/condition, or ameliorates physical or mental performance by means of an added practical ingredient, through processing, modification or biotechnology (Salvo et al. 2022).

FFs and NTs are ordinary foods to which constituents have been added or from which constituents obtained by technological or biotechnological means have been removed in order to achieve targeted consequences; in the case of the class studied in the present chapter, the augmentation of the antioxidant consequence. In the case of antioxidant FFs, such constituents can be natural antioxidants from plants, vegetables and fruits, which can be consumed as such or as constituents of FFs and NTs.

7.3   INTERNATIONAL APPROACHES RELATED TO FUNCTIONAL FOODS

FFs research in Japan began in the 1980s when the government funded 86 specific programs on "Systematic Analysis and Development of Food Functions", then the Ministry of Education sponsored studies focused on "Analysis of Physiological Regulation Functions of Foods" and "Analysis of Functional Foods and Molecular Design", only in 1991 to introduce the hypothesis of "foods for specified well-being uses" (FOSHU).

These foods are included as part of one of the four categories of foods described in the "Food Improvement Act" as "Foods Specially Dietary" (foods that are consumed specifically to ameliorate human well-being and are permitted to display certain consequences they have on well-being).

Due to the convincing results documenting and supporting with scientific theory or hypothesis certain well-being consequences, the Minister of Well-being and Social Assistance has allowed a symbol to appear on the label, according to which the product has government approval. Foods identified as FOSHU must exert a certain physiological consequence on well-being, must be in the form of ordinary foods (not in pill or capsule form) and are supposed to be consumed as part of a normal diet (not as highly rare, consumed only in case of ailments) (Ardahanlı et al. 2022).

Most FOSHU-authorized bio-compounds contain oligosaccharides or lactic bacteria to maintain gut well-being. In the US, FFs are believed to help decrease the Rkd. They contain ingredients that the United States Food and Drug Administration (FDA, or USFDA) has acknowledged as objective evidence of a correlation between nutrients or foods in the diet and certain sicknesses based on the totality of publicly available scientific theory or hypothesis and substantial agreement that exists among qualified experts.

The FDA has recognized FFs since 1997 based on the declarations of the Federal Scientific Body such as the National Institutes of Well-being and the Center for Disease Control or the National Academy of Sciences. In the EU, there is no harmonized legislation on these hypotheses and the consequences of food on well-being, which means that work is done at a national level. It is recognized that the competitive position of food and beverage manufacturing in Europe should be strengthened by a better understanding of the scientific basis of food functionality.

Sweden, since 1990, introduced a program on well-being claims, and in the 1996 version, the program comprises two parts: information on one of the eight authorized diet-well-being relationships, followed by information on the configuration of the product (functionality-based claims) (Sharma et al. 2021).

Acknowledged conditions are obesity (energy), blood cholesterol (lipid quality), blood pressure (sodium), atherosclerosis (blood pressure, serum cholesterol, long-chain polyunsaturated fatty acids

[PUFAs] from fish), constipation (dietary fibre), systemic skeletal disorder (calcium), tooth decay (readily fermentable carbohydrates) and iron (iron) deficiencies.

The food manufacturing and retail organizations behind the scheme have recently suggested an extension to cover claims for specific physiological consequences characteristic of FFs and NTs.

7.4 WELL-BEING CLAIMS FOR FUNCTIONAL FOODS

According to the traditional hypothesis of nutrition, the primary role of diet is to provide adequate amounts of nutrients to meet metabolic demands and maintain optimal well-being. However, epidemiological, clinical and experimental studies have shown that certain categories of food and specific food constituents can influence a diversity of qualities and provide the body with specific well-being interests. Based on scientific data, it is now acknowledged that diet can have beneficial physiological and psychological consequences, beyond the well-known nutritional consequences, by modulating specific goal qualities in the body.

However, diet not only helps to reach epidemiologic, experimental, optimal development, but it can promote better well-being and play an important role in sickness obstruction by reducing the possibility of certain chronic sicknesses. As such, we can consider that the development of the hypothesis of FFs and NTs was made to obtain an optimal configuration of the diet in order to promote well-being and decrease the possibility of chronic sickness. The evaluation of well-being claims for FFs and NTs may take into account that a practical consequence may be provided by essential or non-essential nutrients (Wei et al. 2022).

However, FFs and NTs must be formalistic or everyday foods consumed as part of the regular diet. They should be composed of natural constituents, but one or more constituents may be added, removed and/or adjusted, and/or the bioavailability of one or more constituents may be altered. These foods may be practical for all members of a community or for a determined section of the community. Distinct categories of food claims can thus be consumed to promote the interests of FFs and NTs. Practical and well-being claims are of great importance because they constitute claims that influence the behavior of users, and thus, can influence their well-being.

7.4.1 DISTINCT CATEGORIES OF CLAIMS: NUTRITIONAL AND WELL-BEING

European experts suggest the following attestation of the well-being claim corresponding to FFs and NTs:

A claim is any direct or indirect statement, symbol, suggestion, implication or any other form of communication (including the brand name), by which it is understood that the food in question presents better special characteristics related to: its origin, properties, consequence, nature, method of production, processing, configuration or any other quality.

For FFs, the distinct categories of claims are determined and classified by international bodies such as Codex Alimentarius Commission (CAC) or the European Commission (EC) or by national organizations/commissions/authorities such as the FDA in the United States or the Food Standards Agency (FSA). There are mentions in two subclasses:

- Nutritional information concerning the nutrient content, comparative of well-being eating patterns (following certain dietary guidelines), regarding nutritional qualities or structural qualities.
- Well-being claims of consolidated or ameliorated function and reducing the Rkd.

Nutrition claims have been determined as "any representation that specifies, suggests or implies that a EBcs has special nutritional properties, but is not limited to energy value, protein, fat and carbohydrate content, or vitamin and mineral content". The claim supporting the nutrient content refers to the level of nutrients in a EBcs/food component (Yu et al. 2022).

These claims may be expressed as "low fat source", "low in saturated fat", "high in fibre", "low in cholesterol" "rich in calcium". CAC defines comparative claims, which compare the levels of nutrients in distinct foods, by using words like "more", "less", "decreased", "increased content". An example: "contains 50% more calcium than regular milk". Well-being eating-pattern statements refer to dietary guidelines and recommendations from national or international authorities on well-being eating. Examples: "diet low in saturated fat is recommended by", "recommends a daily dose of 800 mg of calcium", "recommends an increased dose of fibre".

The nutrient statement describes the physiological role of the nutrient and its relationship to normal body qualities but must not refer to abnormal (pathological) conditions. Examples include "calcium is necessary for bone structure", "calcium contributes to the development of strong bones and teeth", "Alpha-Tocopherol protects the oxidation of fats". The CAC stated that the nutrient statement should be related to the essential nutrients for which the reference value has been established and to the nutrients that are mentioned in official dietary guidelines or recommendations. EBcs for which the nutrient claim is obtained should contain an important source of nutrients from the usual diet. All these categories of nutrition claims are based on knowledge of nutrients and their physiological qualities, which must be widely acknowledged by the network of researchers (Kamioka et al. 2017). So, the so-called "enhanced qualities" (assume practical properties) and Rkd-reduction claims are well-being claims and are particularly important for FFs and NTs. These categories of specific claims refer to the beneficial consequences of foods or constituents, nutrients and non-nutritive substances. Enhanced function or "functional" claims describe the beneficial consequences of essential bio-compounds (EBcs) on physiological or psychological qualities, metabolic activities, biochemical and cellular processes beyond the established role of these foods in normal body qualities. These claims do not directly refer to well-being interests or reduction of Rkd (Kamioka et al. 2019).

Examples: "calcium supplementation ameliorates bone density", "antioxidants decrease the possibility of oxidative stress", "folic acid contributes to the reduction of homocysteine plasma concentrations", "digestible non-oligosaccharides ameliorate the growth of intestinal bacterial microflora".

Claims suggesting that foods have well-being-impacting or well-being-enhancing constituents or are related to a sickness condition have been called well-being claims (Hollmann et al. 2020).

Rkd-reduction claims state that a food or its constituents can help decrease the Rkd. Examples: "adequate calcium intake can help decrease the possibility of systemic skeletal disorder", "adequate folic acid intake in pregnant women can decrease the possibility of new-borns with neural tube defects", "low fat and cholesterol dietary intake can decrease the possibility of coronary heart disease". Nutrition and well-being claims must meet specific standards to ensure users are not misled or confused. They are based on scientific documentation and information, validated, supported by complete, objective and verifiable evidence (Suarez-Torres, Jimenez-Orozco, & Ciangherotti, 2020). The claims must be clear and easy to understand by users. It is essential that FFs and NTs claims meeting these standards are given objective scientific validation.

7.4.2 The Scientific Theory or Hypothesis Required to Obtain a Well-Being Claim for FFs and NTs

In order to obtain well-being claims, a scientific theory or hypothesis is required for the consequences of FFs and NTs. Evidence of the consequences of FFs must be based on objective standards developed and acknowledged by the network of researchers. FFs and NTs must favorably modulate the body's goal qualities, thus becoming significant for improving well-being or establishing a state of well-being or for reducing the Rkd. Based on current knowledge, the goal function to be modulated must be clearly determined. A set of markers (MKs) can be displayed to define this function, demonstrating the modulation consequences. Such distinct categories of evidence are needed, including biochemical, biological, epidemiological, observational data and data from human intervention studies. Data are required to describe molecular, tissue and organ consequences as well as at the level of individuals and also at the community level. Evidence must be based on studies that consumed MKs to track goal qualities or biological response or MKs of intermediate sickness endpoints.

The basic data of studies, even at the cellular level, data from animal studies and various biochemical measurements have the role of explaining the mechanism of action of the constituents of FFs and NTs, or earmarking important data concerning the mechanism of action. Epidemiological studies, prospective or cross-sectional studies must provide data on the relationship between food consumption and distinct outcomes. Meta-analysis of epidemiological studies can be very useful. Also, the data obtained from human intervention studies are very important. In all studies, acceptance of a set of bio-MKs must be seriously considered. The study community should be almost identical to the community for which the FFs and NTs are intended. For most EBcs, this will be the general community. However, the general community consists of some well-being subjects, others at high possibility for certain conditions and others already influenced by these conditions (Esquivel-Alvarado et al. 2022).

The efficacy and safety of a FFs and NTs product must be studied for all these distinct community categories. Where FFs and NTs are targeted at a subcategory of the general community – for example, a high-possibility category – the subcategory must be clearly determined and explained in a way that is easy for users to understand. Data can document the consequence of individual EBcs separately, but they must also demonstrate that the final FFs and NTs product will impact physiological and well-being consequences. All requested data must be consistent, meet appropriate scientific standards and biological standards and have statistical significance in order to be acknowledged by an objective body (Alonso-Miravalles et al. 2022).

In 2002, the Food and Drug Administration described a new initiative, called the "Nutrition for Better Well-being Consumer Information Initiative", to encourage formalistic food and dietary supplement decision makers to try to report, up-to-date and as accurately as possible, scientific conclusions concerning the well-being interests of bio-compounds and to help eliminate false labeling by tracking MKs in human dietary supplements that mislead through false claims concerning well-being interests or other manufacturing defects.

7.5 FUNCTIONAL FOODS: KNOWLEDGE, MANUFACTURING, LEGISLATION

7.5.1 THE KNOWLEDGE OF FUNCTIONAL FOODS

Knowing the mechanisms through which FFs and NTs can modulate the goal qualities and the relevance of these foods on the well-being status of the community and the reduction of the possibility of some sickness will start from the knowledge of the basics of biological knowledge. The relevance of FFs and NTs can also be supported by epidemiological data that could demonstrate a clear and statistically supported relationship between the consumption of separate EBcs (supported by the values of a serum, fecal, urinary or tissue marker of the consumption of substances subjected to study) and their specific interests (Zeng et al. 2022).

Moreover, the existence of evidence linking the regular consumption of certain EBcs with the reduction of the possibility of certain sickness, which may appear over time, will be of particular importance. The goals of FFs and NTs knowledge are as follows:

- Identifying the beneficial interactions between a practical component of a EBcs and one or more of the goal qualities in the body and obtaining evidence concerning the mechanisms of these interactions (results of studies done in vitro, in cell cultures, of the use of animal models in vitro and in vivo; results of human studies conducted will also be included).
- Identification and validation of significant MKs of these qualities and their modulation by these EBcs.

- Assessing the safety of the required amount of a certain food component for it to be practical. This will require evidence that is equally applicable to all substantial community categories, including those who are behaviorally indulgent and who are expected to compromise the anticipated interests of the FFs and NTs. It is quite possible that this will involve post-commercialization monitoring, including consequences on the entire diet.
- The formulation of hypotheses to be tested in humans, the purpose of which is to show the association between the significant consumption of specified compounds and the improvement of one or more goal qualities, either directly or via a significant marker for ameliorated well-being status, or to decrease the possibility of certain sickness (Wojdyło et al. 2021).

7.5.2 The Functional Food Manufacturing

As for the FFs and NTs manufacturing, its genesis occurred for a series of reasons. First of all, users are aware of the possible positive role that diet can play in various sicknesses. Despite the lack of coherence of information received, users, perhaps as they advance beyond middle age, become increasingly interested in the relationships between EBcs and quality of life. Indeed, a recent survey conducted in the USA proved that 95% of the community believe that food has the possibility to ameliorate well-being by doing more than earmarking nutrients. Several of those surveyed were interested in learning concerning foods that have these practical abilities. On the one hand, the increase in educational level can be responsible for this fact; on the other hand, the increase in interest in the general area of preventive well-being. Public well-being regulatory bodies have begun to endorse the interests of FFs and NTs. Consequently, the legislative frameworks are now well developed in countries such as Japan, which allows more than 200 FFs to be shared under the FOSHU brand, and in the USA, the FDA grants the prerequisites for some mentions concerning well-being to be done on 15 categories of EBcs (Kamioka et al. 2021).

Also, governments consider positive these regulatory aspects for FFs and NTs being aware of the economic possibility of these bio-compounds as part of preventive public well-being strategies; however, there is data on the cost savings that could be achieved through use of these foods. Processes have been developed for a systematic investigation of existing data linking FFs and NTs to physiological mechanisms influencing Rkd, but the seriousness of this process varies considerably from country to country. The FDA agreed to convene a panel of independent scientists to weigh all clinically significant data on well-being claims on product labels (Kong et al. 2022). The development of this exhaustive examination process ameliorated the authenticity of well-being claims, which led to the development of the FFs and NTs manufacturing.

7.5.3 Legislation, Projects, and Scientific and Legislative Forums in the Field of Functional Foods in Europe

The creation and development of FFs and NTs is a key issue and also a challenge for knowledge, which should be based on basic scientific knowledge significant to key qualities and their possible modulation by EBcs. FFs and NTs are not universal, and a food-focused approach should be influenced by local considerations. A scientific approach to food is universal and therefore very suitable for a pan-European approach. The food-practicality approach has scientific foundations to bring a better understanding of the interactions between diet and well-being.

Emphasis is placed on the importance of the consequences of EBcs on well-identified and characterized goal-qualities in the body, related to well-being aspects, more approximately than strictly oriented toward reducing the Rkd occurrence. Particular attention is now paid to well-being claims for EBcs, including ameliorated function, Rkd reduction and nutrient function claims. There are already many FFs products and NTs on the market with claims for well-being consequences beyond simply earmarking nutrients. An important basis for the well-being claim is the growing series of reports of the consequences of dietary constituents on body qualities. There is no scientific consensus on how actions based on these reports should be evaluated at a European level. In the absence of such a consensus, distinct national and international bodies apply distinct approaches in their attempt to regulate an evolving market. The resulting fragmentation of the regulatory framework for well-being claims leads to diverse and possibly conflicting information vs. message for users concerning diet and well-being as well as uncertainty for the manufacturing (Zanchini, Di Vita, & Brun 2022).

In this context, International Life Sciences Institute Europe (ILSI Europe) initiated the concerted action "Process for the Assessment of Scientific Support for Claims on Foods" (PASSCLAIM). Its objective is to define the standards for evaluating scientific support for claims made in relation to EBcs. Reasons for scientific evaluation:

- To provide truthful information and support consumer confidence in EBcs with claims.
- To satisfy regulatory requirements.
- To maintain fair and balanced competition on the market.

The validation of agreed standards for this process should facilitate the achievement of these objectives in a harmonized manner. It was suggested that any "enhanced function" and "decreased Rkd" claims should be scientifically justified, and the importance of validated exposure of MKs demonstrate ameliorated function/decreased Rkd claims. Particularly with regard to Rkd reduction claims, it has been found that the end goal – the sickness itself – often cannot be measured directly, for ethical or practical reasons (Plasek & Temesi 2019).

Therefore, the identification and validation of suitable MKs were considered as key issues. The MKs were classified as being related to exposure, goal function or a biological response and an appropriate intermediate goal of good well-being or reduction of Rkd or both.

Safety is an essential condition for all EBcs. Nutritional safety considerations are particularly significant for foods for which nutrition and well-being claims are made. Enhanced function support has been determined in the EC Concerted Action on Functional Food Science in Europe (FUFOSE), where specific beneficial consequences of nutrients on physiological and psychological qualities or biological activity beyond their usual meaningful role in growth and development of other normal body qualities are presented.

In the CAC working categories, they support the function of nutrients in accordance with well-being claims, referring to the normal physiological consequences of nutrition in the growth, development and normal qualities of the body. In Codex terms, "Other Feature Claims" are more or less equivalent to well-being claims for "Enhanced Feature". In the proposed EU regulation, "Well-being claims describing a generally acknowledged role for a nutrient or other substance" would include claims for both nutrient function and other qualities (Plasek, Lakner, & Temesi 2021).

A substantial legislative problem so far has been the fact that claims concerning the obstruction, reduction and cure of sickness are limited to being attributed only to medicines. Accordingly, the mention of consequences for EBcs in relation to the sickness on food labels or in other promotional material was regarded as a claim. Any diet based on reducing the Rkd through healthy eating is a well-established hypothesis in nutrition and forms the basis of the Journal of Dietary Guidelines. Elaboration of standards for the scientific substantiation of the claims are based on intermediate standards, which were tested by practical application on two categories of experts. The measures taken by the experts were:

- To correlate examples of categories of possibility for mentions in distinct areas from the point of view of physiological qualities and, if it was the case, in distinct stages of the sickness.
- To describe the scientific requirements for the quality of the data needed to support these claims and to assess the relevance of the scientific support (Lusk 2019).

A common feature in all these approaches is the requirement for sound scientific substantiation, with a procedure for reviewing evidence in support of claims, a protocol for extracting data from individual research papers in a systematic and consistent manner, and a template for documentation of evidence. Standards for scientific argumentation of the mentions:

a) The food or component to which the said consequence is attributed should be clearly characterized.
b) The justification for a claim must be based on human data, primarily from intervention studies which should include the following aspects:
   • characterization of the study category's eating habits and other significant lifestyle aspects;
   • adequate control;
   • the study categories should be representative of the goal category;
   • monitoring the subjects' cooperation regarding the consumption of food or EBcs with the tested component;
   • an adequate duration of exposure and follow-up to demonstrate the intended consequence;
   • statistical power to test the hypothesis;
   • be allocated a sufficient quantity of the food component or product in accordance with its intended consumption pattern;
   • to consider the influence of the food matrix and the dietary context on the practical consequence of the component.
c) When the true objective of a claimed benefit cannot be measured directly, the study should use MKs.
d) MKs should be:
   • biologically validated in the sense that they have a known relationship on the final response and have a known variability within the goal community;
   • methodologically validated in terms of their analytical characteristics.
e) Within a study, the goal variables should evolve in a statistically significant way and the evolution should be biologically meaningful for the goal category for which the claim is made.
f) A claim should be scientifically justified by considering the body of available data and weighing all the evidence.

Thus, this document presents this consensus picture of standards, provides reasonable assurance that the scientific data underlying well-being claims for EBcs are appropriate for this purpose and can be validated. From the point of view of a partnership formed by many scientific experts, these standards are necessary to provide a basis for the harmonization of claims as well as for the evaluation of scientific supporting well-being data on EBcs, which have the possibility to have a positive impact on stakeholders, including on interest categories (users, well-being professionals and manufacturing) and in the aggregate (national and international regulatory agencies), by geographic regions (Bryła 2020).

The current state of European research in the field of FFs and NTs enriched with natural antioxidants and the authorization of their use in studies on human subjects are also presented in the recommendations of the British Nutrition Foundation (after the analysis of 52 projects on the program Antioxidants in Food AN04/N04, 1999–2002 in framework FP5) for setting standards for FFs and NTs:

• Testing FFs and NTs in multi-center interventional studies is not usually recommended.
• Bioavailability studies of some plant derivatives, including polyphenols, vitamins and minerals, are needed at this stage to determine their action in vivo.
• The consequences of plant-derived nutrients at the cellular and tissue level must be studied in human subjects, anticipating a consequential response (degenerative sickness, senescence).

- Multidisciplinary collaboration is necessary to study the factors that influence the effective modification of selected foods to become FFs and NTs as well as to understand the influence of the preparation and processing of FFs and NTs on their bioavailability (Franco-Arellano et al. 2020).

7.6 USE OF FUNCTIONAL FOOD PRODUCTS: NEW DIRECTIONS IN THE DIET

Regarding the extent to which *functional foods reach at-possibility communities*, certain considerations can be made following some studies and surveys done in this regard in Western Europe. Several surveys have shown that a higher socio-economic status is associated with a healthy diet; that their diet is closer to the recommendations. Users with a low or middle socio-economic status would therefore gain the most from FFs and NTs. It has been suggested that FFs and NTs would appeal to the healthiest, most educated and affluent users, but this does not appear to be true: a Dutch community survey of 1,183 users, aged 19–91, found that the factors of use of FFs products and NTs depend on the type of food. Stanol-enriched margarine was most consumed by smokers and poorer users. A Finnish study showed a higher consumption of such margarine for users with a higher socio-economic status.

Educating healthcare providers in the following aspects of FFs and NTs will be an important task for non-commercial nutritionists. A uniform attestation of the term "functional food" and clear legislation on well-being claims would further strengthen the acceptance and success of FFs and NTs now and in the future (Kraus, Annunziata, & Vecchio 2017).

Substitution of trans, saturated fats with non-hydrogenated, unsaturated fats. Replacing saturated or trans fats in the diet with carbohydrates or other categories of fat decreases the possibility of cardiovascular sickness (CVD). Margarine has been a rich source of trans fat for nearly a decade, but food manufacturers have significantly decreased trans-fat content as reports of negative well-being consequences surfaced (Iqbal et al. 2021).

Eating a diet rich in fruits, vegetables, nuts and whole grains and low in refined grain products. In the US, vegetable consumption is close to the recommended daily allowance, but fruit consumption is less than half the recommended amount. In Europe, fruit and vegetable consumption is lower than recommended. As a result, many users do not meet dietary recommendations for fibre, folic acid, ascorbic acid and other vitamins. For example, it has been estimated that around 50% of Dutch users do not meet the dietary recommendations for folate. Ready-made fruit and vegetable salads can increase consumption for users who have limited time to prepare their daily meals. Foods enriched with fibre and vitamins can be an alternative to fruits and vegetables, but only up to a certain point. Distinct dietary fibres have distinct consequences on CVD possibility: water-soluble dietary fibres such as pectin and guar gum appear to have stronger consequences than insoluble fibres such as wheat bran. A mixture of distinct dietary fibres naturally found in fruits and vegetables appears to be necessary for a CVD protective consequence. Adding vitamins to foods to compensate for decreased fruit and vegetable consumption may not have the intended consequence. β-carotene was thought to decrease the possibility of malignant diseases in smokers because intake of carotene-rich foods was associated with decreased malignant diseases possibility. However, carotene supplements have been found to increase the possibility of malignant lung diseases for smokers. And other substantial clinical studies on antioxidants have had disappointing results.

It was thus concluded that other BCs of fruits and vegetables may protect against CVD. Therefore, fortifying food with known vitamins and minerals may not be enough (Popoola-Akinola, Raji, & Olawoye 2022).

The consumption of FFs and NTs in CVD and diabetes can make an important contribution through the intake of specific nutrients. Consumption of micronutrient-enriched cereals was associated with significantly increased intakes of iron, B vitamins, vitamin D and fibre in the Irish adult community.

Consumption of an oat bran-rich diet. Dietary fibre is classified as soluble and insoluble. Soluble fibre is found in foods such as beans, oats, legumes, barley and prunes. The use of oat bran fibre in the control (management) of CVD possibility was the first requirement raised by the US Dietary Supplement Well-being and Education Act (DSHEA) back in 1990.

The message written in languages of international circulation is authorized to appear on the package and contain information. This supports the consumption of 25 g/day of oats contained in food to decrease the possibility of CVD, this being a more sophisticated way of translating the message that has resonated in North America for several decades; namely, "Eat your porridge – it is bravo to you" (Soliman 2019).

The essential quality of this message was authorized by the extensive content of mass epidemiological studies, which showed that a significant daily intake of fibre (25–50 g) was associated with a modest but decreased possibility of CVD by lowering the level of low-density lipoprotein (LDL) and total cholesterol. However, high dietary fibre intake by mass has been shown in Finland to be associated with a decreased possibility of death from coronary heart sickness. Men who reported an average intake of 27 g/day of fibre showed a possibility factor relative to death due to coronary heart sickness of 0.83 compared to men in the same community whose average reported fibre intake was 10 g lower. Soluble fibre intake lowers LDL cholesterol levels through a series of processes that alter glucose and cholesterol metabolism. The mechanism of action is by increasing the elimination of bile acids in the feces and by interfering with the reabsorption of bile acids.

More precisely, this consequence of fibres can be attributed to their binding and diluting action of bile acids and lowering of intestinal pH, thus inhibiting the conversion of primary bile acids to secondary bile acids, ultimately resulting in a reduction in fat and cholesterol absorption. Fermentation of fibre in the colon by the action of intestinal microflora leads to the production of short-chain fatty acids and gas. These short-chain fatty acids not only provide fuel for colon lining cells but their production is linked to lower serum cholesterol and malignant diseases possibility.

Due to the undigested fibres, there are also increases in the volume and dry weight of the wet feces, the speed of intestinal transit increases, which decreases the possibility of an interaction with the intestinal epithelium of both nutrients and mutagenic feces. It is likely that other non-digestible polysaccharides and oligosaccharides with BCs properties in the control of cholesterol and carbohydrate metabolism will be discovered in the future. Mannan, a non-digestible carbohydrate complex from the konjac plant, has been discovered that could gluco-control glycemic values and lipid profile in the curative meaning of insulin resistance syndrome (Dahl, & Stewart 2015).

Soy protein consumption. The "healthy" claim for soy protein consumption is associated with a reduction in the possibility of coronary heart sickness, allowing it to appear on the packaging of bio-compounds containing soy protein under the DSHEA brand. The FDA concluded that soy protein that is included in a diet low in saturated fat and cholesterol can decrease the possibility of coronary heart-sickness by lowering blood-cholesterol levels. This consequence is conferred, at least in part, by the amino acid profile that differs from that of animal proteins in such a way as to lead to the desirable lowering of circulating LDL cholesterol. A meta-analysis of the consequences of soy protein intake on serum lipids found, in most studies, that energy intake, fat, saturated fat and cholesterol were almost identical in subjects who ingested soy protein versus the control category. In the control, soy proteins were ingested in an average daily intake of 47 g.

The mode of action by which soy protein is seen to lower cholesterol concentrations is through activation of the LDL receptor pathway (Robbani et al. 2022). Soy protein contains a series of estrogenic compounds called isoflavones (Figure 7.1).

These isoflavones, especially genistein and daidzein, exist as constituents in soy proteins that possess antioxidant properties, being implicated in both the regulation of circulating lipid levels and malignant diseases possibility. Studies conducted with isoflavone-free soy indicate a loss of the consequences of the soy protein-supplemented diet; however, an isoflavone-enriched extract has been

genistein or 5,7,4'-trihydroxyisoflavone

($C_{15}H_{10}O_5$)

daidzein or 7,4'-dihydroxyisoflavone

($C_{15}H_{10}O_4$)

17-β-estradiol or (17β)-estra-1,3,5(10)-

triene-3,17-diol ($C_{18}H_{24}O_2$)

Glycitin or glycitein 7-O-glucoside

($C_{22}H_{22}O_{10}$)

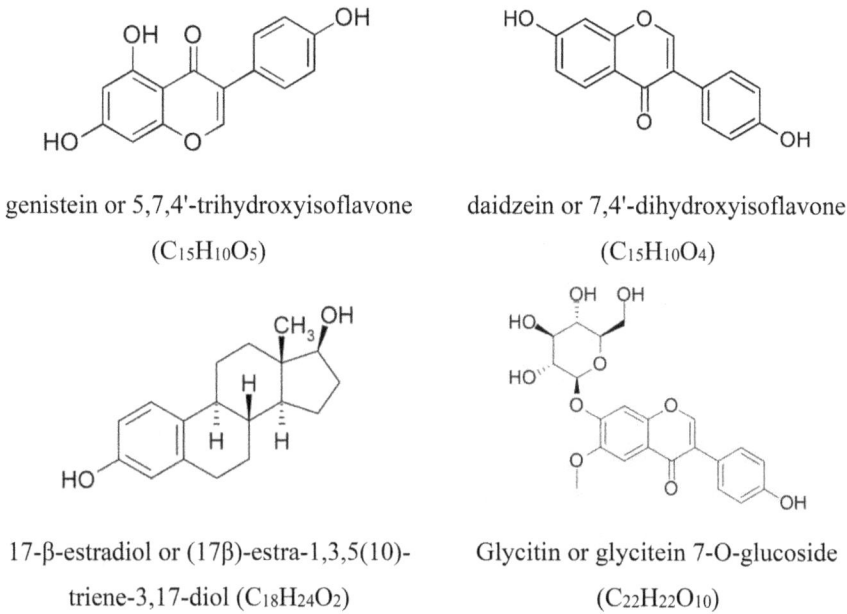

FIGURE 7.1 Structure and chemical formula of some isoflavones.

shown to have no hypocholesterolemic activity, so it would be important to consume soy proteins that contain at least a minimal amount of isoflavones.

There is also some suggestion that isoflavones ingested via soy protein undergo biotransformation by intestinal microflora and are absorbed into the circulation where they influence endogenous estrogenic levels. These phytoestrogens and their metabolites exhibit several hormonal and nonhormonal activities that could explain some of the biological consequences of phytoestrogen-rich diets. The mechanisms by which soy isoflavonoids can inhibit the development of the atherosclerotic process independent of the consequences of plasma lipoproteins could include antioxidant, antiproliferative and antimigratory consequences on smooth muscle cells, with an effect on thrombus formation and the maintenance of normal vascular reactivity (Jia et al. 2022).

Consumption of certain soy proteins has been hypothesized to increase circulating genistein levels that would inhibit the activity of tyrosine kinase, an enzyme associated with the development of atherosclerotic plaque.

A complete description of the ingredients responsible for the action of soy proteins, the mechanisms of action and the data obtained from human and animal research can be found in the documents that argue the position of the FDA (Singh et al. 2015).

The soy-based food chapter certainly remains an area of particular interest for future FFs and NTs research.

Increasing consumption of omega-3 fatty acids from fish, fish oil supplements or plant sources. Fish fatty acids and fish oils have gained interest and publicity for their role in the obstruction and control of CVD in humans. Fish oils are listed as FFs and NTs ingredients because of their remarkable consequence in preventing sudden cardiac death. The recommended consumption of fish in Western countries is one or two servings per week (Venugopalan et al. 2021).

The average consumption varies a lot between countries; there are countries in Europe where this consumption is six–seven times higher than in others, but it is still lower than this recommendation. Instead of increasing the amount of fish in the diet, FFs and NTs enriched with n–3 fatty eicosapentaenoic acid (EPA) and docosahexaenoic acid (DHA) can be consumed. Several foods can be enriched with fish oil; for example, margarine, dairy bio-compounds, cold cuts, meat.

The addition of these bio-compounds to an *"Ad libitum"* diet significantly increased EPA and DHA in plasma and platelets. Omega-3 fatty acids were recognized several decades ago as also important in maintaining the integrity of the nervous system, especially during its development. Indeed, the fatty acids contained in retinal membrane phospholipids are over 50% omega–3 polyenoic fatty acids, which means that there is a need for a minimal amount of such essential fatty acids at a given stage of development (Ahmmed et al. 2020).

A diet high in $C_{18}H_{30}O_2$-linoleic acid (an omega–6 fatty acid) but low in $C_{18}H_{30}O_2$ (an omega–3 fatty acid) has been shown to lead to episodes of numbness, paresthesias, weakness, inability to walk, leg pain, vision in fog in a six-year-old girl maintained on total parenteral nutrition for five months. When $C_{18}H_{30}O_2$ was reintroduced into the diet, the child's neurological symptoms disappeared. It is estimated that the requirement of $C_{18}H_{30}O_2$ is 0.54% of energy intake (Neggers et al. 2020). Only in the last few years has the evidence been substantial to now state with certainty that the intake of omega-3 fatty acids relative to omega-6 and non-essential fatty acids can decrease the possibility of disorders that, until recently, were not associated with fatty acid status.

In the US, the "healthy" status of omega-3 fatty acids in relation to CVD has been re-evaluated but is not usually acknowledged. The FDA concluded that there are still insufficient significant scientific theories or hypotheses to support the relationship between the two omega-3 fatty acids EPA and DHA and the reduction of coronary heart Rkd, but it allows the following statement to be consumed: "The scientific theory or hypothesis that that omega–3 fatty acids may decrease CHD possibility are suggestive but not conclusive. It is not known what consequence omega 3 fatty acids have on CHD possibility in the general community". The recommended intake level of fish oil fatty acids consistent with well-being interests is 2–4 g/day omega–3 (Martínez et al. 2022). The importance of omega-3 fatty acids in modulating the possibility of various sicknesses is usually highly appreciated (Table 7.1).

Chicken eggs enriched with omega-3 fatty acids can provide an alternative source of EPA and DHA. In particular, in communities where egg consumption is higher than fish consumption, this

TABLE 7.1

Sickness Influenced by Omega-3 Fatty Acid Intake and Possible Mechanisms of Action

Sickness	Possibility mechanisms of action of omega–3 fatty acids	References
Coronary heart sickness (CHD) and cerebrovascular accident (CVA)	Prevents arrhythmias (ventricular tachycardia and fibrillation); precursors of prostaglandins and leukotrienes; have anti-inflammatory properties; inhibits the synthesis of cytokines and mitogens; stimulates endothelial nitric oxide derivatives; have hypolipidemic properties with consequences on triglycerides and very low-density lipoprotein (VLDL); inhibits atherosclerosis.	(Zhou et al. 2022)
Essential fatty acid deficiency during growth	Essential fatty acids essential fatty acids (EFA) are important constituents of phospholipids membranes and a part of membranes in the brain and retina.	(Kwasek, Thorne-Lyman, & Phillips 2020)
Autoimmune sickness (including lupus and nephropathy)	Are involved in eliminating the cell-mediated immune response; inhibits the function of monocytes; inhibits the production and action of cytokines and eicosanoids; stabilizes renal function.	(Ruggeri et al. 2021)
Inflammatory bowel sickness	Have anti-inflammatory properties; inhibits interleukin-1ß (leukocytic pyrogen); inhibits the production of tumor necrosis factor; free radicals bind to necrophages; decreases the platelet response.	(Martin et al. 2015)
Breast, colon, prostate malignant diseases	Inhibits tumor growth.	(Accardi et al. 2019)
Rheumatoid arthritis	Alters eicosanoid metabolism; relieves inflammation.	(Zorgetto-Pinheiro et al. 2022)

could be an effective strategy to increase n–3 fatty acids. Eggs can be enriched with n–3 fatty acids if hens are fed bio-compounds rich in linseed or fishmeal.

It has been shown that a consumption of two to four enriched eggs/day significantly increased the concentration of PUFAs in platelet phospholipids. Beneficial consequences on blood lipids have been shown to be absent. Fortified omega–3 oils can be a successful source of n–3 fatty acids only if they are acknowledged by users. In a sensory evaluation with 78 untrained volunteers, no difference in taste was found, and shelf life was not distinct for enriched and "normal" pots (Tian et al. 2022).

Although three enriched eggs must be consumed to provide approximately the same amount of n–3 fatty acids as a single meal of fish, they may be a good source of n–3 fatty acids for users who do not like fish (Lyu et al. 2022). Further research in this area will certainly clarify and reveal the mechanisms that accompany these diet–sickness associations.

Probiotics and prebiotics. An area of research that is ongoing now and will remain in the future is that of probiotics and prebiotics. Probiotics are foods that contain bacteria, such as milk and milk bio-compounds – yogurt and kefir – which can favorably modify the configuration of the intestinal flora through the competition of one type of culture with another.

The gastro-intestinal tract is inhabited by a multitude of distinct microorganisms, a mixture that varies depending on the type of bacteria consumed (Khan et al. 2022).

Instead, prebiotics change the intestinal bacterial configuration not by adding bacteria but by changing the substrate offered to the existing mixture. Specific attestations are presented in Table 7.2.

The positive well-being outcomes of probiotics and prebiotics, including lowering cholesterol levels, protection against gastrointestinal sickness, and improving immunomodulation and sickness resistance are the subject of ongoing and future research. Fermented milk has been shown to cause an increase in the bacterial content of the human gut.

These bacteria, once present in the large intestine, are thought to ferment indigestible carbohydrates derived from food. This fermentation causes increased production of short-chain fatty acids that lower the concentration of circulating cholesterol either by inhibiting its hepatic synthesis or by redistributing cholesterol from plasma to the liver. In addition, increased bacterial activity in the large intestine results in the consolidation of bile acids.

Deconjugated bile acids are not well absorbed by the intestinal mucosa and are excreted. Consequently, cholesterol, being a precursor of bile acids, is consumed to accelerate the "de novo" synthesis of bile acids. It has been suggested that these combined actions are the mechanism that explains the association of fermented milk consumption with a decrease in the concentration of circulating cholesterol (Kumar et al. 2022).

TABLE 7.2

Attestations and Examples of Probiotics and Prebiotics

Probiotics	A food supplement with live microbes that interests the animal's metabolism by improving its intestinal microbial balance.
	A microbial preparation containing live cells and/or dead cells, including their metabolites, which is intended to ameliorate the microbial or enzymatic balance of the mucosa or to stimulate defense mechanisms.
	Examples: fermented vegetables, yogurt, kefir.
Prebiotics	A non-digestible food ingredient that favorably influences the host by selectively stimulating the growth or activity, or both, of bacteria or a limited series of bacteria in the colon, resulting in ameliorated host well-being.
	Examples: neosaccharides, inulin, soy oligosaccharides, isomalto-oligosaccharides, galacto-oligosaccharides, xylo-oligosaccharides, oligosaccharides, lactulose, raffinose, sorbitol, xylitol, palatinose, lactosucrose.

Several strains of bacteria have been studied as probiotics. *Lactobacillus* and *Bifidobacterium*, which are usually found in yogurts, are the bacteria most commonly consumed for the curative meaning of gastro-intestinal sickness by improving the ability of the intestine to prevent the invasion of pathogens. The well-being and immunity of the intestine largely depends on the presence of microflora. Probiotic therapy is supposed to provide a defense barrier to the gut by normalizing gut permeability and modifying the gut microenvironment. Such therapy also strengthens the intestinal immune barrier, particularly through intestinal immunoglobulin A and the inflammatory response. In addition, some probiotics have been shown to decrease the fecal concentration of enzymes, mutagens, and secondary bile salts that may be involved in colon carcinogenesis. Short-chain fatty acids such as acetate, propionate and butyrate, produced during intestinal fermentation, may also have promising uses in the curative meaning of colon malignant diseases. Increased production of short-chain fatty acids was accompanied by a decrease in the pH of the colonic contents and an increase in the proliferation of normal cells concomitant with suppression of the proliferation of transformed cells, which, in turn, was associated with a lower incidence of colon malignant diseases in distinct communities (Davachi et al. 2022).

A case-control study of black and white South Africans showed a significant inverse correlation between fecal pH and total fecal short-chain fatty acid concentration. The authors concluded that a high concentration of short-chain fatty acids in feces in the study category may provide protection against chronic intestinal sickness.

Although traditional thinking has been that the presence of one bacterium more than another in the gut is sufficient to produce these actions, more recent evidence suggests that by-bio-compounds of the flora are responsible for the bioactivity with real well-being interests. These by-bio-compounds include short-chain fatty acids such as short BCs peptides resulting from the cleavage of milk or other proteins in the intestine (Ho et al. 2022).

This change in mindset will likely stimulate active research exploring the mechanisms that might explain the well-being interests of probiotics and prebiotics.

Plant sterols and stanols and their esters are other FFs and NTs that are the subject of growing interest. These substances are not chemically distinct but are not found in quantities in eukaryotic cells (according to the following structures). Plant sterols [$C_{17}H_{28}O$] and their derivatives act in the small intestine by competitively inhibiting the intestinal absorption of cholesterol (Figure 7.2).

Recent data show that $C_{17}H_{28}O$ and stanols are equally effective with or without a fatty acid ester attached to the sterol ring in their ability to lower LDL cholesterol.

$C_{17}H_{28}O$ and their derivatives have a unique property compared to other FFs and NTs in that the chemical modification of the BCs is followed by obtaining a final component distinct from the normal form found in food.

Future areas of research on plant $C_{17}H_{28}O$ will likely also include inverse links between β-sitosterol [$C_{29}H_{50}O$] consumption and malignant diseases possibility. Compared to a cholesterol control – $C_{29}H_{50}O$ from lymph-node carcinoma of the prostate – LNCaP (a human prostate malignant diseases cell line) decreased the cell growth rate by 24% (Molska et al. 2022).

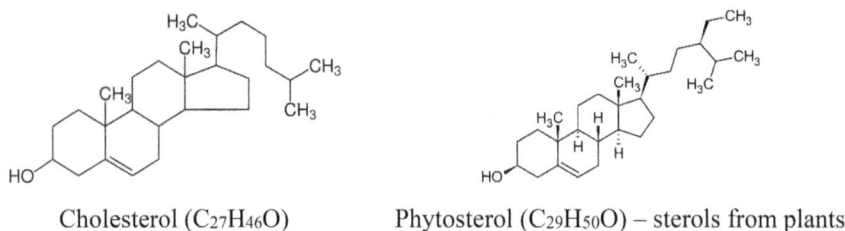

Cholesterol ($C_{27}H_{46}O$)   Phytosterol ($C_{29}H_{50}O$) – sterols from plants

FIGURE 7.2   Structure and chemical formula of cholesterol and phytosterol.

The phytosterol diet also exerts protective consequences on colonocyte growth proliferation by inhibiting the growth of HT-29 cells, a human colon malignant diseases cell line, compared to control curative meanings. Moreover, in the curative meaning of men with benign prostatic hyperplasia, $C_{29}H_{50}O$ produced improvement in urological symptoms and urinary flow rates. As prostate malignant diseases occur worldwide and are the second leading cause of malignant-disease death in men, future research will certainly focus on this area (Cofán & Ros 2019).

7.7 CONCLUSIONS AND RECOMMENDATIONS

In the last decades, the dietary recommendations for reducing cardiovascular possibility have aimed at limiting the intake of fats, especially saturated ones. The predominant role of fat type over total intake in reducing possibility is now evident. It has been shown that there are human communities with relatively low cardiovascular possibility, despite the traditional consumption of high-fat meat bio-compounds. Although there is no doubt concerning the association between saturated fat intake and increased LDL levels, a diet rich in PUFAs, and to some extent, monounsaturated fatty acids (MUFA), has been shown to have protective consequences. Substitution of saturated fats with unsaturated fatty acids is usually a desirable part of cardioprotective diets. The optimal MUFA/PUFAs ratio in the diet to ensure such an effect is not yet clear. The goal of these diets is to ensure a high omega-3/PUFAs and omega-6/PUFAs ratio through the consumption of fish, shellfish and vegetable oils. The hypothesis that LDL oxidation is the substantial mechanism involved in the pathogenesis of atherosclerosis has led to the idea that antioxidants can prevent atherosclerosis by limiting this process. Numerous natural antioxidants, predominantly of vegetable origin, have been identified. Flavonoids and antioxidant vitamins are two substantial categories of these.

REFERENCES

Accardi, G., Shivappa, N., Di Maso, M., Hébert, J. R., Fratino, L., Montella, M., La Vecchia, C., Caruso, C., Serraino, D., Libra, M., & Polesel, J. 2019. Dietary inflammatory index and cancer risk in the elderly: A pooled-analysis of Italian case-control studies. *Nutrition (Burbank, Los Angeles County, Calif.)*, *63–64*, 205–210. https://doi.org/10.1016/j.nut.2019.02.008

Ahmmed, M. K., Ahmmed, F., Tian, H. S., Carne, A., & Bekhit, A. E. 2020. Marine omega-3 (n-3) phospholipids: A comprehensive review of their properties, sources, bioavailability, and relation to brain health. *Comprehensive Reviews in Food Science And Food Safety*, *19*(1), 64–123. https://doi.org/10.1111/1541-4337.12510

Alonso-Miravalles, L., Barone, G., Waldron, D., Bez, J., Joehnke, M. S., Petersen, I. L., Zannini, E., Arendt, E. K., & O'Mahony, J. A. 2022. Formulation, pilot-scale preparation, physicochemical characterization and digestibility of a lentil protein-based model infant formula powder. *Journal of the Science of Food and Agriculture*, *102*(12), 5044–5054. https://doi.org/10.1002/jsfa.11199

Ardahanlı, İ., Özkan, H. İ., Özel, F., Gurbanov, R., Teker, H. T., & Ceylani, T. 2022. Infrared spectrochemical findings on intermittent fasting-associated gross molecular modifications in rat myocardium. *Biophysical Chemistry*, *289*, 106873. https://doi.org/10.1016/j.bpc.2022.106873

Bryła P. 2020. Selected predictors of the importance attached to salt content information on the food packaging (a study among polish consumers). *Nutrients*, *12*(2), 293. https://doi.org/10.3390/nu12020293

Cofán, M., & Ros, E. 2019. Use of plant sterol and stanol fortified foods in clinical practice. *Current Medicinal Chemistry*, *26*(37), 6691–6703. https://doi.org/10.2174/0929867325666180709114524

Dahl, W. J., & Stewart, M. L. 2015. Position of the academy of nutrition and dietetics: Health implications of dietary fibre. *Journal of the Academy of Nutrition and Dietetics*, *115*(11), 1861–1870. https://doi.org/10.1016/j.jand.2015.09.003

Davachi, S. M., Dogan, B., Khazdooz, L., Zhang, S., Khojastegi, A., Fei, Z., Sun, H., Meletharayil, G., Kapoor, R., Simpson, K. W., & Abbaspourrad, A. 2022. Long-term *Lacticaseibacillus rhamnosus GG* storage at ambient temperature in vegetable oil: Viability and functional assessments. *Journal of Agricultural and Food Chemistry*, *70*(30), 9399–9411. https://doi.org/10.1021/acs.jafc.2c02953

Esquivel-Alvarado, D., Zhang, S., Hu, C., Zhao, Y., & Sang, S. 2022. Using Metabolomics to identify the exposure and functional biomarkers of ginger. *Journal of Agricultural and Food Chemistry*, 10.1021/acs.jafc.2c05117. Advance online publication. https://doi.org/10.1021/acs.jafc.2c05117

Franco-Arellano, B., Vanderlee, L., Ahmed, M., Oh, A., & L'Abbé, M. 2020. Influence of front-of-pack labelling and regulated nutrition claims on consumers' perceptions of product healthfulness and purchase intentions: A randomized controlled trial. *Appetite*, 149, 104629. https://doi.org/10.1016/j.appet.2020.104629)

Ho, S. W., El-Nezami, H., Corke, H., Ho, C. S., & Shah, N. P. 2022. L-citrulline enriched fermented milk with *Lactobacillus helveticus* attenuates dextran sulfate sodium (DSS) induced colitis in mice. *The Journal of Nutritional Biochemistry*, 99, 108858. https://doi.org/10.1016/j.jnutbio.2021.108858

Hollmann, S., Kremer, A., Baebler, Š., Trefois, C., Gruden, K., Rudnicki, W. R., Tong, W., Gruca, A., Bongcam-Rudloff, E., Evelo, C. T., Nechyporenko, A., Frohme, M., Šafránek, D., Regierer, B., & D'Elia, D. 2020. The need for standardisation in life science research – an approach to excellence and trust. *F1000Research*, 9, 1398. https://doi.org/10.12688/f1000research.27500.2

Iqbal, S., Ayyub, A., Iqbal, H., & Chen, X. D. 2021. Protein microspheres as structuring agents in lipids: Potential for reduction of total and saturated fat in food products. *Journal of the Science of Food and Agriculture*, 101(3), 820–830. https://doi.org/10.1002/jsfa.10645

Jia, Y., Yan, X., Huang, Y., Zhu, H., Qi, B., & Li, Y. 2022. Different interactions driving the binding of soy proteins (7S/11S) and flavonoids (quercetin/rutin): Alterations in the conformational and functional properties of soy proteins. *Food Chemistry*, 396, 133685. https://doi.org/10.1016/j.foodchem.2022.133685

Kamioka, H., Origasa, H., Kitayuguchi, J., & Tsutani, K. 2021. Compliance of clinical trial protocols for foods with function claims (FFC) in Japan: Consistency between clinical trial registrations and published reports. *Nutrients*, 14(1), 81. https://doi.org/10.3390/nu14010081

Kamioka, H., Tsutani, K., Origasa, H., Yoshizaki, T., Kitayuguchi, J., Shimada, M., Tang, W., & Takano-Ohmuro, H. 2017. Quality of systematic reviews of the Foods with Function Claims registered at the Consumer Affairs Agency Web site in Japan: A prospective systematic review. *Nutrition Research (New York, N.Y.)*, 40, 21–31. https://doi.org/10.1016/j.nutres.2017.02.008

Kamioka, H., Tsutani, K., Origasa, H., Yoshizaki, T., Kitayuguchi, J., Shimada, M., Wada, Y., & Takano-Ohmuro, H. 2019. Quality of systematic reviews of the foods with function claims in Japan: Comparative before- and after-evaluation of verification reports by the consumer affairs agency. *Nutrients*, 11(7), 1583. https://doi.org/10.3390/nu11071583

Khan, F. F., Sohail, A., Ghazanfar, S., Ahmad, A., Riaz, A., Abbasi, K. S., Ibrahim, M. S., Uzair, M., & Arshad, M. 2022. Recent innovations in non-dairy prebiotics and probiotics: Physiological potential, applications, and characterization. *Probiotics and Antimicrobial Proteins*, 10.1007/s12602-022-09983-9. Advance online publication. https://doi.org/10.1007/s12602-022-09983-9

Kong, F., Kang, S., Zhang, J., Jiang, L., Liu, Y., Yang, M., Cao, X., Zheng, Y., Shao, J., & Yue, X. 2022. The non-covalent interactions between whey protein and various food functional ingredients. *Food Chemistry*, 394, 133455. https://doi.org/10.1016/j.foodchem.2022.133455

Kraus, A., Annunziata, A., & Vecchio, R. 2017. Sociodemographic factors differentiating the consumer and the motivations for functional food consumption. *Journal of the American College of Nutrition*, 36(2), 116–126. https://doi.org/10.1080/07315724.2016.1228489

Kumar, D., Lal, M. K., Dutt, S., Raigond, P., Changan, S. S., Tiwari, R. K., Chourasia, K. N., Mangal, V., & Singh, B. 2022. Functional fermented probiotics, prebiotics, and synbiotics from non-dairy products: A perspective from nutraceutical. *Molecular Nutrition & Food Research*, 66(14), e2101059. https://doi.org/10.1002/mnfr.202101059

Kwasek, K., Thorne-Lyman, A. L., & Phillips, M. 2020. Can human nutrition be improved through better fish feeding practices? A review paper. *Critical Reviews in Food Science and Nutrition*, 60(22), 3822–3835. https://doi.org/10.1080/10408398.2019.1708698

Lusk J. L. 2019. Consumer beliefs about healthy foods and diets. *PloS One*, 14(10), e0223098. https://doi.org/10.1371/journal.pone.0223098

Lyu, S., Pan, F., Ge, H., Yang, Q., Duan, X., Feng, M., Liu, X., Zhang, T., & Liu, J. 2022. Fermented egg-milk beverage alleviates dextran sulfate sodium-induced colitis in mice through the modulation of intestinal flora and short-chain fatty acids. *Food & Function*, 13(2), 702–715. https://doi.org/10.1039/d1fo03040j

Martin, F. P., Lichti, P., Bosco, N., Brahmbhatt, V., Oliveira, M., Haller, D., & Benyacoub, J. 2015. Metabolic phenotyping of an adoptive transfer mouse model of experimental colitis and impact of dietary fish oil intake. *Journal of Proteome Research*, 14(4), 1911–1919. https://doi.org/10.1021/pr501299m

Martínez, R., Mesas, C., Guzmán, A., Galisteo, M., López-Jurado, M., Prados, J., Melguizo, C., Bermúdez, F., & Porres, J. M. 2022. Bioavailability and biotransformation of linolenic acid from basil seed oil as a novel source of omega-3 fatty acids tested on a rat experimental model. *Food & Function*, *13*(14), 7614–7628. https://doi.org/10.1039/d2fo00672c

Molska, M., Reguła, J., Grygier, A., Muzsik-Kazimierska, A., Rudzińska, M., & Gramza-Michałowska, A. 2022. Effect of the addition of buckwheat sprouts modified with the addition of *Saccharomyces cerevisiae* var. *boulardii* to an atherogenic diet on the metabolism of sterols, stanols and fatty acids in rats. *Molecules (Basel, Switzerland)*, *27*(14), 4394. https://doi.org/10.3390/molecules27144394

Neggers, Y. H., Kim, E. K., Song, J. M., Chung, E. J., Um, Y. S., & Park, T. 2009. Mental retardation is associated with plasma omega-3 fatty acid levels and the omega-3/omega-6 ratio in children. *Asia Pacific Journal of Clinical Nutrition*, *18*(1), 22–28.

Plasek, B., Lakner, Z., & Temesi, Á. 2021. I believe it is healthy-impact of extrinsic product attributes in demonstrating healthiness of functional food products. *Nutrients*, *13*(10), 3518. https://doi.org/10.3390/nu13103518

Plasek, B., & Temesi, Á. 2019. The credibility of the effects of functional food products and consumers' willingness to purchase/willingness to pay-review. *Appetite*, *143*, 104398. https://doi.org/10.1016/j.appet.2019.104398

Popoola-Akinola, O. O., Raji, T. J., & Olawoye, B. 2022. Lignocellulose, dietary fibre, inulin and their potential application in food. *Heliyon*, *8*(8), e10459. https://doi.org/10.1016/j.heliyon.2022.e10459

Puttasiddaiah, R., Lakshminarayana, R., Somashekar, N. L., Gupta, V. K., Inbaraj, B. S., Usmani, Z., Raghavendra, V. B., Sridhar, K., & Sharma, M. 2022. Advances in nanofabrication technology for nutraceuticals: New insights and future trends. *Bioengineering (Basel, Switzerland)*, *9*(9), 478. https://doi.org/10.3390/bioengineering9090478

Robbani, R. B., Hossen, M. M. M., Mitra, K., Haque, M. Z., Zubair, M. A., Khan, S., & Uddin, M. N. 2022. Nutritional, phytochemical, and *in vitro* antioxidant activity analysis of different states of soy products. *International Journal of Food Science*, *2022*, 9817999. https://doi.org/10.1155/2022/9817999)

Ruggeri, R. M., Giovinazzo, S., Barbalace, M. C., Cristani, M., Alibrandi, A., Vicchio, T. M., Giuffrida, G., Aguennouz, M. H., Malaguti, M., Angeloni, C., Trimarchi, F., Hrelia, S., Campennì, A., & Cannavò, S. 2021. Influence of dietary habits on oxidative stress markers in Hashimoto's thyroiditis. *Thyroid: Official Journal of the American Thyroid Association*, *31*(1), 96–105. https://doi.org/10.1089/thy.2020.0299

Salvo, E. D., Conte, F., Casciaro, M., Gangemi, S., & Cicero, N. 2022. Bioactive natural products in donkey and camel milk: A perspective review. *Natural Product Research*, 1–15. Advance online publication. https://doi.org/10.1080/14786419.2022.2116706

Sharma, S., Singh, A., Sharma, S., Kant, A., Sevda, S., Taherzadeh, M. J., & Garlapati, V. K. 2021. Functional foods as a formulation ingredients in beverages: Technological advancements and constraints. *Bioengineered*, *12*(2), 11055–11075. https://doi.org/10.1080/21655979.2021.2005992

Singh, A., Meena, M., Kumar, D., Dubey, A. K., & Hassan, M. I. 2015. Structural and functional analysis of various globulin proteins from soy seed. *Critical Reviews in Food Science and Nutrition*, *55*(11), 1491–1502. https://doi.org/10.1080/10408398.2012.700340

Soliman G. A. 2019. Dietary fibre, atherosclerosis, and cardiovascular disease. *Nutrients*, *11*(5), 1155. https://doi.org/10.3390/nu11051155

Suarez-Torres, J. D., Jimenez-Orozco, F. A., & Ciangherotti, C. E. 2020. Drug excipients, food additives, and cosmetic ingredients probably not carcinogenic to humans reveal a functional specificity for the 2-year rodent bioassay. *Journal of Applied Toxicology: JAT*, *40*(8), 1113–1130. https://doi.org/10.1002/jat.3971

Tian, Y., Zhu, H., Zhang, L., & Chen, H. 2022. Consumer preference for nutritionally fortified eggs and impact of health benefit information. *Foods (Basel, Switzerland)*, *11*(8), 1145. https://doi.org/10.3390/foods11081145

Venugopalan, V. K., Gopakumar, L. R., Kumaran, A. K., Chatterjee, N. S., Soman, V., Peeralil, S., Mathew, S., McClements, D. J., & Nagarajarao, R. C. 2021. Encapsulation and protection of omega-3-rich fish oils using food-grade delivery systems. *Foods (Basel, Switzerland)*, *10*(7), 1566. https://doi.org/10.3390/foods10071566

Wei, M., Ma, T., Cao, M., Wei, B., Li, C., Li, C., Zhang, K., Fang, Y., & Sun, X. 2022. Biomass estimation and characterization of the nutrient components of thinned unripe grapes in China and the global grape industries. *Food Chemistry: X*, *15*, 100363. https://doi.org/10.1016/j.fochx.2022.100363).

Wojdyło, A., Nowicka, P., Turkiewicz, I. P., Tkacz, K., & Hernandez, F. 2021. Comparison of bioactive compounds and health promoting properties of fruits and leaves of apple, pear and quince. *Scientific Reports*, *11*(1), 20253. https://doi.org/10.1038/s41598-021-99293-x

Yu, J. C., Hlávka, J. P., Joe, E., Richmond, F. J., & Lakdawalla, D. N. 2022. Impact of non-binding FDA guidances on primary endpoint selection in Alzheimer's disease trials. *Alzheimer's & Dementia (New York, N. Y.)*, *8*(1), e12280. https://doi.org/10.1002/trc2.12280

Zanchini, R., Di Vita, G., & Brun, F. 2022. Lifestyle, psychological and socio-demographic drivers in functional food choice: A systematic literature review based on bibliometric and network analysis. *International Journal of Food Sciences and Nutrition*, *73*(6), 709–725. https://doi.org/10.1080/09637486.2022.2048361).

Zeng, X., Li, H., Jiang, W., Li, Q., Xi, Y., Wang, X., & Li, J. 2022. Phytochemical compositions, health-promoting properties and food applications of crabapples: A review. *Food Chemistry*, *386*, 132789. https://doi.org/10.1016/j.foodchem.2022.132789

Zhou, C., Zhao, W., Zhang, S., Ma, J., Sultan, Y., & Li, X. 2022. High-throughput transcriptome sequencing reveals the key stages of cardiovascular development in zebrafish embryos. *BMC Genomics*, *23*(1), 587. https://doi.org/10.1186/s12864-022-08808-x

Zorgetto-Pinheiro, V. A., Machate, D. J., Figueiredo, P. S., Marcelino, G., Hiane, P. A., Pott, A., Guimarães, R., & Bogo, D. 2022. Omega-3 fatty acids and balanced gut microbiota on chronic inflammatory diseases: A close look at ulcerative colitis and rheumatoid arthritis pathogenesis. *Journal of Medicinal Food*, *25*(4), 341–354. https://doi.org/10.1089/jmf.2021.0012

8 Markers of Functional Foods and Nutraceuticals in Health Maintenance

Monica Butnariu

8.1 INTRODUCTION

Food products whose nutritional value is enriched and that provide specific health benefits beyond basic nutrition are known as functional foods. The concept of functional food refers to "a food product that, in addition to the basic nutritional impact, will have beneficial effects on one or more functions of the human body, improving the general condition, implicitly the physical one, and reducing the risk of developing some ailments". This concern offers great opportunities for the food industry; there is great potential to transform classic foods, consumed daily, into functional foods. Functional foods represent one of the most intensively discussed and widely promoted research topics in the food and nutritional sciences. They are not miracle foods, nor do they represent a use of them to continue unhealthy habits. Functional foods support a healthy and balanced lifestyle.

Functional foods can be from the category:

- Natural foods.
- Foods to which a component has been attached.
- Foods from which a component has been removed.
- Foods where the bioavailability of some components has changed.
- Or, a combination of the foregoing.

According to the American Dietetic Association, functional foods include:

- Conventional (whole) foods: fruits, vegetables, nuts, peanuts, dark chocolate, yogurts.
- Modified foods: fortified (iodized salt, orange juice with added calcium).
- Enriched (bread enriched with folate) with enhancers (nutritional bars, yogurts, tea, foods with bioactive ingredients such as lutein, fish oils, ginko biloba).
- Medical food: products intended for enteral nutrition, under medical supervision, used for the nutritional approach specific to a condition (for example, products without phenylalanine for patients with phenylketonuria).
- Foods for special diets: prepared for children, for weight loss, products without gluten (for celiac disease) or without lactose (for those with lactose intolerance).

Looking at it as a whole, it may seem that, in fact, all foods are functional because they provide nutrients and energy to support growth or vital processes. But, in reality, functional foods are those considered to offer additional benefits that can reduce the risk of disease or promote optimal health (scientifically proven benefits) through their content of biologically active compounds.

DOI: 10.1201/9781003361497-9

8.2 ATTESTATIONS, CLASSIFICATIONS AND CURRENT LEGISLATIVE CONSIDERATIONS RELATING TO MARKERS

The ultimate goal of functional foods (FFs) and nutraceutical (NTs) studies is really that, whenever possible, the said benefit is directly measured. However, even if the ideal goal for human intervention studies, performance and well-being, can be identified, they may not be measurable in practice. There are several reasons that cause this:

- There may be an extended period of time between the introduction of the intervention and the occurrence of the desired result (for example, a lower incidence of a sickness as evidence of a reduction in the possibility of occurrence of this sickness).
- It would not be feasible or ethical to access the appropriate goal tissues or biochemical processes (e.g., vascular wall or bronchial mucosa).

Other times, although it is possible to measure the desired outcome, such as constituents or processes resulting from energy metabolism, protein consumption, lipid and lipoprotein metabolism and glucose kinetics, doing so in a large-scale study would be prohibitively expensive dependent on expertise and resources, which would be impractical (Zheng et al. 2022).

FUFOSE recommended that, when the definitive endpoint cannot be determined, a more readily measurable set of markers (MKs) can be consumed. The strength and relevance of MKs to measure the key objective or goal must be ensured. The FUFOSE consensus indicated how this could be achieved. If MKs represent an aspect directly involved in the process, then they should be considered factors, and if they represent correlated aspects, then they should be considered indicators. In the following, certain standards will be presented, which define MKs, consumed to measure certain blood constituents and at the same time to measure subjective behavioral experiences.

There are several categories of MKs that can be chosen: biochemical, physiological or behavioral. MKs can directly represent the unfolding of an event of interest or related events. They must be specific, sensitive, reproducible, validated and biologically meaningful. MKs must also have the following characteristics: be linked to goal qualities, indicate amelioration or enhancement of biological response function or be appropriate for intermediate points to be able to accurately describe the process of improving well-being or reducing risk of disease (Rkd). MKs should record the short- and extended-term impact of essential bioactive compounds (EBCs). It should also be possible to use these MKs in the safety assessment of FFs and NTs. All MKs must meet standard quality control standards. Using a determined set of MKs, it should be possible to document the modulation of goal qualities in the biological process in a significant way. Practical consequences must be proven in human nutrition studies for all members of a community or for a special category clearly determined by specific MKs; for example, for distinct age categories, sex (Fan et al. 2022).

Based on data on dose-dependent consequences, it must be possible to demonstrate the cumulative practical consequences for foods actually consumed as part of the daily diet. Safety must also be assessed for the amount of food required to show practical consequences and then documented and presented according to acknowledged standards. In the path of producing a sickness, one can distinguish: MKs of exposure to danger (dietary intake), MKs of biological response, MKs of sickness and MKs of susceptibility. All categories of MKs are significant for antioxidants.

For example, the level of alpha-tocopherol in the blood, as a marker of exposure, can be studied in relation to the oxidation resistance of LDL, which is a marker of biological response. It can also be associated with the thickening of the carotid wall, an indicator of sickness, in subjects with hypercholesterolemia or with specific categories, representatives of susceptibility MKs (Zhang et al. 2022).

FUFOSE classifies as a practical outcome significant MKs if they:

a) Refer to exposure to the constituents of the EBcs being studied, such as the marker in serum, feces, breath, urine or tissue. Examples:

- the level of folic acid in red blood cells – marker for exposure to folic acid from EBcs;
- blood tryptophan level – marker for exposure to tryptophan from EBcss.

MKs of food component exposure may provide some indication, but not absolute proof, of the bioavailability of the food component or its presence or a practical derivative or metabolite at the goal site (or function) in the body.

b) Refer to the goal function or biological response, such as changes in body fluids, levels of a metabolite, the presence of proteins or enzymes or changes in a given function. Examples:
   - reduction of plasma homocysteine levels is a possible response to the folic acid diet;
   - blood pressure, a response to the caffeine diet.
c) Refer to a specific objective, characteristic of good well-being, sickness possibility reduction or both, such as the measure of biological processes that directly relate to the ultimate objective. Examples:
   - the degree of narrowing of the carotid artery as evidence of CVD;
   - change in bone mineral density, an indicator for the possibility of bone fractures.

The end objective itself, if attainable, should be measured in some way. If this is possible, such measurement can be consumed as a basis for validating intermediate endpoint MKs for use in further studies.

As the MKs are further from the final objective, they become more attenuated and less specific, more insignificant and can even induce confusion in the studies (Zahoor et al. 2022).

Instead, they become more specific and more quantitatively related the closer they are to the end goal in question. Characterization of the mechanisms and pathways leading to outcomes refines the identification of MKs and informs how they can be selected.

The generation of this knowledge, including approaches based on genomic and post-genomic molecular biology, the biological and physiological validity of MKs, is fundamental for the development of "foods with claims" (with requirements to have a nutritional function, to support the improvement of body qualities and the reduction Rkd).

As such, a new generation of assays using validated and acknowledged indicators as intermediate points could be consumed to test the efficacy of antioxidants. In practice, to date, *in vivo* measurement of prooxidants harmful to human well-being has been difficult. It is essential to use viable MKs with damaging oxidant consequences to fix non-damaging body structures that can be morally consumed and acknowledged by human volunteers. In the case of Rkd reduction, it is important to demonstrate the clear link of the indicators to those phenomena. MKs must represent relatively immediate results or, at least, over a reasonable period of time in order to be consumed to evaluate interventions. In this way, results obtained over an extended period of time can be substituted, where possible. Epidemiological studies are included here. In order to be consumed without possibility, MKs must undergo standard quality control procedures and rigorous validation testing.

MKs must be clearly linked to certain phenomena involved in the biological process studied. This fact is essential in preventing the execution of increasingly detailed measurements that involve an extended period of time and high costs. Single-track studies are needed to determine the sensitivity and specificity of these indicators. Studies, such as the frequency of the negative test when the process is present or the frequency of the positive test when the process is absent, are consumed for this purpose (Fathy et al. 2022).

The legislative authorities in the field require the use of ethical and minimally invasive procedures to measure the indicators in question. Both dynamic and static measurements are consumed. Static and dynamic MKs can be chosen based on objective assessments of physiological and psychological performance and subjective assessments of quality of life and other almost identical outcomes.

8.2.2   Marker Validation

The MKs must be:

- Biologically valid in the sense that they must have a known relationship with the outcome taking into account their variability within the goal community.
- Validate methodologically, in terms of their analytical characteristics.

There should be evidence that any marker, by itself, reflects a biologically significant consequence and can be accurately and reproducibly measured. The validation of a marker includes two aspects: biological validation and technical or methodological validation. While biological validation is common to all laboratories, methodological validation must be established for each laboratory.

Biological validation does not refer to the extent to which a marker reflects a particular well-being outcome of interest but to the process that leads to that outcome. It depends on the technical competence of each individual laboratory. Biological validation of the marker derives from its relationship to the biological processes leading to the beneficial consequence in well-being and involves a change reaction in accordance with a changing event or circumstances (You et al. 2022).

In addition to the perspective from the biological process, there is a need to have knowledge concerning the sensitivity and specificity of the marker according to the state of well-being; a marker does not mean reaching the ultimate well-being goal. Therefore, the appropriateness of a marker must be considered on a case-by-case basis. A single marker may not meet all the standards necessary to fully justify a well-being consequence. However, the marker can contribute to the totalization of evidence.

8.2.2.1   Methodological Validation and Quality Control

Any laboratory that performs measurements must be competent to perform measurements and to certify that the product value can be trusted and that the method is technically performing. Studies for documentation and control in terms of good laboratory practice (GLP), good clinical practice (GCP) and good epidemiological practice (GEP) should not be confused with the technical requirements of the analyses.

Quality control (QC) is important for mentions in terms of technical validation of measurements and includes aspects such as accuracy, precision, repeatability, linear reproducibility. Requirements for these can be found on the web sites of chemical societies and national and international assay validation committees (e.g., www.fasor.com/iso25/, www.aoac.org, www.nmkl.org, www.ich.org). During method development, validation data can be collected and compiled into a test method file that is unique to each laboratory (Rabail et al. 2022).

After method validation, routine analyses can be performed. For this, quality control is usually performed by running control samples simultaneously and checking the actual results against their means and standard deviation. In conclusion, total validation in the measurement of any parameter of interest is an integration of biological validation and methodological validation. Bioindicators now exist to assess DNA and PUFAs oxidative damage; there are also indicators that measure damage caused by protein oxidation. However, there are many anomalies regarding these bio-MKs because there are both internal contradictions in measuring the same material by distinct procedures and external contradictions that refer to obtaining results that differ according to the laboratory, although the same procedures are consumed.

Validation studies are needed in which the methodology is tested within the same laboratory, and especially between distinct laboratories whose results must coincide with those of other laboratories when using the same material. The predictive value of bioindicators in assessing their relevance in the etiology of a specific sickness also requires validation. Only when this type of validation is performed and all experts agree on the methodology will it be possible to use these procedures in new studies, which will establish the quantitative relationship between antioxidant consumption and the interests of consumption in human subjects. Thus, the most urgent request for the deepening of studies for MKs of oxidative processes in the human body is the validation of MKs for damage caused by oxidation. Before these MKs can be consumed as bioindicators to assess the level at which antioxidants are beneficial to well-being, it is necessary to engage them in validation programs. These validation studies also involve analyses of antioxidants and their metabolites (Beheshtizadeh et al. 2022). In general, three categories of validations are essential:

- Comparing the results obtained in the same laboratory.
- Comparison of the results obtained in distinct laboratories.
- Various supplementary validations.

Studies done on an identical biological material, using a distinct but complementary methodology, are compared in the same laboratory; in this way, the numerical differences in the obtained results can be eliminated or at least decreased.

Distinct procedures seem to give distinct results for what, at first sight, should give the same result using distinct means. If, after data processing, numerical differences remain, there must be clear reasons for the scientific explanation of the difference. For example, distinct procedures may measure slightly distinct aspects of the same oxidation damage. To assess the degree of oxidation damage for a given set of samples, as many established procedures as possible are consumed. The results are compared by as many laboratories as possible. Distinct validations are consumed to demonstrate that the measurements taken are related to those phenomena that led to the onset of the sickness (Flórez-Martínez et al. 2022).

For example, DNA damage caused by oxidation is an indicator in the mutagenesis process and a possible occurrence of carcinogenesis. Oxidation of LDL is an indicator for arterogenesis and vascular sickness. Therefore, evidence from human studies, based on MKs of biological response, or intermediate MKs of sickness endpoints can provide a scientific basis for FFs and NTs Information vs. Message and indications.

8.3 EXAMPLES OF USUALLY ACKNOWLEDGED MARKERS

The need to characterize and establish relationships between categories of people, the consequences and impact of various diets and possible MKs is felt in various branches of medicine such as:

- Regarding the impact of diet in **cardiovascular sickness**, usually, it has been concluded that LDL cholesterol and blood pressure are acknowledged and established as MKs being linked to changes in the possibility of CVD so that mentions can be made both for the consolidated function of and reducing the Rkd. HDL cholesterol, preprandial triacylglycerol and plasma homocysteine are established as examples of MKs sensitive to dietary factors and are methodologically validated, but it is still unclear to what extent the change in these MKs reflects enhancement of function (emphasized in nutrition) in reducing the Rkd. As such, there is a need to develop and validate MKs (of ameliorated function) sensitive to dietary changes in correlation with decreased Rkd in hemostatic function and oxidative degradation (Hadjimbei, Botsaris, & Chrysostomou 2022).
- For **systemic skeletal disorder**, although bone well-being problems encompass many disorders of the skeleton, this condition has been considered in particular, as it is a substantial public well-being problem in the EU. Bone mineral density (BMD), a measure of bone calcium content, has been identified as an example of a marker of ameliorated function in correlation with bone strength for individuals of all ages and sexes. For people over 50

living in countries with a high possibility of fractures, BMD was considered to be a good marker of fracture possibility, accepting that, if a dietary component provides evidence of a reduction in Rkd through changes in BMD, it can be considered to have an impact in reducing the possibility of fractures (Asfha, Mishra, & Vuppu 2022).

- With regard to **physical and fitness parameters**, mentions of muscle strength and power, body resistance to exercise, energy supply and supplementation, hydration status, flexibility, tissue growth and general immune qualities have led to the examination of several procedures of measurement of these fitness parameters (including tests of muscle strength, energy metabolism, food intake, body configuration, gastrointestinal function and immune function). For most, the reliability and shelf life of EBcs were considered adequate. On the other hand, regarding immune qualities, in correlation with physical and fitness performance, the interpretation of the available MKs were considered problematic, remaining as a basis for future studies (Unterberger et al. 2022).

- For **the regulation of body weight**, insulin sensitivity and diabetes, the biological qualities underlying these three conditions have been characterized in relation to the corresponding sickness: obesity, metabolic syndrome and diabetes. Good MKs and reliable measurement procedures were identified for the modulation of each key objective function with its range of associated qualities. In terms of body weight regulation, the goal function is adipose tissue deposition, which can be measured by both laboratory and field procedures. A series of associated qualities involved in the regulation of adipose tissue in the body can also be measured. Insulin sensitivity, the goal function in the metabolic syndrome, has several validated procedures available for its measurement (lipotoxicity, body fat configuration, oxidative stress, inflammation and vascular function). In diabetes, the goal function is the regulation of blood glucose levels, associated with qualities such as: the release of glucose into the bloodstream, the use of glucose and the secretion and sensitivity of insulin (Wagner et al. 2022).

- In the diet-**malignant diseases** relationship, it has been suggested that approximately one-third of all malignant diseases cases are caused by improper doses and imbalances of dietary constituents. Therefore, it is of key importance to develop clear standards to support malignant diseases possibility reduction claims in relation to foods or categories of EBcs. The focus was on colon, lung, breast and prostate tumors. Eighteen MKs have been identified that represent distinct events and points in the chain from initial exposure to carcinogens to overt malignancy. The true end goal in this field – human malignancy – usually cannot be measured as a basis for mentions. Pre-malignant, diseased lesions such as polyps in the colon were thus considered a solid marker, and polyp recurrence in humans was considered the only good marker usually available on which to base Rkd reduction claims. Therefore, it is essential to develop MKs for the events in the pathogenic process, which can substitute the final objectives (respectively the formation of the tumor at the end) (Gomes et al. 2022).

- For **mental well-being and performance,** it has been found that food and drink can influence brain qualities. Claims regarding several aspects of mental function can be proven using validated scientific instruments (tests, questionnaires, etc.). Mood, arousal (including activation, alertness, attention and sleep), motivation and effort, perception, memory and intelligence were examined. In the area of mental consequences, the final goal (improvement of qualities) can often be directly assessed by appropriate tests, unlike physiological qualities or other intermediate MKs (Kose et al. 2022).

- In terms of **intestinal well-being**, many parameters of digestion can be measured, such as absorption and secretion, intestinal behavior and transit time, intestinal flora, gastric emptying and motility, but interpretation is complicated because there is great individual variability in the term of what are considered to be normal limits. The recognized but under-determined hypothesis of well-being and the hypothesis of gastrointestinal well-being were also discussed and identified as an important area for future development (Zengin et al. 2022).

- Regarding the **immune system**, it is considered that a single test cannot define the immune function, but the measurement of several parameters, in integration, can be consumed to assess the practical capacity of this system (Ojueromi, Oboh, & Ademosun 2022).

8.4 BIOMARKERS OF OXIDATIVE STRESS

A general problem in studying oxidative stress in biological systems and in evaluating the consequences of antioxidants in vivo – i.e., in patients – arises regarding strategies for reliable measurements of oxidative parameters. Several MKs and procedures have been consumed to assess the oxidation bio-compounds (oxidation MKs) of various biomolecules in vitro, in biological systems and in vivo. In vitro measurements, although quite effective in assessing antioxidant possibility, being done in a controlled system, are not very predictive of possible in vivo activities. It should also be added that, since distinct antioxidants act by distinct mechanisms and distinct categories of bio-compounds may appear on distinct oxidative substrates, as such, tests should goal distinct oxidative measurement techniques using distinct categories of support.

For example, in vivo measurements are often consumed in connection with the assessment of oxidative processes in pathological conditions, but in some cases, some changes may occur artifactually during sample collection (e.g., cells, plasma preparation). In vivo measurements are made directly from samples taken without any manipulation – for example, urine – but, nevertheless, the reflection of the processes taking place in the body does not exactly imitate the processes at the place of these events (Dai et al. 2022).

The measurement of isoprostanes (IsoPs), a non-enzymatic product, as an oxidative metabolite of arachidonic acid $[C_{20}H_{32}O_2]$ is considered to be, with the limitations mentioned earlier, a valid indicator (biomarker) of lipid peroxidation. The increase of this marker has been observed in conditions where consolidated lipid peroxidation can be predicted (in people who smoke or who have diabetes or hyper-cholesterolemia). With particular regard to measurements of lipid peroxidation MKs, ideal assays should have the following characteristics:

- Quantification of the substantial bio-compounds of the peroxidation process.
- Low coefficients of variation of the analyses.
- No interference with other biomolecules.
- Reliable chemical procedures of analysis (e.g., mass spectroscopy, MS or high-performance liquid chromatography, HPLC) or other validated procedures.
- The possibility of not confusing the oxidation of ingested lipids with the diet.
- Knowledge of the steady states of peroxidation bio-compounds and the total rate of lipid peroxidation for ongoing processes.
- The measured parameters must be stable during storage (Tabrizi et al. 2022).

Measuring the consequences of antioxidants by means of validated bio-MKs for oxidative processes should be feasible before starting human studies.

8.5 THE IMPACT OF ANTIOXIDANT NUTRITIONAL CONSTITUENTS FROM FUNCTIONAL FOODS AND NUTRACEUTICALS IN SOME DEGENERATIVE SICKNESS

8.5.1 FUNCTIONAL NUTRITION ENRICHED WITH ANTIOXIDANTS AND CARDIOVASCULAR SICKNESS

8.5.1.1 Cardiovascular Sickness and their Impact in the Global Community

Considering the enormous impact of CVD worldwide, we must emphasize that even very modest reductions in the influence of possibility factors, through the design and use of appropriate FFs and NTs, can have very important links with well-being and a profound economic significance.

The statistics from the AHA/ASA (American Heart Association) (see www.americanheart.org/statistics/03cardio.html) indicate the enormous impact of CVD. More than 61 million Americans sometimes have more than one type of CVD. CVD is one of the leading causes of death each year; moreover, it is one of the top seven causes of death, and the estimated cost of CVD and stroke care in the United States in 2003 was $352 billion.

In developed countries, childhood obesity has reached epidemic proportions, and this will surely translate into a dramatic increase in type 2 diabetes, which is characterized by high levels of triglycerides, LDL-C (low-density lipoprotein–cholesterol), and decrease in the level of HDL-C (high-density lipoprotein-cholesterol) – i.e., a change in the direction of a highly atherogenic lipid profile (Teimouri et al. 2022).

Furthermore, the World Well-being Organization (see www.who.int/ncd/cvd) makes a very convincing case that the impact of CVD is not limited to Western countries but will reach epidemic proportions in developing countries' development, both due to demographic and lifestyle changes. It has been estimated that, by 2025, CVD will be the series one cause of death in the world.

8.6   DIET AND CARDIOVASCULAR SICKNESS

As shown, CVDs are still a substantial cause of death among Western European communities and are becoming an important cause of morbidity and mortality worldwide. Thanks to advanced knowledge and medical curative meanings, many patients survive an initial event.

For this reason, obstruction of secondary events in CVD is a growing task for nutritionists and other well-being professionals. Cardiovascular possibility can be decreased by changing lifestyle, and one of the coordinates is diet. There is now substantial evidence from epidemiological and clinical studies that a diet rich in fruits, vegetables, whole grains, fish and low-fat dairy bio-compounds and also low in sodium and low in saturated fat can decrease the possibility of coronary heart sickness and hypertension. People who adopted such diets benefited from a much lower possibility of heart sickness. Evidence-based strategies to decrease the possibility of CVD:

- Substitution of trans, saturated fats with non-hydrogenated unsaturated fats.
- Increasing consumption of omega-3 fatty acids from fish, fish oil supplements or other plant sources.
- Eating a diet rich in fruits, vegetables, nuts and whole grains and low in refined grain bio-compounds (Berger &Thorn 2022).

However, such a cautious diet is not typical of what users in Western countries eat. It appears that, today, they are less likely to invest in extended-term well-being if taste and convenience are compromised: in 1998, only 24% of users ate "healthy foods" for extended-term sickness obstruction, as opposed to 45% in 1990. However, almost all users indicated that they sometimes bought food for well-being reasons. The food manufacturing is aware of this, and some EBcs appear on the market with various well-being claims. Indeed, well-being claims on food packaging have been shown to have a positive influence on users' perception of food.

Thus, FFs products and NTs in palatable, ready-to-use form that suggest short-term or extended-term well-being interests have a huge market due to their well-being possibility. Active obstruction of coronary heart sickness (CHD) should be started immediately after its first clinical manifestation. Secondary obstruction focuses on reducing possibility in people with established CAD who are at increased possibility of recurrent cardiac events and death. It is important to remember that the two main causes of death in these patients are sudden cardiac death (SCD) and heart failure (HF), often resulting from myocardial ischemia and subsequent necrosis (Vanegas et al. 2022).

The main mechanism underlying recurrent cardiac events is myocardial ischemia resulting from atherosclerotic plaque rupture or ulceration. Plaque is usually the consequence of intraplaque inflammation combined with a high lipid content at the level of the lesion, with a high concentration of leukocytes and lipid peroxidation bio-compounds. Thus, in patients for whom CVD has been established, the main goals of the preventive strategy are to prevent malignant ventricular arrhythmias and the development of severe ventricular dysqualities (and HF) as well as to minimize the possibility of inflammation and ulceration. This means that the priority in secondary obstruction is somewhat distinct from that of primary obstruction. In the context of primary obstruction, intervention focuses on traditional possibility factors (e.g., blood cholesterol or blood pressure) more than specific clinical complications such as SCD.

This does not mean that traditional CD possibility factors should not also be measured, and if necessary, corrected in secondary obstruction, as they play an important role in the development of CD complications. Because complications such as SCD and associated syndromes are often unpredictable, occur, in most cases, outside a hospital and far from any possibility therapeutic resources and account for approximately 50% of all causes of cardiac mortality, there should be a priority in any curative meaning programs (Zazpe et al. 2016).

For this reason, in the present text, we will focus our dietary recommendations and comments mainly on clinical efficacy and not on surrogate efficacy. Regardless of the specific clinical goals of the program, nutritional assessment and counseling of each individual with CD must be a key point of preventive intervention.

Nutrition is, however, only one component of such a program.

Exercise, behavioral interventions (especially to help the patient abstain from smoking) and drug therapy are of equal importance. Control of possibility factors has traditionally been viewed from the perspective of obstruction. The preventive dietary program is usually initiated during the hospitalization due to the first event of CVD. By shortening the stay in the coronary care unit, the dietary program is initiated in the following days of hospitalization, then continued in secondary obstruction centers and included in cardiac rehabilitation programs (Mata-Fernández et al. 2021).

A diet in the individual obstruction program should be carried out under the guidance of a specialized dietitian and in close collaboration with the patient's cardiologist and primary care physician, so that there is no discontinuity or discrepancy in dietary counseling between the hospitalization and post-hospital phases; hospitalization of the rehabilitation program.

8.7 THE ROLE OF ANTIOXIDANTS IN THE OBSTRUCTION OF CVD

SCD is usually determined as death from a cardiac cause occurring within one hour of the onset of symptoms. However, in many studies, distinct attestations are consumed, with a time interval from three to 24 hours (in the old attestation given by the World Well-being Organization). The magnitude of the problem is considerable because SCD is very common, often being the first manifestation of coronary sickness, and represents approximately 50% of cardiovascular mortality in developed countries. In most cases, SCD occurs without warning symptoms even after leaving the hospital. In fact, this mode of death is a substantial public well-being problem. Since up to 80% of patients influenced by SCD have developed CD, the epidemiology and obstruction possibility should, theoretically, be expressed in parallel with that of CD. In other words, any curative meaning aimed at reducing CVD should decrease the incidence of SCD. Regarding the consequence of dietary antioxidants and their link to the possibility of CD in general and SCD in particular, this is highly controversial. For example, for Alpha-Tocopherol, the most widely studied dietary antioxidant, discordant findings have been published between the interests estimated based on epidemiological observations and the results of clinical trials. In contrast to studies with n–3 PUFAs, the results show that Alpha-Tocopherol supplementation does not support a significant consequence on the primary endpoint; namely, the composite of pain, death and nonfatal AMI (Oda et al. 2022).

However, the secondary analysis provides a clearer view of the clinical consequence of Alpha-Tocopherol in CVD patients, which cannot be readily dismissed. These data suggest that Alpha-Tocopherol may be useful for the primary obstruction of SCD in patients with established CD. The Alpha-Tocopherol study data are not isolated. Such ambivalent reactions to Alpha-Tocopherol may, at least partially, explain why its consequences have been neutral or non-significant in many studies, with negative consequences masking beneficial ones. However, the GISSI study showed that cardiovascular mortality and SCD were significantly decreased with Alpha-Tocopherol supplementation, and the consequence on overall mortality showed a favorable downward trend. Data from the HOPE trial testing the consequence of 400 IU of Alpha-Tocopherol/day in patients at high possibility of CHD (so in the primary obstruction domain) were published, and an apparent lack of consequence for Alpha-Tocopherol was reported, which does not help answer the question of whether or not Alpha-Tocopherol is protective against MSCs. In this study, it is not clear whether the patients took the capsules during meals (an indispensable condition for the intestinal absorption of Alpha-Tocopherol), whether or not the patients were Alpha-Tocopherol deficient, or whether some patients took other vitamin supplements (a common practice nowadays among certain communities), and MSC was apparently not among the predetermined goals (Rychter et al. 2022).

In addition, patients with left ventricular dysfunction, a substantial possibility factor for SCD, were not determined.

8.8   ANTIOXIDANTS, LIPID METABOLISM AND OXIDATIVE MODIFICATIONS OF LDL-CHOLESTEROL

Both lipo- and water-soluble forms of antioxidants present in the blood may be important in the obstruction of CVD due to their ability to prevent oxidation of complex lipoproteins. Lipoproteins are extremely important in CVD because we know for sure that high LDL-C causes atherosclerosis, which is the main cause of the most common CVD. In contrast, high HDL–C levels are a negative possibility factor for CVD. Atherosclerosis involves the gradual creation of "plaque" in the arterial wall. LDL-C is the substantial source of lipids in these plaques.

There is now significant evidence that LDL lipids (primarily cholesterol esters) attach in plaques to cells in the arterial wall called macrophages. These macrophages collect LDL – so much that they become "foamy" in essential quality and are therefore called "foam" cells. This is the first step in the atherosclerosis process that begins in childhood. Surprisingly, however, LDL incubated in macrophages does not turn into foam cells. After LDL is oxidized, oxLDL will cause macrophages to transform into foam cells (Xian et al. 2022).

Macrophages have receptors for native LDL, and the downregulation of these receptors is regulated by intracellular cholesterol accumulation. Unlike native LDL, the chemically adjusted form of LDL can be taken up by certain macrophage monocyte receptors (scavenger receptors) whose degradation is not regulated by intracellular cholesterol accumulation. LDL is the main plasma transporter for both Alpha-Tocopherol and CoQ10; both act as LDL antioxidants by inhibiting lipid peroxidation of lipids containing polyunsaturated fatty acid moieties. Some studies indicate that most of the endogenous Alpha-Tocopherol in LDL must be oxidized before it is converted to a highly absorbable form of oxLDL capable of transforming macrophages into foam cells. Since antioxidants, such as Alpha-Tocopherol, prevent the oxidation of LDL, it is logical to suggest that antioxidants could prevent the formation of foam cells and thereby delay the process of atherosclerosis. This suggestion is called the "oxidative modification hypothesis". Although most in vitro experiments support this view, not all evidence is in agreement.

Agree or disagree, oxLDL formation occurs in vivo, and the mechanisms for this oxidation are still open to research. Another important issue in the discussion is the apparent discrepancy between experimental studies and clinical studies on antioxidants, with divergent results.

Most studies with antioxidants in experimental models of atherosclerosis have shown that this curative meaning is able to delay the progression of atherosclerosis, while the results of clinical trials are in conflict with this position, with negative consequences also being reported (Seenak et al. 2021).

Conclusions regarding the role of antioxidants in the obstruction of atherosclerosis arise from observational studies that have proven an inverse relationship between the consumption of antioxidant vitamins and the possibility of cardiovascular events. However, meta-analysis of observational studies indicated that, among antioxidant vitamins, Alpha-Tocopherol was the only one that had a beneficial consequence against atherosclerotic complications.

Based on these data, almost all studies were based on the assumption that Alpha-Tocopherol supplementation would represent a useful approach to prevent CVD. But the profile of candidates for antioxidant curative meaning was not precisely determined: any patient at possibility of cardiovascular events was enrolled indiscriminately in these studies, leading to confusing results. Antioxidant status is considered to be an important marker of oxidative stress, and its determination may be useful for better identification of candidates for antioxidant curative meaning.

To support this hypothesis, inherent data on oxidative stress and antioxidant status in patients at possibility of CVD and in patients included in observational and interventional studies were reviewed. As an antioxidant, Alpha-Tocopherol has been the most important research topic in this field, being the main fat-soluble antioxidant in the body that must be obtained from the diet, since it cannot be synthesized. In vivo research has clearly shown that Alpha-Tocopherol prevents lipid peroxidation in humans. Dietary Alpha-Tocopherol is primarily γ-tocopherol, while Alpha-Tocopherol supplements are predominantly A-tocopherol (natural or synthetic). Alpha-tocopherol has the greatest biological activity in protecting fetal resorption in pregnant female rats (Zuraini et al. 2021).

Synthetic Alpha-Tocopherol is the most common form commonly found in supplements. There are very few studies focusing on the possibility role of vitamin D as an antioxidant in biological systems. One such study found that vitamin D3 can act as an antioxidant in vivo on rat liver with greater efficiency than that seen with Alpha-Tocopherol supplementation. It is unlikely that plasma vitamin D could be an effective antioxidant because its levels are very low. In contrast, plasma levels of Alpha-Tocopherol are at least 250 times higher than typical plasma concentrations of vitamin D.

Usually, there are no data to suggest qualities of vitamin D in the obstruction of CVD by virtue of its possibility role as an antioxidant. However, lack of vitamin D is a possibility factor in the development of CVD and diabetes, but the molecular mechanisms are not yet fully understood. In conclusion, there is convincing evidence that oxidative stress is detectable in patients with possibility factors for classic atherosclerosis, but its impact in the progression of atherosclerosis is still unclear. The reason for this uncertainty is the lack of clear evidence to indicate that MKs of oxidative stress, such as blood–lipid peroxides or urinary–F2–IsoPs, have any value in estimating the progression of atherosclerosis, even though there is some evidence from epidemiological studies suggesting that oxidized LDL antibodies can be consumed (Zhao et al. 2017).

Instead, studies seem to indicate that low-antioxidant status increases the possibility of CVD. The clinical characteristics of patients with low-antioxidant status have not been determined and should be studied in the near future. To date, antioxidant clinical trials have enrolled patients without assessment of either oxidative stress or antioxidant status, and this indiscriminate enrollment may be the motivation for the negative results of antioxidant studies. Subjects were fed normal doses of Alpha-Tocopherol ranging from 200–2000 mg/day for eight weeks. The highest plasma Alpha-Tocopherol dose was increased five-fold, but the urinary excretion of IsoPs and 4-hydroxynonenal (fatty acid breakdown bio-compounds by auto-oxidation) was not influenced. The results suggest that, normally, supplemental Alpha-Tocopherol will not confer any supplementary antioxidant protection to such fed subjects. In contrast, previous studies on smokers have proven an effect on plasma levels of Alpha-Tocopherol and IsoPs, suggesting that consequences are obtained only in subjects with a certain oxidative stress. The protective consequence of Alpha-Tocopherol against coronary events in the SPACE Study may reflect the fact that subjects were known to have increased oxidative stress due to hemodialysis. Similarly, other people with increased oxidative stress (such as smokers, diabetics) might constitute a much more likely community to benefit from antioxidant curative meaning.

In addition, it has been suggested that antioxidants may be effective in the initial stages of inhibiting the atherosclerosis process in humans and ineffective or much less effective in reducing atherosclerotic plaque, instability and rupture.

If this were the case, one might find a way to assess the early stages of the lesion's development (e.g., with high-resolution ultrasound or magnetic resonance imaging) more than relying on clinical endpoints that are usually too late observables. Of course, if the development of early lesions has been successfully inhibited, there should eventually be a decrease in the frequency of clinical events, but in this case, studies may need to be extended beyond the formalistic five years. Another aspect that deserves further attention is choosing the appropriate antioxidant curative meaning (Cao et al. 2019).

Several mechanisms have been proposed to date, including enzymatic and nonenzymatic LDL oxidation, but the exact process leading to LDL accumulation on the vascular wall is still unclear. This fact creates uncertainty concerning the type of antioxidants that might be significant for inhibiting atherosclerotic progression. Thus, future studies with antioxidants should not be discouraged; on the contrary, a better identification of the selection standards of possibility subjects for antioxidant curative meaning should be studied, together with the selection of an appropriate daily antioxidant regimen.

8.9 FUNCTIONAL FOOD ENRICHED WITH ANTIOXIDANTS AND THE METABOLIC SYNDROME

8.9.1 Metabolic Syndrome Constituents

Over time, the metabolic syndrome (MS) has been known under several names such as insulin resistance syndrome, syndrome X, plurimetabolic syndrome, metabolic X syndrome, cardio-metabolic syndrome, etc. Insulin resistance (IR) is the central pathological element of MS. The IR is determined as the need for an abnormally large amount of insulin for a normal biological response leading to a compensatory increase in insulin secretion and hyperinsulinemia. Visceral obesity was first reported by Morgagni in the nobles whose lifestyle was characterized by sedentarism and copious meals. In 1947 Vague described gynoid and android obesity, and IR was reported for the first time in 1936 by Himsworth, who showed that, in obese subjects with diabetes mellitus (DM), there is a decreased uptake of glucose when insulin is administered. In 1988, Raven described metabolic resistance syndrome, or syndrome X, with the following entities: central obesity, hyperinsulinemia, hypertriglyceridemia, hyperuricemia, hypertension, and identified IR as the common pathophysiological disorder of this syndrome (Wang et al. 2022).

The quantitative investigation of IR became possible with the development of procedures for determining insulinemia and after the discovery of the glycemic clamp. Other constituents identified as being associated with IR and increased cardiovascular possibility are polycystic ovary syndrome (PCOS), non-alcoholic fatty liver, acanthosis nigricans, endothelial dysfunction, hyperuricemia, increased prothrombotic factors, leptin, fibrinogen and inflammation MKs (protein C reactive and interleukin 6). Although age is not one of the constituents of MS, it certainly plays an important role, with the prevalence of MS increasing with age. The pathogenic substrate could be the decrease in insulin action, due to changes in the amount and distribution of adipose tissue, which, in many elderly people, increases in amount and is preferentially deposited at the visceral level (Sharma et al. 2022). The main constituents of the SM are shown in Table 8.1.

The importance of MS derives from its association with a greatly increased possibility for ischemic cardiovascular events, with the possibility of developing type 2 DM (if not already present) and with increased overall and cardiovascular mortality, a fact documented by numerous studies conducted in the US and Europe.

8.9.2 Attestation of Metabolic Syndrome in Adults

MS has benefited from – over time – several attestations, each established by an organization or association with authority in the field (Table 8.2): the WHO attestation in 1999, the National

TABLE 8.1
Main Constituents of Metabolic Syndrome

Metabolic deficiencies	Main characteristics
Insulin resistance, hyperinsulinemia	increased beta-cell response to glucose
	basal hyperinsulinemia (appears early)
	hypoinsulinemia and decreased sensitivity of beta cells to glucose (late)
	decrease in glucose consumption mediated by insulin
	decrease in the series of insulin receptors
	decrease in glycogen synthetase activation (in muscles, adipose tissue)
	alteration of Glucose transporter type 4 (GLUT4), expression
	increased expression of protein kinase C isoforms
Impaired Glucose Tolerance (IGT)	DZ type 2
	fasting blood sugar (FBS) or fasting blood glucose (FBG)
	impaired fasting glycemia (IFG)
	the presence of DM type 2 complications: renal, nervous, ocular
Obesity	increase in body fat mass
	increase in visceral adiposity
	central distribution (in the upper half of the body): intra-abdominal fat (IAF) > 0.9 in women, > 1 in men
Dyslipidemia	hypertriglyceridemia (increasing very low-density lipoproteins (VLDL))
	decrease in cholesterol associated with high-density lipoprotein (HDLc)
	increase in LDLc and the series of small and dense particles
	increase in LDL/HDL cholesterol ratio
	increasing free fatty acids (AGL)
Mild, moderate and severe hypertension	increased hypertension (HTN) or thoracic aortic dissection (TAD) or both

TABLE 8.2
Comparative Presentation of the Standards for Defining MS in Adults

WHO in 1999	*IR identified by 1 of the following: DM type 2, FBG, IFG or, in those with blood glucose < 110 mg/dL: glucose uptake below the lowest quartile for the general community established by hyperinsulinemic euglycemic clamp;* + any two of the following:
	Hypertension (≥ 140 mm Hg systolic BP or ≥ 90 mm Hg diastolic blood pressures) or hypotensive curative meaning
	TG ≥ 150 mg/dL (≥ 1.7 mmol/L and/or HDL cholesterol < 35 mg/dL (< 0.9 mmol/L) in men, < 39 mg/dL (< 1.0 mmol/L) in women
	BMI > 30 kg/m2 and/or abdominal mass index > 0.9 in men, > 0.85 in women
	Urinary albumin excretion ≥ 20 µg/min or albumin creatinine ratio ≥ 30 mg/g
NCEP–ATP III in 2001	*At least three of the following:*
	Abdominal obesity: CA > 98 cm in men, > 85 cm in women
	Triglycerides ≥ 150mg/dL or specific curative meaning for this dyslipidemia
	HDLc < 40 mg/dL in men, < 50 mgdL in women or specific curative meaning for this dyslipidemia
	Fasting blood glucose ≥ 110mgdL (later the blood glucose limit was changed by the ADA to 100 mg/dL)*
	Blood pressure ≥ 130/85mmHg
AACE in 2002**	*Overweight/obesity: body mass index (BMI) ≥ 25 kg/m²*
	Total cholesterol (TC) ≥ 150 mg/dL
	High-density lipoprotein cholesterol (HDL-C) < 40 mg/dL in men and < 50 mg/dL in women
	Blood pressure: systolic ≥ 130/85 mmHg

(Continued)

TABLE 8.2 *(Continued)*
Comparative Presentation of the Standards for Defining MS in Adults.

	Fasting blood glucose between 110 and 126 mg/dL*
	Blood glucose at 2 h during Oral glucose tolerance tests (OGTT) > 140 mg/dL
	Supplementary possibility factors: family history of type 2 DM, hypertension or coronary heart sickness, polycystic ovary syndrome, sedentary lifestyle, advanced age, belonging to certain ethnic categories at increased possibility for DM or coronary heart sickness
IDF in 2005	*Abdominal obesity (CA >94 cm, in men and > 80 cm, in women) ***, ***** + any two of the following:
	High triglyceride levels: ≥ 1.7 mmol/l (≥ 150 mg/dl) or specific curative meaning for this type of dyslipidemia
	Low HDL cholesterol: < 1.03 mmol/l (< 40 mg/dl) in men or < 1.29 mmol/l (< 50 mg/dl) in women or specific curative meaning for this type of dyslipidemia
	High BP, systolic BP ≥ 130 mmHg or diastolic BP ≥ 85 mmHg or hypotensive curative meaning
	Elevated fasting blood glucose: ≥ 5.6 mmol/l (≥ 100 mg/dl) or FBG or previously diagnosed type 2 diabetes

*>the lower limit for fasting blood glucose was changed by the ADA in 2003 to 100 mg/dL; **AACE does not specify the series of standards needed to establish the diagnosis of MS, leaving this to the discretion of the clinician; *** in Caucasians **** if BMI ≥ 30 kg/m2, it is considered abdominal obesity.

Cholesterol Education Program (NCEP) Expert Panel attestation from 2001, the attestation from American Association of Clinical Endocrinologists since 2003 (AACE) and that of the International Diabetes Federation since 2005 (Table 8.3).

The particular impact it has on the well-being of the general community determined the need to adopt diagnostic standards that allow, on the one hand, ease of application in practice and, on the other hand, to be unanimously acknowledged. This was achieved by the 2005 Berlin International Diabetes Federation (IDF) consensus. The IDF 2005 attestation contains essentially the same standards but in a distinct order, the mandatory element being central obesity, expressed by abdominal circumference (Malin et al. 2022). When the four distinct attestations were consumed in the same communities, the IDF standards led to higher prevalence than the other three, which yielded almost identical prevalence.

8.9.3 Obesity, Adipose Tissue Distribution and the Metabolic Syndrome

Epidemiological studies have shown a clear association between obesity and mortality, due to the increased incidence of cerebrovascular CVD and diabetes. In moderate obesity, the regional distribution of adipose tissue appears to be an important determinant of cardiovascular and metabolic alteration, as body mass index (BMI) correlates inconsistently with these changes. Over the past 20 years, studies have proven that obesity is not a homogeneous condition and that the regional distribution of adipose tissue is important for understanding the relationship between obesity and disorders of lipid and carbohydrate metabolism. Numerous prospective studies have revealed the fact that excess fat in the upper part of the body (e.g., central or abdominal), considered "male obesity of the android type", correlates more frequently with increased mortality and the possibility of diabetes, dyslipidemia, hypertension arterial and atherosclerosis of the coronary, cerebral and peripheral vessels, than with the "gynoid" type (fat deposit in the lower part of the body and at gluteo-femoral level). (Ivanov et al. 2022).

In these studies, fat distribution was assessed by anthropometric measurements such as skinfold and waist-to-hip ratio (abdominal–buttock index). Although measuring the abdominal–buttock index is a simple and convenient method for epidemiological studies and provides a good estimate

TABLE 8.3
EBcs with a Beneficial Consequence in the Metabolic Syndrome

BCs	Food sources	Physiological consequences
Fatty acids (FA)		
monounsaturated FA (MUFA): oleic acid omega-6; polyunsaturated FA (PUFAs): linoleic acid	olive oil, oil of sunflower, rapeseed oil, nuts, olives, avocado, corn, saffron, sunflower oil	mild hypocholesterolemic consequences, possible lowering of LDL ox, supplementary non-lipid consequences
omega-3 polyunsaturated FA (PUFAs): α-$C_{18}H_{30}O_2$	rapeseed oil, soybean oil, walnuts, hazelnuts	mild hypocholesterolemic consequences, lowering LDL production, adverse consequences on cytokines
Flavonoids		
Flavonols: quercetin Kaempherol, myricetin	apples, onions, broccoli, cabbage, cherries, berries, green tea, red wine	mild hypocholesterolemic consequences, TG lowering, supplementary antiarrhythmic and antithrombotic consequence
Flavanols: catechins	green and black tea, red wine, apples, chocolate, cocoa	mild hypocholesterolemic consequences; antioxidant consequence, prevents the accumulation of LDL ox
Flavanones: naringenin, hesperetin	oranges, grapefruit	mild hypocholesterolemic consequences
Anthocyanins	red wine, berries, cherries	anti-inflammatory consequence, reduction of platelet aggregation
Isoflavones: genistein, daidzein	soy and soy bio-compounds	–
Antioxidant vitamins		
α–tocoferol (viamina E)	vegetable oils, seeds	–
acid ascorbic (vitamina C)	fruits, vegetables	weak estrogenic activity; improving endothelial dysfunction
Carotenoizi		
β – carotene	green vegetables, fruits	experimentally inhibits lipid peroxidation, controversial results in human studies; antioxidant consequence, prevents the accumulation of LDL ox, anti-inflammatory consequence, controversial results in human studies
Lycopene	tomato, watermelon	antioxidant consequence, inhibits lipid peroxidation, cardiovascular protective consequence
Lutein	green vegetables, fruits	antioxidant consequence, inhibits lipid peroxidation, cardiovascular protective consequence; requires confirmation
BCs with sulfur		
Allicin [$C_6H_{10}OS_2$], S-allylcysteine, S-methylcysteine	garlic and preparations	slightly hypocholesterolemic consequences proven in limited experimental and human studies, to be confirmed in trials, inhibition of hepatic cholesterol synthesis, antioxidant consequence, hypotensive, inhibition of platelet aggregation
Dietary fibre		
Psyllium, pectins, guar gum, hemicellulose	cereals, vegetables	slightly well-documented hypocholesterolemic consequences, increase in LDL clearance, bile sequestrant consequence, hypotensive, anti-inflammatory
Proteins		
Vegetable proteins	vegetable proteins, soya, vegetables	hypocholesterolemic consequences, unclear mechanism, difficult to separate from the consequence of isoflavones
Plant stanols and sterols (phytosterols)		
Sitosterol, campesterol, sitostanol, campestanol	pine oil, soybean oil, seeds, nuts (macadamia), margarines enriched with $C_{17}H_{28}O$/stanols	well-documented hypocholesterolemic consequences due to inhibition of cholesterol absorption

of the distribution of adipose tissue in the upper body, it cannot distinguish between visceral and subcutaneous fat. Imaging techniques, especially computed tomography (CT), make a clear distinction between adipose tissue and other categories of tissue and allow measurement of visceral abdominal fat (the area of visceral fat) and subcutaneous fat.

Numerous studies have shown that the alteration of metabolic processes is mediated by intra-abdominal fat storage (Chiou et al. 2022).

For example, the area of visceral fat correlated with glucose intolerance determined by OGTT in the presence of hyperinsulinemia suggests insulin resistance. The consequence of abdominal visceral adipose tissue accumulation on glucose tolerance is independent of total adiposity. If the visceral fat area is restored to normal, there is no extended any association between obesity and glucose tolerance. In addition to influencing glucose-insulin homeostasis, abdominal obesity has been associated with changes in the plasma levels of lipids and lipoproteins, especially with an increase in plasma triglycerides and a decrease in the concentration of HDL-cholesterol, due to the association of insulin resistance with changes in the transport of plasma lipids and the level of lipoproteins.

Although the cause-consequence relationship has not yet been well established, it appears that visceral fat represents an important link between the constituents of the metabolic syndrome: glucose intolerance, hypertension, dyslipidemia and insulin resistance (Sooriyaarachchi et al. 2022).

However, because significant metabolic heterogeneity persists in obese patients with almost identical excess visceral adipose tissue, it is hypothesized that genetic susceptibility plays a substantial role in modulating the possibility associated with excess visceral adipose tissue. In this regard, visceral obesity should be considered a factor that exacerbates the genetic susceptibility of constituents of the metabolic syndrome. Given the consensus regarding the correlation between visceral fat and cardiovascular possibility factors, especially dyslipidemia and hyperinsulinemia, the primary importance of visceral versus subcutaneous abdominal adipose tissue in insulin sensitivity has been disputed by some authors (Khosravipour et al. 2021).

Abdominal subcutaneous fat, as evidenced by magnetic resonance imaging and CT, was found to be at least as strongly correlated with insulin sensitivity as visceral fat.

8.9.4 Metabolic Syndrome and Cardiovascular Possibility

The presence of three or more MS standards increases the possibility of mortality from coronary heart sickness, CVD or any other cause. Review of data from 6,255 patients who participated in the US National Well-being and Nutrition Examination Survey NHANES 2 from 1976–1980 with cause-of-death analysis documented over the past 13 years has proven that MS patients without diabetes had had a 65% higher mortality possibility than those without MS, diabetes or coronary heart sickness. Those with diabetes had a 2.9 times higher possibility; those with coronary heart sickness, 4.2 times higher; and those with diabetes combined with coronary sickness, 6.5 times higher. The difference between the prevalence of MS and its associations with the prevalence of coronary heart sickness by ethnicity and gender was determined.

Participants (aged 40–69) were 2,346 Europeans (76% male), 1,711 South Asians (83% male) and 803 African–Caribbeans (57% male), all London residents. Metabolic syndrome was determined according to WHO and NCEP standards. The diagnosis of coronary artery sickness was made based on history and ECG changes. Anthropometric measurements and biochemical determinations were made from fasting blood and a sample of urine collected/24 h. The highest prevalence of MS was present in South Asians (WHO, men 46%, women 31%; NCEP, men 29 %, women 32%) and the lowest in European women (WHO, 9%; NCEP, 14%). The prevalence of coronary heart sickness was 10% in South Asian men, 9% in European men, 5–6% in Afro–Caribbean and European women and 2% in South Asian women. MS has been associated with coronary heart sickness prevalence in European and South Asian men.

The association with coronary heart sickness was weaker in Afro-Caribbean women and non-significant in European women (Su & Zhang 2022).

The correlation between high prevalence of MS and high prevalence of coronary heart sickness was particularly significant. In another study, conducted by the Association of Silent Coronary Artery Disease and Metabolic Syndrome in Chinese Subjects with Type 2 Diabetes, diabetic patients who were already part of a possibility management program for coronary artery sickness were monitored. Diagnostic coronary angiography was performed to confirm the presence and severity of coronary artery sickness. Age, sex, duration of diabetes, serum uric acid level, smoking and presence of metabolic syndrome diagnosed according to WHO standards were significantly correlated with silent coronary artery sickness. All these studies demonstrate that MS is an important predictor of cardiovascular possibility. Estimation of total cardiovascular possibility is an extremely important measure that has appeared in cardiovascular obstruction guidelines since 1994. Their substantial objective is to decrease mortality and morbidity in subjects with absolute high possibility and to assist subjects with absolute low possibility to maintain it by promoting a healthy lifestyle. For the calculation of the total possibility, the SCORE RiskOGram was validated and is usually consumed and recommended by the European guideline for the obstruction of CVD, 2007 edition (European Society of Cardiology). The SCORE possibility assessment system estimates the possibility for a first fatal cardiovascular event at ten years – acute myocardial infarction, stroke, aortic aneurysm or others – unlike other systems that only assess coronary possibility. The choice of cardiovascular mortality to define the possibility allows the country data to be recalibrated in the sense of an overestimation in countries where mortality has decreased and an underestimation in countries where it has increased. The SCORE possibility chart estimates the possibility of a fatal coronary event at ten years, depending on sex, smoking, age, total cholesterol or the total cholesterol/HDL cholesterol ratio (Chieng & Kistler 2022). The low-possibility risk chart is consumed in countries with low mortality; for example, Belgium, France, Greece, Italy, Luxembourg, Spain, Portugal and Switzerland. All other countries use the high-possibility risk chart. According to the recommendations of the European Guidelines, the management of the patient with MS and cardiovascular possibility involves non-pharmacological measures of lifestyle change that include weight control, diet, physical exercise and pharmacological measures.

8.9.5 Nutrition in the Metabolic Syndrome

The role of nutrition in the etiology and obstruction of CVD, implicitly the metabolic syndrome, is documented by the causal correlations between the consumption of saturated fats, overweightness or obesity, lipidogram alterations and the increased incidence of CVD. In nutritional studies, the decrease in fat intake is usually associated with a relative or absolute increase in carbohydrate intake. In these conditions, a decrease in the level of LDL and HDL cholesterol and an increase in the concentration of triglycerides are observed. The decrease in HDL is mitigated when the patient loses weight or when carbohydrates are derived from high-fibre foods.

Weight loss in MS is recommended because overweightness or obesity is associated with increased absolute cardiovascular possibility, in part by increasing blood pressure and lowering HDL cholesterol but also by increasing the incidence of newly diagnosed diabetes. Weight loss is mandatory for obese people with BMI $\geq$ 30 kg/m^2 and recommended for overweight people with BMI $\geq$ 25 kg/m^2 and < 30 kg/m^2. Men with a waist circumference between 94–102 cm and women with a waist circumference between 80–88 cm should be advised not to gain weight, and for values above these, weight loss is recommended. Body weight control can be achieved through caloric restriction and regular exercise three times a week, which are thought to ameliorate lipid metabolism. General dietary recommendations include the consumption of a wide diversity of foods with an energy intake adjusted to daily needs, which sums up the basal metabolic rate and a series of calories added, depending on the physical effort performed and the type of work performed, calculated in calories/kg body according to the tables.

The daily food ration should contain fruits, vegetables, whole grains and bread, fish, lean meat and low-fat dairy bio-compounds. The total amount of lipids must represent less than 30% of the total, of which less than a third can be saturated, the rest being represented by monounsaturated and polyunsaturated fats from vegetable and marine sources. Salt intake should be decreased in the case of associated hypertension by avoiding the addition of salt in food preparation and by choosing fresh or frozen foods and avoiding canned foods high in NaCl (Muñoz et al. 2022).

The beneficial consequences of many EBcs can be consumed for therapeutic purposes so that the boundary at which a food component becomes a drug is not well determined. Moreover, the relationship between EBcs and the hypolipidemic drug curative meaning recommended in MS has at least two dimensions: first, both the pharmaceutical agent and the food component can have cholesterol-lowering consequences, so their combined consequence can be an example of a synergistic interaction of the type primary. Second, nutritional factors can interfere with the consequences of lipid-lowering medication by influencing its metabolism or the regulatory pathways necessary for their action, causing synergistic or antagonistic consequences – secondary interaction.

8.9.6 NATURAL FOOD CONSTITUENTS WITH LIPID-LOWERING AND CARDIOPROTECTIVE PROPERTIES WITH A BENEFICIAL CONSEQUENCE IN METABOLIC SYNDROME

Current research considering the description and characterization of natural EBcs with lipid-lowering and cardioprotective properties is extremely dynamic and full of controversy.

Dietary constituents with proven lipid-lowering properties are listed in Table 8.3, but often, their beneficial action on cardiovascular possibility reduction is multiple and involves physiological pathways unrelated to lipid transport or metabolism (Mathis, Tanaka, & Hiramatsu 2022).

Many natural bio-compounds contain complex integrations of BCs that act simultaneously through interdependent mechanisms, so the comprehensive analysis of such a complicated situation is difficult and presents the possibility of simplistic or erroneous conclusions. However, several categories of substantial nutritional factors can be readily identified.

8.10 CONCLUSIONS AND RECOMMENDATIONS

Numerous studies have proven an inverse correlation between flavonoid intake and cardiovascular possibility, while others have detected no consequence. Although the lipid-lowering consequences of isolated flavonoids are being researched, the specific action of each BCs present in natural foods is impossible at the current level of knowledge. Attempts to find a simple solution to this problem are illustrated by the use of antioxidant vitamin supplements in cardiovascular obstruction. Epidemiological and experimental studies have suggested that daily intake of antioxidant vitamins E, C and beta-carotene may be associated with decreased cardiovascular possibility. The idea has been applied in numerous controlled trials investigating the consequence of antioxidant vitamin supplements on cardiovascular possibility.

The results of these studies were negative and concluded that there is no evidence to recommend antioxidant supplements in the obstruction of coronary heart sickness. Controversies also persist regarding the use of garlic as a lipid-lowering and cardioprotective agent. Garlic preparations and supplements on the market have variable amounts of allicin – considered the main substance responsible for the bioactivity of garlic, making it difficult to conclude concerning their effectiveness as lipid-lowering agents. Two recent meta-analyses have shown that garlic preparations, in amounts roughly equal to the equivalent of half to one clove of garlic per day, lower total cholesterol and LDL-cholesterol by concerning 10% in subjects with elevated plasma levels. The results of many studies have been conflicting, even though they consumed the same type of garlic powder, in the same amounts. Although there is evidence that garlic can lower LDL-cholesterol, the cholesterol-lowering consequence appears to be limited to certain compounds in garlic. The beneficial consequences of antioxidant diets rich in fruits and vegetables and bio-compounds derived from these sources are evident and are widely recommended for reducing cardiovascular possibility. It seems that the diet rich in natural bio-compounds containing various antioxidants that act synergistically can be much more effective for cardioprotection than the action of isolated supplements.

The mild cholesterol-lowering consequence of soluble dietary fibre is well documented, although its mechanisms are not clear and may be due to other constituents in grains and vegetables. Increased fibre consumption, especially from whole grains, is part of the Western nutritional strategy in cardiovascular obstruction. The amount of protein in the diet is closely related to the issue of fat intake. Substituting soy for animal protein resulted in lower LDL and triglycerides, although this consequence may be due to the impact of soy isoflavones.

The configuration of food is much more important than the type of protein in the diet for ensuring serum lipid balance. It has been suggested that consumption of animal protein itself is not harmful, unless it is associated with increased intake of saturated fat.

To avoid this unhealthy association, the source of protein in the diet can be replaced with nuts, soy, vegetables, chicken and fish. Using the lipid-lowering properties of plant sterols and stanols by inhibiting intestinal cholesterol absorption is an attractive strategy to correct the lipid profile, especially in moderate hypercholesterolemia. New polyunsaturated margarines enriched with sterols and stanols have been introduced, but their extended-term consequence is not fully known, especially that of inhibiting the absorption of fat-soluble vitamins.

Caution is advised in their use. Moderate alcohol consumption decreases cardiovascular possibility. This association, which can be partially explained by alcohol's ability to raise HDL cholesterol, occurs not just with a particular alcoholic drink but with the action of alcohol itself. The foregoing EBcs are widely consumed in the prescription of cardioprotective diets for patients in cardiovascular obstruction and metabolic syndrome.

Research into new, natural constituents with hypolipidemic properties is ongoing – e.g., policosanol, a mixture of alcohols isolated from sugar cane, guggulipids (extracted from *Commiphora mucul*) or red yeast rice (rice fermented with *Monascus ruber* yeast) are in the testing phase. The analysis of these constituents demonstrates that the expected consequence is average and that, for a marked consequence, it is necessary to combine it with lipid-lowering medication. A beneficial alternative to these researches is the concern for the development of FFs and NTs, which, through the synergistic activity of the bioconstituents and through the design oriented to obtain the consequences, can offer a wide range of action in the reversibility of the metabolic syndrome and in cardiovascular obstruction.

REFERENCES

Asfha, D., Mishra, T., & Vuppu, S. 2022. Teff grain-based functional food for prevention of osteoporosis: Sensory evaluation and molecular docking approach. *Plant Foods for Human Nutrition (Dordrecht, Netherlands)*, 10.1007/s11130–022–01012-y. Advance online publication. https://doi.org/10.1007/s11130-022-01012-y

Beheshtizadeh, N., Gharibshahian, M., Pazhouhnia, Z., Rostami, M., Zangi, A. R., Maleki, R., Azar, H. K., Zalouli, V., Rajavand, H., Farzin, A., Lotfibakhshaiesh, N., Sefat, F., Azami, M., Webster, T. J., & Rezaei, N. 2022. Commercialization and regulation of regenerative medicine products: Promises, advances and challenges. *Biomedicine & Pharmacotherapy = Biomedecine & Pharmacotherapie*, 153, 113431. https://doi.org/10.1016/j.biopha.2022.113431

Berger, A., & Thorn, E. 2022. Can low-carbohydrate diets be recommended for reducing cardiovascular risk? *Current Opinion in Endocrinology, Diabetes, and Obesity*, 29(5), 413–419. https://doi.org/10.1097/MED.0000000000000750

Cao, S. Y., Zhao, C. N., Gan, R. Y., Xu, X. Y., Wei, X. L., Corke, H., Atanasov, A. G., & Li, H. B. 2019. Effects and mechanisms of tea and its bioactive compounds for the prevention and treatment of cardiovascular diseases: An updated review. *Antioxidants (Basel, Switzerland)*, 8(6), 166. https://doi.org/10.3390/antiox8060166

Chieng, D., & Kistler, P. M. 2022. Coffee and tea on cardiovascular disease (CVD) prevention. *Trends in Cardiovascular Medicine*, 32(7), 399–405. https://doi.org/10.1016/j.tcm.2021.08.004

Chiou, W. C., Lai, W. H., Cai, Y. L., Du, M. L., Lai, H. M., Chen, J. C., Huang, H. C., Liu, H. K., & Huang, C. 2022. Gut microbiota-directed intervention with high-amylose maize ameliorates metabolic dysfunction in diet-induced obese mice. *Food & Function*, *13*(18), 9481–9495. https://doi.org/10.1039/d2fo01211a

Dai, Y., Quan, J., Xiong, L., Luo, Y., & Yi, B. 2022. Probiotics improve renal function, glucose, lipids, inflammation and oxidative stress in diabetic kidney disease: A systematic review and meta-analysis. *Renal Failure*, *44*(1), 862–880. https://doi.org/10.1080/0886022X.2022.2079522

Fan, Z., Jia, W., Du, A., Xia, Z., Kang, J., Xue, L., Sun, Y., & Shi, L. 2022. Discovery of Se-containing flavone in Se-enriched green tea and the potential application value in the immune regulation. *Food Chemistry*, *394*, 133468. https://doi.org/10.1016/j.foodchem.2022.133468

Fathy, H. M., Abd El-Maksoud, A. A., Cheng, W., & Elshaghabee, F. 2022. Value-added utilization of citrus peels in improving functional properties and probiotic viability of *Acidophilus-bifidus-thermophilus* (ABT)-type synbiotic yoghurt during cold storage. *Foods (Basel, Switzerland)*, *11*(17), 2677. https://doi.org/10.3390/foods11172677

Flórez-Martínez, D. H., Contreras-Pedraza, C. A., Escobar-Parra, S., & Rodríguez-Cortina, J. 2022. Key drivers for non-centrifugal sugar cane research, technological development, and market linkage: A technological roadmap approach for Colombia. *Sugar Tech: An International Journal of Sugar Crops & Related Industries*, 1–13. Advance online publication. https://doi.org/10.1007/s12355-022-01200-9

Gomes, S., Teixeira-Guedes, C., Silva, E., Baltazar, F., & Preto, A. 2022. Colon microbiota modulation by dairy-derived diet: New strategy for prevention and treatment of colorectal cancer. *Food & Function*, *13*(18), 9183–9194. https://doi.org/10.1039/d2fo01720b

Hadjimbei, E., Botsaris, G., & Chrysostomou, S. 2022. Beneficial effects of yoghurts and probiotic fermented milks and their functional food potential. *Foods (Basel, Switzerland)*, *11*(17), 2691. https://doi.org/10.3390/foods11172691

Ivanov, S. V., Ostrovskaya, R. U., Koliasnikova, K. N., Alchinova, I. B., Demorzhi, M. S., Gudasheva, T. A., & Seredenin, S. B. 2022. Low molecular weight NGF mimetic GK-2 normalizes the parameters of glucose and lipid metabolism and exhibits a hepatoprotective effect on a prediabetes model in obese Wistar rats. *Clinical and Experimental Pharmacology & Physiology*, *49*(10), 1116–1125. https://doi.org/10.1111/1440-1681.13693

Khosravipour, M., Khanlari, P., Khazaie, S., Khosravipour, H., & Khazaie, H. 2021. A systematic review and meta-analysis of the association between shift work and metabolic syndrome: The roles of sleep, gender, and type of shift work. *Sleep Medicine Reviews*, *57*, 101427. https://doi.org/10.1016/j.smrv.2021.101427

Kose, J., Paz Graniel, I., Péneau, S., Julia, C., Hercberg, S., Galan, P., Touvier, M., & Andreeva, V. A. 2022. A population-based study of macronutrient intake according to mental health status with a focus on pure and comorbid anxiety and eating disorders. *European Journal of Nutrition*, *61*(7), 3685–3696. https://doi.org/10.1007/s00394-022-02923-x

Malin, S. K., Remchak, M. E., Smith, A. J., Ragland, T. J., Heiston, E. M., & Cheema, U. 2022. Early chronotype with metabolic syndrome favours resting and exercise fat oxidation in relation to insulin-stimulated non-oxidative glucose disposal. *Experimental Physiology*, 10.1113/EP090613. Advance online publication. https://doi.org/10.1113/EP090613

Mata-Fernández, A., Hershey, M. S., Pastrana-Delgado, J. C., Sotos-Prieto, M., Ruiz-Canela, M., Kales, S. N., Martínez-González, M. A., & Fernandez-Montero, A. 2021. A Mediterranean lifestyle reduces the risk of cardiovascular disease in the "Seguimiento Universidad de Navarra" (SUN) cohort. *Nutrition, Metabolism, and Cardiovascular Diseases: NMCD*, *31*(6), 1728–1737. https://doi.org/10.1016/j.numecd.2021.02.022

Mathis, B. J., Tanaka, K., & Hiramatsu, Y. 2022. Factors of obesity and metabolically healthy obesity in Asia. *Medicina (Kaunas, Lithuania)*, *58*(9), 1271. https://doi.org/10.3390/medicina58091271

Muñoz, S. E., Díaz, M., Reartes, G. A., Aballay, L. R., Niclis, C., Román, M. D., Coquet, J. B., Carrillo, M., & Canale, M. G. 2022. The "diet model" and metabolic syndrome components: Results from the Cordoba Health and Dietary Habits Investigation. *Nutrition (Burbank, Los Angeles County, Calif.)*, *102*, 111739. https://doi.org/10.1016/j.nut.2022.111739

Oda, M., Fujibayashi, K., Wakasa, M., Takano, S., Fujita, W., Kitayama, M., Nakanishi, H., Saito, K., Kawai, Y., & Kajinami, K. 2022. Increased plasma glutamate in non-smokers with vasospastic angina pectoris is associated with plasma cystine and antioxidant capacity. *Scandinavian Cardiovascular Journal: SCJ*, *56*(1), 180–186. https://doi.org/10.1080/14017431.2022.2085884

Ojueromi, O. O., Oboh, G., & Ademosun, A. O. 2022. Black Seed (*Nigella sativa*): A favourable alternative therapy for inflammatory and immune system disorders. *Inflammopharmacology*, *30*(5), 1623–1643. https://doi.org/10.1007/s10787-022-01035-6

Rabail, R., Sultan, M. T., Khalid, A. R., Sahar, A. T., Zia, S., Kowalczewski, P. Ł., Jeżowski, P., Shabbir, M. A., & Aadil, R. M. 2022. Clinical, nutritional, and functional evaluation of chia seed-fortified muffins. *Molecules (Basel, Switzerland)*, *27*(18), 5907. https://doi.org/10.3390/molecules27185907

Rychter, A. M., Hryhorowicz, S., Słomski, R., Dobrowolska, A., & Krela-Kaźmierczak, I. 2022. Antioxidant effects of vitamin E and risk of cardiovascular disease in women with obesity – A narrative review. *Clinical Nutrition (Edinburgh, Scotland)*, *41*(7), 1557–1565. https://doi.org/10.1016/j.clnu.2022.04.032

Seenak, P., Kumphune, S., Malakul, W., Chotima, R., & Nernpermpisooth, N. 2021. Pineapple consumption reduced cardiac oxidative stress and inflammation in high cholesterol diet-fed rats. *Nutrition & Metabolism*, *18*(1), 36. https://doi.org/10.1186/s12986-021-00566-z

Sharma, P., Gupta, V., Kumar, K., & Khetarpal, P. 2022. Assessment of serum elements concentration and polycystic ovary syndrome (PCOS): Systematic review and meta-analysis. *Biological Trace Element Research*, *200*(11), 4582–4593. https://doi.org/10.1007/s12011-021-03058-6

Sooriyaarachchi, P., Jayawardena, R., Pavey, T., & King, N. A. 2022. Shift work and the risk for metabolic syndrome among healthcare workers: A systematic review and meta-analysis. *Obesity Reviews: An Official Journal of the International Association for the Study of Obesity*, *23*(10), e13489. https://doi.org/10.1111/obr.13489

Su, Y., & Zhang, X. 2022. Association of metabolic syndrome with adverse outcomes in patients with stable coronary artery disease: A meta-analysis. *Hormone and Metabolic Research = Hormon- und Stoffwechselforschung = Hormones et metabolisme*, 10.1055/a-1946–4823. Advance online publication. https://doi.org/10.1055/a-1946-4823

Tabrizi, R., Ostadmohammadi, V., Akbari, M., Lankarani, K. B., Vakili, S., Peymani, P., Karamali, M., Kolahdooz, F., & Asemi, Z. 2022. The effects of probiotic supplementation on clinical symptom, weight loss, glycemic control, lipid and hormonal profiles, biomarkers of inflammation, and oxidative stress in women with polycystic ovary syndrome: A systematic review and meta-analysis of randomized controlled trials. *Probiotics and Antimicrobial Proteins*, *14*(1), 1–14. https://doi.org/10.1007/s12602-019-09559-0

Teimouri, M., Homayouni-Tabrizi, M., Rajabian, A., Amiri, H., & Hosseini, H. 2022. Anti-inflammatory effects of resveratrol in patients with cardiovascular disease: A systematic review and meta-analysis of randomized controlled trials. *Complementary Therapies in Medicine*, *70*, 102863. https://doi.org/10.1016/j.ctim.2022.102863

Unterberger, S., Aschauer, R., Zöhrer, P. A., Draxler, A., Franzke, B., Strasser, E. M., Wagner, K. H., & Wessner, B. 2022. Effects of an increased habitual dietary protein intake followed by resistance training on fitness, muscle quality and body composition of seniors: A randomised controlled trial. *Clinical Nutrition (Edinburgh, Scotland)*, *41*(5), 1034–1045. https://doi.org/10.1016/j.clnu.2022.02.017

Vanegas, P., Zazpe, I., Santiago, S., Fernandez-Lazaro, C. I., de la O, V., & Martínez-González, M. Á. 2022. Macronutrient quality index and cardiovascular disease risk in the Seguimiento Universidad de Navarra (SUN) cohort. *European Journal of Nutrition*, *61*(7), 3517–3530. https://doi.org/10.1007/s00394-022-02901-3

Wagner, L., Veit, R., Fritsche, L., Häring, H. U., Fritsche, A., Birkenfeld, A. L., Heni, M., Preissl, H., & Kullmann, S. 2022. Sex differences in central insulin action: Effect of intranasal insulin on neural food cue reactivity in adults with normal weight and overweight. *International Journal of Obesity (2005)*, *46*(9), 1662–1670. https://doi.org/10.1038/s41366-022-01167-3

Wang, S., Du, Q., Meng, X., & Zhang, Y. 2022. Natural polyphenols: A potential prevention and treatment strategy for metabolic syndrome. *Food & Function*, 10.1039/d2fo01552h. Advance online publication. https://doi.org/10.1039/d2fo01552h

Xian, C., Lai, D., Liu, J., Li, S., Cao, J., Chen, K., Liang, D., Fu, N., Wang, Y., & Xiao, M. 2022. Protein-enriched extracts from housefly (*Musca domestica*) maggots alleviates atherosclerosis in apolipoprotein E-deficient mice by promoting bile acid production and consequent cholesterol consumption. *Archives of insect Biochemistry and Physiology*, *111*(2), e21951. https://doi.org/10.1002/arch.21951

You, H., Abraham, E. J., Mulligan, J., Zhou, Y., Montoya, M., Willig, J., Chen, B. K., Wang, C. K., Wang, L. S., Dong, A., Shamtsyan, M., Nguyen, H., Wong, A., & Wallace, T. C. 2022. Label compliance for ingredient verification: Regulations, approaches, and trends for testing botanical products marketed for "immune health" in the United States. *Critical Reviews in Food Science and Nutrition*, 1–20. Advance online publication. https://doi.org/10.1080/10408398.2022.2124230

Zahoor, H., Watchaputi, K., Hata, J., Pabuprapap, W., Suksamrarn, A., Chua, L. S., & Soontorngun, N. 2022. Model yeast as a versatile tool to examine the antioxidant and anti-ageing potential of flavonoids, extracted from medicinal plants. *Frontiers in Pharmacology*, *13*, 980066. https://doi.org/10.3389/fphar.2022.980066

Zazpe, I., Santiago, S., Gea, A., Ruiz-Canela, M., Carlos, S., Bes-Rastrollo, M., & Martínez-González, M. A. 2016. Association between a dietary carbohydrate index and cardiovascular disease in the SUN (Seguimiento Universidad de Navarra) Project. *Nutrition, Metabolism, and Cardiovascular Diseases: NMCD, 26*(11), 1048–1056. https://doi.org/10.1016/j.numecd.2016.07.002

Zengin, M., Sur, A., İlhan, Z., Azman, M. A., Tavşanlı, H., Esen, S., Bacaksız, O. K., & Demir, E. 2022. Effects of fermented distillers grains with solubles, partially replaced with soybean meal, on performance, blood parameters, meat quality, intestinal flora, and immune response in broiler. *Research in Veterinary Science, 150*, 58–64. https://doi.org/10.1016/j.rvsc.2022.06.027

Zhang, J., Chai, X., Zhao, F., Hou, G., & Meng, Q. 2022. Food Applications and potential health benefits of hawthorn. *Foods (Basel, Switzerland), 11*(18), 2861. https://doi.org/10.3390/foods11182861

Zhao, C. N., Meng, X., Li, Y., Li, S., Liu, Q., Tang, G. Y., & Li, H. B. 2017. Fruits for prevention and treatment of cardiovascular diseases. *Nutrients, 9*(6), 598. https://doi.org/10.3390/nu9060598

Zheng, Z., Li, J., Chen, Y., Sun, H., & Liu, Y. 2022. Preparation and characterization of lipophilic antioxidative peptides derived from mung bean protein. *Food Chemistry, 395*, 133535. https://doi.org/10.1016/j.foodchem.2022.133535

Zuraini, N., Sekar, M., Wu, Y. S., Gan, S. H., Bonam, S. R., Mat Rani, N., Begum, M. Y., Lum, P. T., Subramaniyan, V., Fuloria, N. K., & Fuloria, S. 2021. Promising nutritional fruits against cardiovascular diseases: An overview of experimental evidence and understanding their mechanisms of action. *Vascular Health and Risk Management, 17*, 739–769. https://doi.org/10.2147/VHRM.S328096

9 Plant-Based Short and Cyclo-Peptides

Ebenezer I. O. Ajayi, Olorunfemi R. Molehin, Adeniyi S. Ohunayo, Aderonke E. Fakayode, Abraham Nkumah, Olabimpe Olayinka, and Alaba A. Adebayo

9.1 INTRODUCTION

Plant-based peptides (PBP) have been previewed to be one of the reservoirs of natural therapy, and as such, attentions have been focused on exploration of these groundbreaking proteins. Drug development and testing originating from natural products such as plants are currently gaining tremendous attention because of their pharmacological and cytopathological potential coupled with their little or no side effects. In many instances, PBP such as short and cyclic peptides have been studied to have delivery potential because of their great stability, despite their short structures. The scientific discovery of PBPs have opened up many other plant-based compounds with a view to determining their potential for drug discovery and delivery from natural products-based proteins and their bioavailability in primary and secondary metabolites (Attah et al., 2016). Peptides are structurally composed of a minimum of two and above types of amino acids; in that regard, oligopeptides are mostly termed a short peptide because of their short chains of amino acids, while a long chain of amino acids are called polypeptide; regardless, there are not too many differentiating entities or borderlines to describe or give a better understanding of them other than their weight, atomic mass and, most importantly, sizes of protein, peptides, oligopeptides and polypeptides. However, according to the biological dictionary, proteins composed of two to 40 amino acids are termed oligopeptides, while, on the other hand, International Union of Pure and Applied Chemistry (IUPAC) stipulates that polypeptide are composed of 50 or more of such amino acids (Schmidt et al., 2011).

Peptides are an exceptional group of bio-molecules that have presented much potential in pharmacology and pharmacodynamics due to their well-defined biological and cytopathological features. Their discovery has shown how important the small chemical molecules can be to biological systems because of their atomic mass and weight. Plant-based peptides possess the transitional nature encompassing "beyond size", having major advantages for being small compounds such as penetrability and highly potent proteins, which includes selective toxicity and target potentials while excluding their drawbacks of similar molecules; such drawbacks, observed in similar molecules, may include the following: side effects, drug to drug compatibility and impermeability of the membrane. Hence, short and cyclic peptides of plant origin are increasingly gaining attention as an important and promising platform of many diverse applications either in diagnosis or therapies (Fosgerau and Hoffmann, 2015).

Disulfide-rich cyclopeptides originating or sourced from natural products are structurally composed of 30 amino acids with a configuration of a head-to-tail cyclized backbone serving as a basic structure and then a knotted prearrangement of its three disulfide bonds. Plant-based peptides are naturally occurring but not available in all plants; their bioavailability is found in few plants but wide among the plant tissues such as bark, seeds, leaves, roots, flowers and stems. Before their medicinal exploration, they are known to be part of a plant's innate defensive apparatus, highly potent against pests (flies) and nematodes. For this purpose, they can be regarded as innate toxins of plants, hence becoming very toxic to certain plant pests such as insects. Nevertheless, interest

DOI: 10.1201/9781003361497-10

in cyclotides has been aided by their incomparable firmness and their being a possible tool in drug development and designs (Fosgerau and Hoffmann, 2015).

Short and cyclic peptides have many advantages when compared to large peptides. Some of the advantages include their flexibility to be synthesized on large or small scale, chemical variabilities, cost of processing, easy of structural modifications, biocompatibility, selective toxicities and safety, all as a result of composition of harmless amino acids and the very little likelihood for buildup in tissues through biomagnification (Soudy et al., 2019). In general, peptides are multifunctional, having high binding affinities and potential for a wide range of biological targets; however, limitations of short peptides cannot be underemphasized, as they are found to lack some of selectivity for receptors; some ease of its flexibility could be a problem. Other disadvantages of short peptides may include permeabilities, susceptibilities to proteolytic enzymes present in the biological systems and their activities might be reduced following the metabolism (Haggag et al., 2018)

9.2   DISCOVERY OF CYCLOPEPTIDES

The first cyclopeptide to be discovered was named kalata B1; these short sequences of amino acids drew the attention of Lorents Gran, who was servicing on a Red Cross mission within the African communities – more precisely, DR Congo during the early 1960s (Figure 9.1). During his mission, he observed that Congolese women were given concoctions of leaves of *Oldenlandia affinis*; after being boiled, the concoctions were taken as tea by women in labor, when he noticed that, following ingestion of these leaves, the labor process was accelerated, with reduced pain. Those were the reasons why the Norwegian physicians took some of the plant materials for study and characterization. Interestingly, Lorents Gran discovered that the uterotonic potential was as a result of peptides; after characterization, the peptides were found to be composed of 30 amino acids (Gran, 1973). Structural representation for the first cyclo-peptide remained impossible until the middle of 1990s, long after NMR and mass spectrophotometry were available to analyze cyclic ang-knotted plan of its disulfide links, respectively (Saether et al., 1995).

9.3   CLASSIFICATION OF PLANT-BASED PEPTIDES

Cyclopeptides were originally classified into two main plant subfamilies of short proteins; namely, the Mobius and the Bracelet; classification is structurally based on the occurrence or absence of

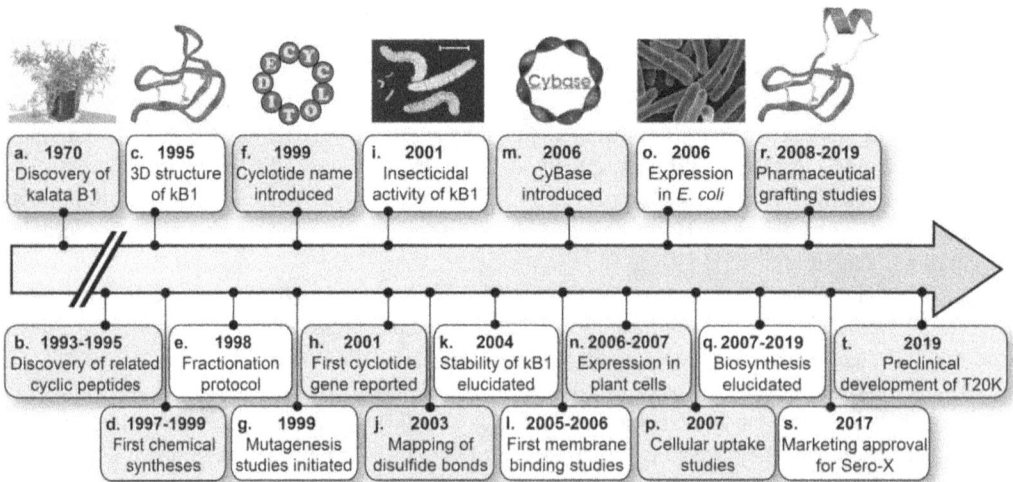

FIGURE 9.1   Timeline of cyclopeptide discovery (de Veer et al., 2019).

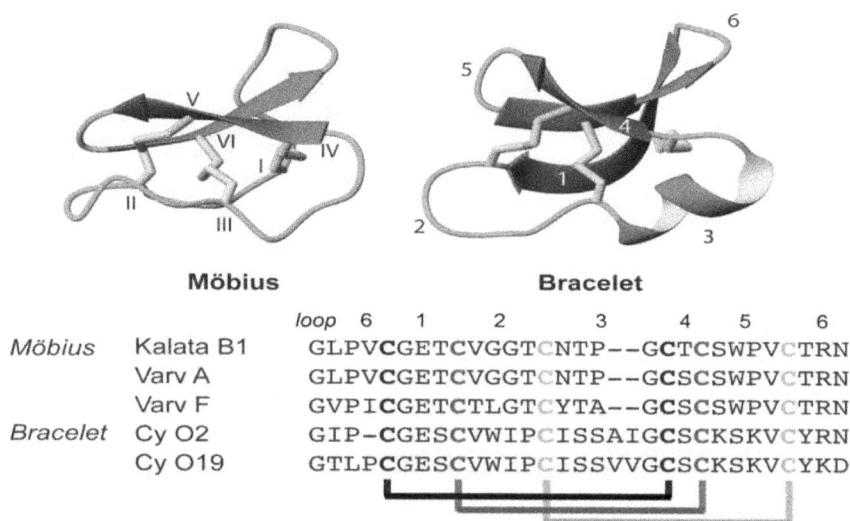

		loop 6	1	2	3	4	5	6
Möbius	Kalata B1	GLPVCGETCVGGTCNTP--GCTCSWPVCTRN
	Varv A	GLPVCGETCVGGTCNTP--GCSCSWPVCTRN
	Varv F	GVPICGETCTLGTCYTA--GCSCSWPVCTRN
Bracelet	Cy O2	GIP-CGESCVWIPCISSAIGCSCKSKVCYRN
	Cy O19	GTLPCGESCVWIPCISSVVGCSCKSKVCYKD

FIGURE 9.2 Sequences and 3-D structures of major subfamilies of cyclopeptides (Burman et al., 2010).

cis-proline in loop 5 of their circular backbone. The nomenclature originates from its peptide connections of the cyclopeptide that occur in its typical *trans* arrangement; the mainstay structures can assume the shape of a bracelet. Nevertheless, a 3-D molecular structure comprising a *cis*-proline results in a 180° intangible twist in the circular backbone, which can then be viewed as a Möbius strip (Jennings et al., 2001) (Figure 9.2). Aside from the first two subclass classification families, a third family of cyclopeptide was discovered; these peptides are thought to have been smaller than those earlier mentioned, and their discoveries were not possible until the discovery of MCoTI-one and MCoTI-two *Momordica cochinchinensis*. Both MCoTI-one and MCoTI-two have been discovered to be different from many other cyclopeptides when those sequencies were being compared, although all the cyclopeptides share almost the same structural compounds of three intertwined disulfide linkages with a cyclic backbone; these structural arrangements are mostly called the cyclic knottins (Hernandez et al., 2000; Chiche et al., 2004).

Cyclopeptides' availability in plants are gene coded; structurally, these protein structures are composed of N and C terminus joined by a peptide bond. The sequences of cyclopeptides are about 30-amino-acids long, while its unique structures force the peptide hydrophobic residues to be exposed on the surface of the protein, making them amphipathic proteins (Burman et al., 2010). In the foregoing figure, the two major cyclopeptide subfamilies were illustrated with examples. Kalata B1, which is the foremost cyclopeptide discovered, belongs to the Mobius subfamily; Cy O2 and O9 are abbreviated as cycloviolacin, both of which are typical examples of the Bracelet subfamily. Many other hundreds of cyclopeptides have been described but are classified into the major subfamilies (Figure 9.3); however, the subfamilies differ in number of amino acid content and also in size. Most cyclotides possess some residues in common, and while some residues are variable, there are quite a few amino acids in a cyclotide sequence and variations are immense (Burman et al., 2010).

9.4 DISTRIBUTION AND OCCURRENCE OF CYCLOPEPTIDES IN PLANTS

Cyclopeptides have been discovered in many plants, but they have been discovered to be restricted to five major families; namely, Violaceae, Cucurbitaceae, Fabaceae, Solanaceae and Rubiaceae families (Attah et al., 2016). Meanwhile, following the discovery of *Oldenlandia affinis* (the first cyclotide-containing plant), cyclotides have since been isolated in various plant species. Patterns of incidence have unraveled that violet (Violaceae) and coffee (Rubiaceae) families have the most

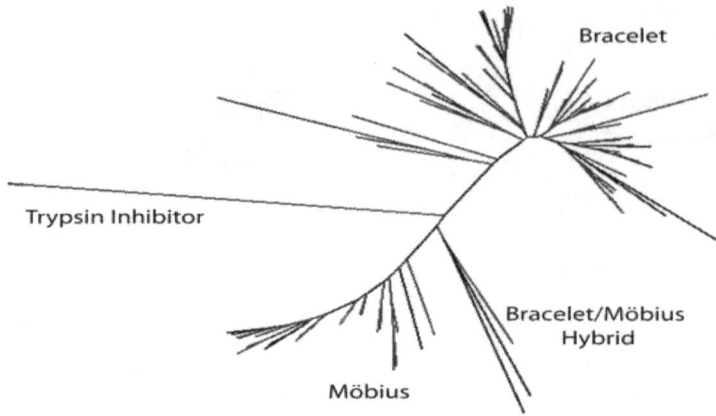

FIGURE 9.3 Clustering and sequence relatedness illustrating the subfamilies of cyclopeptides (Burman et al., 2010).

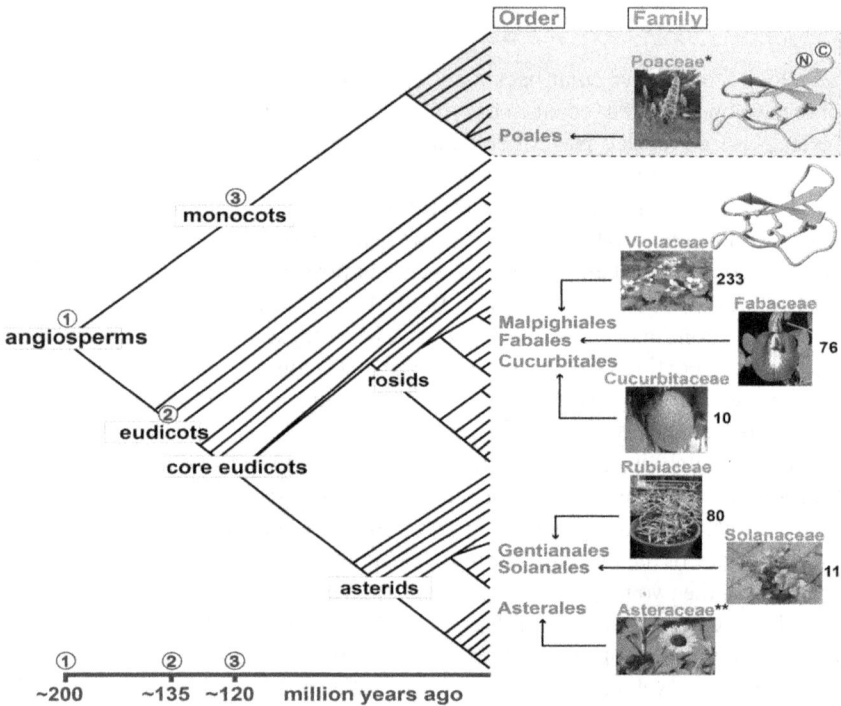

FIGURE 9.4 Cyclopeptide-bearing families (Burman et al., 2010).

described cyclotides (Burman et al., 2010). Plant family Violaceae has more than 900 known distinct species that are scattered within tropical and temperate regions of the world; their dispersion among the few identified plant families is tremendously variable. If not all, most of the Violaceous plant has been studied to contain cyclotides, which signifies that cyclotides are abundant within this family. On the contrary, only about 5% of the Rubiaceae family has been studied to have cyclopeptides. Aside from violet (Violaceae) and coffee (Rubiaceae), only a few members of the families earlier listed are composed of cyclopeptides (Figure 9.4).

The violet (Violaceae) and coffee (Rubiaceae) are phylogenetically distant from one another, but the predominant occurrence of cyclotides between them is remarkable. While the reason is yet unknown or studied, their distribution among violet (Violaceae), coffee (Rubiaceae) and other plant kingdoms are possibly broader than the current knowledge suggests. Screenings and other means of investigation are already in progress; the studies are aimed at finding cyclotides in other plant families. Other than the Violaceae and Rubiaceae, cyclopeptide-bearing plant and sequences have been recognized in cereal crops of Poaceae, such as rice, wheat and maize (Basse, 2005).

9.5   ISOLATIONS OF PLANT-BASED PEPTIDES

Methods of isolation of cyclopeptides have changed over time; extraction and characterization processes of plant-based peptides are time- and resource-consuming. Knowledge of scientific extraction has improved over the years regarding isolation of short cyclopeptides from plants. Until recently, pre-extraction with dichloromethane (DCM) was followed by extraction proper with 50% and 60% of aqueous ethanol and methanol (MeOH), respectively. The process is then subjected to liquid-liquid dichloromethane extraction where it will be filtered (Herrmann et al., 2008).

In recent research, isolation of cyclopeptides from plant material is done following drying and crushing of the desired plant. The powder obtained from the crushed plant will be treated with DCM and MeOH in a 1:1 ratio with continuous stirring at room temperature for 1 day. The solution will be filtered from solid particles, the liquid portion will be collected and 0.5 volume of double distilled water (dd H_2O) will be added to produce the liquid-liquid extraction phase aiding the separation of peptides from the organic phase. The extract will then be enriched by processing it through a solid-phase extraction (SPE) with octadecyl-modified silica gel. The peptide-enriched extract will be further purified with reverse-phase high-performance liquid chromatography (RP-HPLC). The dried extract will be dissolved in solvent A (100% ddH O/0.1% TFA, v/), while extract fractionation and purification of cyclotides will all be carried out on a preparative and semi-preparative scale using a Kromasil C column (Koehbach et al., 2013). HPLC fractions will further be analyzed by MALDI-TOF mass spectrometry (MS) to determine the molecular mass of sample if it ranged between 2,500 to 4,000 Da.

9.6   ACTIVITIES AND BIOLOGICS OF PLANT-BASED PEPTIDES

Plants are a major reservoir of natural drugs that can be used to combat many infectious diseases and other constantly growing health challenges facing humans (Ohunayo et al., 2020). Plant-based peptides such as cyclopeptides were first discovered to have uterotonic activities (Gran, 1973); however, over the years, other important biological properties of plant-based short cyclopeptides have been discovered. Some of those biological activities include hemolytic, antimicrobial, anticancer, anti-HIV, antitumor, nematocidal, immunosuppressive and many others (Attah et al., 2016). According to many reports, cyclic peptides have a biological activity due to their configurations; short, cyclic peptides are more rigid when compared to most short peptides; this gives an advantage of allowing easy of receptor attachment. Furthermore, cyclopeptides are redundant to exopeptidase – a degrading enzyme that breaks the peptide linkages of polypeptides, thus affecting the structural arrangement. The resistance to this group of enzymes is as a result of the composition of amino/carbonyl terminus in their basic structure, which in turn, exerts more structurally and biologically stable binding capabilities than many other peptides such as linear peptides (Zhang et al., 2021).

Cancer is generally regarded as one of the leading causes of human death; anticancer therapies have been used over the years to treat and manage this disease; however, resistance to many of the commercially available synthetic drugs have surfaced, making the treatment more difficult (Houshdar et al., 2021). Plant-based cyclopeptides possess many important advantages over other drugs because of their selective toxicity and low immunogenicity; coupled with that, another major advantage is the ease of flexibility of several changes in their sequences. Cyclopeptides and many other natural products have created new hope of developing more friendly compounds to challenge cancer diseases (Houshdar et al., 2021).

Plants and their products have been important to man not only for food but also for medicinal purposes. Long before now, plant extracts have been studied to inhibit the growth of microorganisms – most especially those housing various resistant genes (Ohunayo et al., 2021). Plant-based short cyclopeptides have been considered as new remedies for combating antibiotic-resistant microorganisms. These structures are increasingly used to design newer antimicrobial molecules due to their innate characteristics. Cyclopeptides are known for their extraordinary firmness, which allows them to withstand breakdown during digestion and also makes them appropriate molecules for combating antibiotic resistance. Cyclic peptides present numerous added advantages such as the huge surface area, which offers a high affinity and selectivity for their targets; a restricted configurational flexibility, which increases binding properties; and low toxicity. Furthermore, they have the capacity to target protein-protein relations because they are able to fill the accessible chemical space and may signify an alternative to small molecules (Zorzi et al., 2017).

9.7 EXAMPLES OF PLANT-BASED PEPTIDES ISOLATED FROM PLANT

Segetalin is a type of cyclopeptide isolated from the seeds of *Vaccaria segetalis*, which was discovered in 1994; the first segetalin discovered was called segetalin A; the sequence composed in its structure was found to be a cyclo (Ala-Gly-Val-Pro-Val-Trp) having estrogenic activity (ES) on the uterine weight of ovariectomized rats when analyzed. Later on, several derivatives of segetalins were discovered; namely, Segetalin A, Segetalin B, Segetalin C and Segetalin D – all isolated from the plant also having estrogenic activities (Morita et al., 1995). The ES activity of segetalin A is lower than that of segetalin B, of which other derivatives such as segetalin C and segetalin D do not have much ES activity when compared to segetalin A and segetalin B. The ES activity relatedness of segetalin A and segetalin B was due to sequence similarities between the two (Houshdar et al., 2021).

After the discovery of segetalin A, B, C and D, *Vaccaria segetalis* was also reported to be the basis of discovery for segetalin E (Figure 9.5), segetalin F, segetalin G and segetalin H. Available report suggests that segetalin H ang segetalin G both possess biological activity, similar to A and B, while segetalin E has an anticancer effect on the growth of lymphocytic leukemia cells (Morita et al., 1996). With advancement in molecular biology, it has been verified that the bioavailability of cyclopeptides in plants are gene coded; hence, peptide-bearing plants possess genes that encode the ability for the plants to synthesize cyclic proteins. This observation was demonstrated first in *Saponaria vaccaria*; presently, the gene responsible for this trait has been isolated and cloned from the root of *Saponaria vaccaria* (Condie et al., 2011).

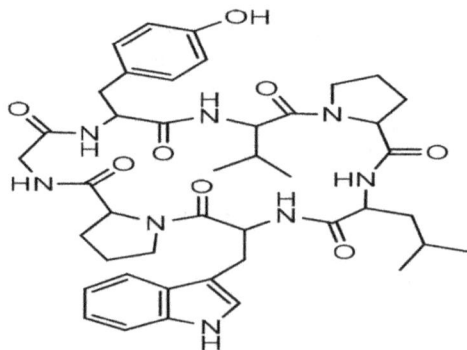

FIGURE 9.5 Typical structure of segetalin E.

Isolation of plant-based cyclopeptides have also been identified from *Stellaria yunnanensis*; these cyclic, short peptides are known to be active against tumor cells while also inhibiting their proliferation. The cyclic peptide isolated from this plant is called Yunanin, having several derivatives (Morita et al., 1996). As elucidation of proline residues in plants gained attention, cycloleonuripeptides were discovered from the fruit of a plant called *Leonurus heterophyllus*. Cycloleonuripeptides have a unique structure because their peptide backbones could assume several configurations owing to their cis-trans isomerization peptide linkages connecting the proline residues. The biological activities of cycloleonuripeptides is thought to have antitumor activity as well as the ability to inhibit abnormal lymphocytic cells (Morita et al., 1996).

9.8 CONCLUSION

Plants play an enormous role in the ecosystem, as they serve as a great source and template for drug development. Since its first discovery, most attention has been focused on drug development from these molecules, leaving its drug delivery potential less or unattended to. Since short and cyclic peptides have all the needed features of delivery drugs or related compounds to target tissues, attention should be drawn to the exploration of this potential.

REFERENCES

Attah AF, Hellinger R, Sonibare MA, Moody JO, Arrowsmith S, Wray S, Gruber CW. Ethobotanical survey of Rinorea dentata (Violaceae) used in South-Western Nigerian ethnomedicine and detection of cyclotides. J Ethnopharmacol. 2016;179:83–91.

Basse CW. Dissecting defense-related and developmental transcriptional responses of maize during *Ustilago maydis* infection and subsequent tumor formation. Plant Physiol. 2005;138(3):1774–1784.

Burman R, Gruber CW, Rizzardi K, Herrmann A, Craik DJ, Gupta MP, Göransson U. Cyclotide proteins and precursors from the genus *Gloeospermum*: Filling a blank spot in the cyclotide map of Violaceae. Phytochemistry. 2010;71(1):13–20.

Chiche L, Heitz A, Gelly JC, Gracy J, Chau PT, Ha PT, Hernandez JF, Le-Nguyen D. Squash inhibitors: From structural motifs to macrocyclic knottins. Curr Protein Pept Sci. 2004;5:341–349.

Condie JA, Nowak G, Reed DW, Balsevich JJ, Reaney MJT, Arnison PG, et al. The biosynthesis of Caryophyllaceae-like cyclic peptides in Saponaria vaccaria L. from DNA-encoded precursors. Plant J. 2011;67:682–690. doi:10.1111/j.1365-313X.2011.04626.x

De Veer SJ, Kan MW, Craik DJ. Cyclotides: From structure to function. Chem Rev. 2019 Dec 26;119(24):12375–12421. doi: 10.1021/acs.chemrev.9b00402. Epub 2019 Dec 12. PMID: 31829013.

Fosgerau K, Hoffmann T. Peptide therapeutics: Current status and future directions. Drug Discov Today. 2015;20:122–128. doi:10.1016/j.drudis.2014.10.003.

Gran L. On the effect of a polypeptide isolated from "Kalata-Kalata" (Oldenlandia affinis DC) 744 on the oestrogen dominated uterus. Acta Pharmacol Toxicol (Copenh.). 1973;33:400–408.

Haggag YA, Donia AA, Osman MA, El-Gizawy SA. Peptides as drug candidates: Limitations and recent development perspectives. Biomed J Sci Tech Res. 2018;8:6659–666.

Hernandez JF, Gagnon J, Chiche L, Nguyen TM, Andrieu JP, Heitz A, Trinh Hong T, Pham TT, Le Nguyen D. Squash trypsin inhibitors from Momordica cochinchinensis exhibit an atypical macrocyclic structure. Biochemistry. 2000;39:5722–5730.

Herrmann A, Burman R, Mylne JS, Karlsson G, Gullbo J, Craik DJ, Clark RJ, Göransson U. The alpine violet, *Viola biflora*, is a rich source of cyclotides with potent cytotoxicity. Phytochemistry. 2008;69(4):939–952.

Houshdar Tehrani MH, Gholibeikian M, Bamoniri A, Mirjalili B. Cancer treatment by caryophyllaceae-type cyclopeptides. Front Endocrinol. 2021;11:600856. doi:10.3389/fendo.2020.600856

Jennings C, West J, Waine C, Craik D, Anderson M. Biosynthesis and insecticidal properties of plant cyclotides: The cyclic knotted proteins from Oldenlandia affinis. Proc Natl Acad Sci USA. 2001;98:10614–10619.

Koehbach J, Attah AF, Berger A, Hellinger R, Kutchan TM, Carpenter EJ, et al. Cyclotide discovery in gentianales revisited-identification and characterization of cyclic cystine-knot peptides and their phylogenetic distribution in rubiaceae plants. Biopolymers. 2013;100(5):438–452. doi:10.1002/bip.22328

Morita H, Yun YS, Takeya K, Itokawa H, Segetalins B. C and D, three new cyclic peptides from Vaccaria segetalis. Tetrahedron. 1995;51(21):6003–6014. doi:10.1016/0040-4020(95)00278-G

Morita H, Yun YS, Takeya K, Itokawa H, Shirota O. A cyclic heptapeptide from Vaccaria segetalis. Phytochemistry. 1996;42(2):439–441. doi:10.1016/0031-9422(95)00911-6

Ohunayo AS, Adekeye DK, Dauda OS, Odeniyi IO, Popoola O, DandAkinwunmi O. Microbial profile of the phyllosphere and the antimicrobial potency of Ficus vogelii extracts. J Pharm Sci Res. 2020;12(1): 191–195.

Ohunayo AS, John-Mese OJ, Dauda OS, Oyinlade PO, Afolabi AT. Antimicrobial assay of methanolic extracts of selected plants on multiple antibiotics resistance Escherichia coli. J Res Pharm Sci. 2021;7(9):7–12.

Saether O, Craik DJ, Campbell ID, Sletten K, Juul J, Norman DG. Elucidation of the primary and three-dimensional structure of the uterotonic polypeptide kalata B1. Biochemistry. 1995; 34:4147–4158.

Schmidt A, Teeter M, Weckert E, Lamzin VS. Crystal structure of small protein crambin at 0.48 A resolution. Acta Cryst F. 2011;67:424–428. doi:10.1107/S1744309 1.vcx110052607.

Soudy R, Kimura R, Patel A, Fu W, Kaur K, Westaway D, Yang J, Jhamandas J. Short amylin receptor antagonist peptides improve memory deficits in Alzheimer's disease mouse model. Sci Rep. 2019;9:10942–10953. doi:10.1038/s41598-019-47255-9.

Zhang JN, Xia YX, Zhang HJ. Natural cyclopeptides as anticancer agents in the last 20 years. Int J Mol Sci. 2021 Apr 12;22(8):3973. doi:10.3390/ijms22083973. PMID: 33921480; PMCID: PMC8068844.

Zorzi A, Deyle K, Heinis C. Cyclic peptide therapeutics: Past, present and future. Curr Opin Chem Biol. 2017;38:24–29. [CrossRef] [PubMed]

Part II

Applications

10 Role of Dietary Fibre and Phytonutrients in Human Health and Nutrition

Rukayat A. Oyegoke, Johnson Olaleye Oladele,
Oluwaseun Titilope Oladele, and Adenike Temidayo Oladiji

10.1 INTRODUCTION

There are very important constituents of food that are very beneficial for the maintenance of human health and that need to be researched. Some of these include dietary fibre, vitamins and minerals. Research has shown that they have numerous health benefits that are yet to be explored. Therefore, the understanding of their constituents, how these constituents interact with each other and other biomolecules and how they elicit their health benefits requires to be understood.

10.2 DIETARY FIBRES

The adoption of the term "dietary fibre" was originally stated by Hipsley in the year 1953 to illustrate the cell wall composition of plants used in food (Gray, 2006). According to Codex 2005, dietary fibre is described as a carbohydrate polymer with several monomeric units ranging from ten and above and is mainly not hydrolyzed (non-digestible and non-absorbable) by the endogenous enzymes in the human small intestine; likewise, it undergoes incomplete and sometimes complete fermentation in the duodenum and is classified under the following categories:

a. Unrefined carbohydrate polymers present naturally in the food consumed.
b. Refined carbohydrate polymers gotten from food raw material either by physical, enzymatic or chemical means; have been shown to exhibit a physiological effect and of great benefit to health, as stated by major scientific literatures and findings.
c. Carbohydrate polymers synthetically produced; these types of carbohydrate polymers are known to have some physiological importance that is profitable to human health, as confirmed by most scientific bodies of competent authority.

The foregoing definition encompasses both natural and synthetic carbohydrate polymers, but the major pointers are that they are found only in plant foods, non-digestible/absorbable in the small intestine, incomplete or sometimes complete fermentation in the duodenum and they are profitable to human health. Because of everyday advances in research on dietary fibre, especially on its classification and constituents, which incorporates many additions constantly, it is now defined as consisting of "intrinsic" plant cell wall polysaccharides.

10.2.1 Types of Fibres and Dietary Sources

10.2.1.1 Classification/Types of Fibres

There is no rigid classification of fibres, as there are many properties that can be used to classify them, but the boundaries of these properties are not absolutely defined. In fact, the mode of

DOI: 10.1201/9781003361497-12

classification is abundant; these include their functions in plants, type of polysaccharides they possess, solubility in their gastrointestinal tract, site and products of digestion, etc. (Tungland and Meyer, 2002). However, the classification that has gained the highest acceptance is the one that classifies dietary fibre on the basis of two things, which are:

i. Its solubility potential in buffer at a specified pH.
ii. Its ability to ferment in vitro using an aqueous enzyme solution as a model for the human alimentary system.

The foregoing means of classification therefore leads to the two major classifications, which are:

i. Soluble and well-fermented fibres.
ii. Insoluble and less-fermented fibres.

10.2.1.2 Sources of Fibres

The major food sources of dietary fibre include but are not limited to cereal grains and brans, woody plants, legumes, fruits, vegetables and nuts (Clifford *et al.*, 2015). They are widely spread in different species of the previously mentioned sources, although their composition varies from one food to another.

10.2.1.2.1 Soluble and Well-Fermented Fibres

This group includes pectin, gums and mucilages.

i. Pectin: This is a complex polysaccharide in which D-galacturonic acid is the principal component – i.e., the polysaccharide is comprised mostly of esterified D-galacturonic acid in alpha – (1–4) linkage (Kay, 1982). This is the reason they are chemically called polygalacturonic acid. The acid-side chain units are esterified with that of the methoxy groups in the natural product. The side chains linked to pectin include arabinose, galactose, xylose, rhamnose and glucose (Figure 10.1).

   This group of fibre serves as the structural components of cell walls and intracellular tissues of plants. They are of high water-solubility (most widely soluble dietary fibre) and form gels easily (Gray, 2006). Natural sources of pectin include fruits, vegetables, legumes, nuts, sugar beets and potatoes.

ii. GUM: Gum is comprised of a Dmannopyranosyl backbone and it is linked by a β-(1→4) linkage; also, there is a A-D-galactose side chain linked (1→6) to the mannose backbone (galactose, glucuronic acid-mannose and galacturonic acid-rhamnose) with xylose, fructose and galactose as side chains (Figure 10.2). It consists of a broad mixture of gelatinous

PECTIN

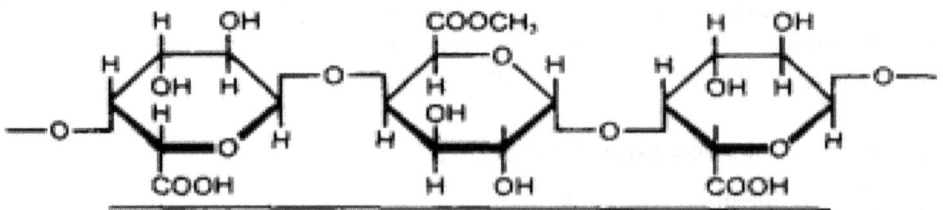

FIGURE 10.1   Structure of pectin. (Major component is D-galacturonic acid.)

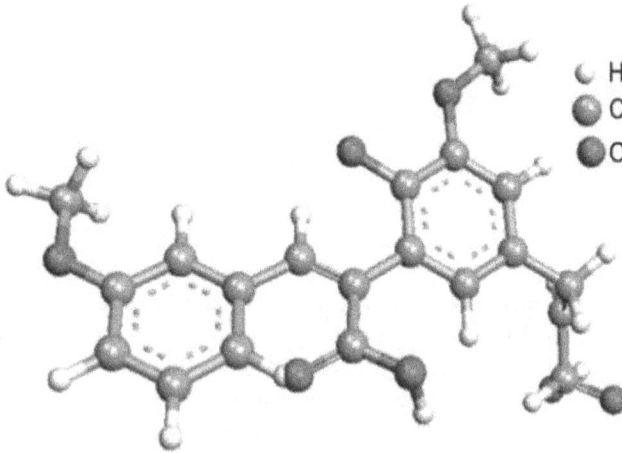

FIGURE 10.2   Structure of gum.

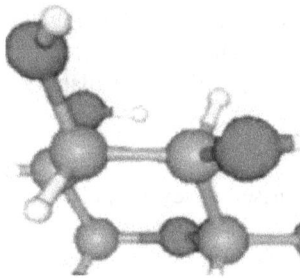

FIGURE 10.3   Structure of mucilage.

polysaccharides and is formed from specialized secretory cells of plant origin, mostly at the site of injury or trauma (Devinder *et al.*, 2012). The degree and pattern of galcto-syl determines its physical characteristics. They are mainly two constituents: leguminous seed gum and gum Arabic; another, less common, one is locust bean gum. Guar gum and locust bean gum are gums from leguminous seed plants hauled out from *Cyamopsis tetragonolobus* and *Ceratonia siliqua* seeds, respectively, while Arabic gum is extracted from the acacia tree (Devinder *et al.*, 2012). The sources of gum include oatmeal, dried beans, legumes, fruits, vegetable, seawort, microbial gum, etc. They are mainly for food and pharmaceutical uses.

iii. Mucilages: The main chain of this fibre consists of several disaccharide units, notable among which are a linkage between galactose and mannose, glucose and mannose, arabi-nose and xylose, galacturic acid-rhamnose with galactose at its side chain (Kay, 1982) (Figure 10.3). These clear, colorless, gel-like fibres are synthesized by plants with the sole aim of protecting the seeds from extreme dehydration. Mucilages are produced in large concentration from psyllium (plantain) and are utilized in minute quantity as gel/thickener, stabilizers and emulsifying agents. Examples include the gum acacia, gum karaya, gum tragacanth, ispaghula, etc.

10.2.1.2.2 Insoluble and Less-Fermented Fibres

These include cellulose, hemicellulose and lignin (Devinder *et al.*, 2012).

10.2.1.2.2.1 Cellulose
Cellulose is a polysaccharides whose monomers are joined by a β-(1→4) glycosidic linkages; this is differentiated from most polysaccharides whose linkages are A-(1→4), as in amylase (Figure 10.4). It is a major component of the plant cell wall and has an un-unbranched polymer of glucose comprised of long, straight chains which are linked by β-(1→4) glycosidic linkages (Devinder *et al.*, 2012). This linkage gives it the rigid nature that is due to the presence of multiple hydrogen bonds. Humans cannot digest cellulose because they lack the enzyme cellulase in their digestive system; hence, it is of no nutritional value to them. However, ruminant animals make good use of it due to the presence of some microorganisms in their system that are capable of breaking it down into smaller molecules. Studies have shown that the presence of dietary fibre from cellulose origin has been implicated in the management or treatment of most frontline diseases such as cardiovascular diseases, diabetes, colon cancer, etc. It is present in unrefined cereals, vegetables, sugar beets, various brans, fruits. The majority of the fibre found in cereal and fruits is mainly cellulose, whereas one-third of it is found in vegetables and nuts (Gray, 2006).

10.2.1.2.2.2 Hemicellulose
Hemicellulose is also a part of the cell wall component of most plants; it differs from cellulose in that it contains a backbone of *β*-(1,4)–linked pyranoside sugars such as xylose, mannose, galactose and glucose and a branched chain of mainly arabinose, galactose and glucuronic acid (Figure 10.5). They are of two types – xylans and galactans – and are mainly found in grains, although they might also be available in fruits, vegetables, nuts and legumes in small amounts (Gray, 2006).

10.2.1.2.2.3 Lignin
Ligin is comprised of several polymers, cross linked to each other with different chemical bonds (Figure 10.6), which are mainly of phenylpropane units. It is not a polysaccharides; however, due to its reactions with hemicelluloses in the cell wall of plants, it is most times allied with plant cell-wall polysaccaharides (Gray, 2006), though realistically, it is the only non-polysaccharide fibre that occurs as a result of pairing of three primary precursors (monolignols p-coumaryl, coniferyl and sinapyl alcohols) (Kay, 1982). The side chain is a three-dimensional structure. Lignin is very inert due to the strong intramolecular bonding. It is insoluble in 72% sulfuric acid. Its variations lie in its molecular weight and the methoxyl content. It resists bacterial degradation. It is a major component of foods with "woody" composition – for instance, celery – and in the outer layers of cereal grains, rice and legume hulls (Gray, 2006).

CELLULOSE

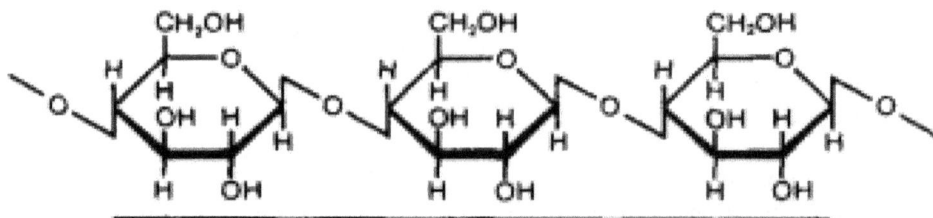

FIGURE 10.4   Structure of cellulose.

HEMICELLULOSE (major component sugars)
a) Backbone Chain

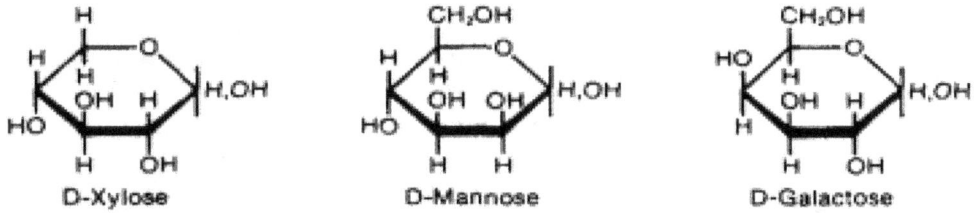

| D-Xylose | D-Mannose | D-Galactose |

b) Side Chains

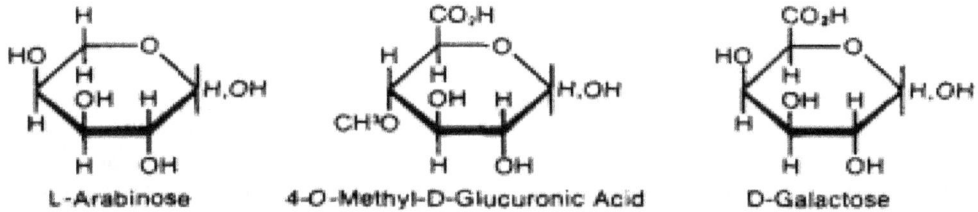

| L-Arabinose | 4-O-Methyl-D-Glucuronic Acid | D-Galactose |

FIGURE 10.5   Structure of hemicellulose.

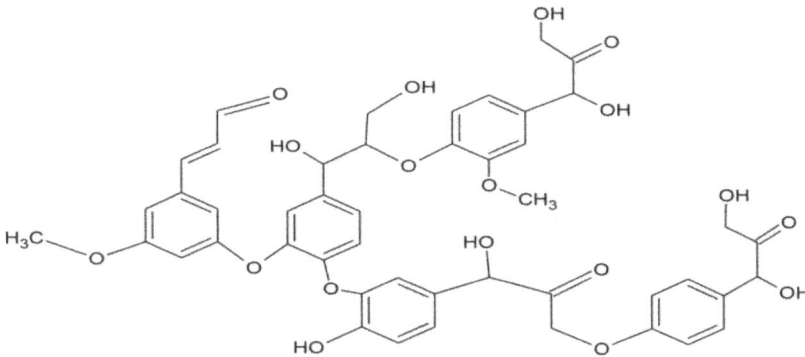

FIGURE 10.6   Structure of lignin.

10.2.2   HEALTH BENEFITS OF DIETARY FIBRES AND MECHANISMS OF ACTIONS

Most dietary fibre that possesses profitable physiological potential and is useful to human health is tagged to be functional fibre (Clifford *et al.*, 2015). Findings from several studies have indicated that free radical production in the human system either during stress, exercise or even digestion contributes greatly to most disease conditions. Thus, it is of crucial importance to look at the anti-inflammatory and antioxidant properties of these fibres to unveil the secret behind its curative actions on most of these pathological disease conditions.

10.2.2.1   Anti-Inflammatory Effects of Dietary Fibre

The human metabolic system works in conjunction with its immune system (Lotternberg *et al.*, 2010), and inflammation can be triggered by several factors as a result of interactions within the human system; notable substances responsible for such actions are: hormones, cytokines, signaling proteins, transcription factors and bioactive lipids. All these substances act in way that fatty tissue generates pro-inflammatory substances, which formerly are taught to be connected only with the immune system – for example, interleukin 6 (IL-6), tumor necrosis factor alpha (TNF-A) (Bullo *et al.*, 2007), C-reactive protein (CRP) and plasma plasminogen activator inhibitor (PAI1) (Xu *et al.*, 2003). This pro-inflammatory activity of fat tissue, generated in the course of immune response or metabolic processes, denotes a likeable risk toward the progression of some acute or chronic disease and its complications (Wellen and Hotamisligil, 2005).

Evidence from several scientific researches shows that consumption of fibres reduces inflammation that occurs due to some chronic disorder; for instance, a diet containing a good amount of fibre can potentially lower inflammation by altering both the pH and the permeability of the gut. The resultant reduction in inflammatory compounds may also adjust the neurotransmitter concentrations to reduce symptoms of depression.

10.2.2.2 Antioxidant Effects of Dietary Fibre

Antioxidants are known to mopped up free radicals generated in the human system that occur either during metabolic processes or exercise (Velioglu *et al.*, 1998). Phytochemical studies have shown that most dietary fibre contains compounds capable of mopping up reactive oxygen species generated in most diseases. For instance, most polyphenol compounds that are attached to diverse polysaccharide complexes are detached in the cause of metabolic processes in the gut, thereby exhibiting their antioxidant potentials.

10.2.2.3 Biological Activities/Effects of Dietary Fibre

10.2.2.3.1 *Irritable Bowel Disease*

This is a general term for many gastrointestinal disorders, and this include diarrhea, constipation, ulcerative colitis, etc. Laxation is a biological process that is often underrated or taken for granted until it is abused, resulting in the constipation process (AACC, 2001). Constipation is a physiological effect that brings unease to the body system, and it has been defined as a condition in which there is need to strain on defecation, resulting in abdominal pain and bloating (AACC, 2001). Constipation is related to stool weight and consistency as well regularity of bowel movement (Gray, 2006). There is no gainsaying in understating the discomfort in constipation as well as the risk it potentiates in development of other diseases such as diverticular diseases and hemorrhoids. High dietary fibre nutrition has been scientifically proven to boost the laxation and thereby relief of constipation through different mechanisms exhibited by various types of fibres. Fibres have been confirmed to have an established effect on bulk and consistency of stool as well as the lowering of intestinal mobility (Heredia *et al.*, 2002). This might be due but not limited to hydration aptitude of the existing residues, generation of osmotically active metabolites but also the initiation of bacterial output and growth as well as species distribution due to the increase in low colonic pH and thereby improving/increasing the frequency, regularity of defecation as well as reduction of transit time. Diverticula are purses on the intestinal wall that can become inflamed and painful. This inflammatory condition, which arises due to bacterial infection, is called diverticultis, which is mainly due to reduced fecal bulk. Studies have shown that this effect can be ameliorated by the regular intake of dietary fibre through the previously mentioned mechanisms. Cellulose is of high effectiveness in this respect, as it has a high bran content, and this protective effect may involve increase in stool weight and decrease in transit time and intracolonic pressure (Gray, 2006).

10.2.2.3.2 *Cancer*

Consumption of dietary fibre has been scientifically confirmed to be effective in the management of various types of cancer – most especially breast and colon cancer. Several mechanisms of action of these fibres have been have proposed particularly for colon cancer and is mainly attributed to the antioxidant component present in them, as in their ability to mop up reactive oxygen species in the cells.

This finding is based on the awareness that insoluble fibre increases the time at which wastes are evacuated from the body. Therefore, the body has less exposure to toxic substances produced during digestion. Phenolic compounds present in lignin are also well known to assist in the mopping of reactive oxygen species. Dietary fibre also regulates the colonic pH, thus moderating the metabolic end-products of human intestinal flora, thus helping reduce the risk of cancer. Similarly, butyric acid, a volatile fatty acid, is a metabolic by-product produced after fermentation of most dietary fibre by the microflora in the colon stimulates apoptosis of cancerous colon cells in vitro and even provides the mechanism for inhibiting multiplication of cancerous cells.

10.2.2.3.3   Diabetes

It is widely accepted that inclusion of dietary fibre in the diet minimizes the risk of being diabetic to a great extent, and likewise, helps regulate the blood sugar level. Several successes have been recorded in the management of diabetics when dietary fibre is introduce to foods, which, in turn, leads to the reduction of the administration of insulin in the situation of a type 1 condition and also sulfonylurea drugs for the type 2 (Rivellese *et al.*, 1980). Higher intake of fibre, especially that in whole grains when compared to refined, has been shown to modestly lessen the glycemic index and enhance insulin sensitivity, which, in turn, results in a decreased risk for developing type 2 diabetes. Also, fibre exhibits its action by delaying the uptake of glucose from the small intestine, thus causing the rise in blood glucose, and in so doing, putting it at a minimal level, which, in turn, attenuates the insulin response, resulting in a slower decline in blood glucose level. Other possible mechanisms of fibre action include delayed gastric emptying, lessening the release of gastric inhibitory polypeptide, improved glucose tolerance, reduced insulin requirements and increased peripheral tissue insulin sensitivity (AACC, 2001).

10.2.2.3.4   Obesity, Satiety and Weight Loss

The rate at which obesity is becoming pronounced is alarming, both in the Western world and in developing countries. Consumption of fibres are known to caused fullness due to its bulky nature and low energy-density; likewise, its water-absorbing ability (AACC, 2001).

Therefore, due to its promotion of satiety, it's performed a crucial function in the control of energy balance and body weight. It has also been reported that foods with a low glycemic index are more satiating than the ones with a high glycemic index. Dietary fibres delay gastric emptying, and more importantly, by forming gels, slow down the absorption of carbohydrates from the small intestine in such a way that it is less accessible to digestive enzymes, thereby reducing the contact with the intestinal mucosa (Gray, 2006).

10.2.2.3.5   Coronary Heart Diseases and Related Disorders

High cholesterol level in the system has been a culprit in most heart-related disease and disorder. The consumption of fibres that are water soluble tends to bind to bile acids, thereby increasing the excretion of cholesterol from the system (Clifford *et al.*, 2015). A variety of foods loaded with dietary fibre have been verified to reduce the atherogenicity of semi-synthetic diets with or without added fat and sterol. It has also been ascertained that the hypolipidic effect in humans lowers both serum cholesterol and triglycerides (Takahashi *et al.*, 1993). It should also be noted that dietary fibre may reduce total body cholesterol, even when a significant reduction in serum cholesterol does not occur (Oda *et al.*, 1993).

10.3   MICRONUTRIENTS AND HEALTH BENEFITS

Micronutrients are vital elements necessary for growth and healthy living for both humans and other organisms. It is required to coordinate a series of physiological functions for health maintenance (Awuchi *et al.*, 2020). The essential micronutrients required by humans are vitamins and minerals, and they are required in amounts less than 100 mg daily (Ormsbee *et al.*, 2014). They are referred to as essential nutrients since they are either synthesized in minute amount in the body or not synthesized at all and therefore must be taken in from our diet.

10.3.1   Vitamins and Health Benefits

Vitamins play a key role in the prevention of most frontline diseases that are nutritionally related; they are required to prevent the nutritional deficiency disease "beriberi" because of its vital need (Naik, 2012). Vitamins are grouped into two based on their solubility (Figure 10.7). These are:

   i) Fat-soluble vitamins (vitamins A, D, E and K).
   ii) Water-soluble vitamins (vitamins $B_{complex}$ and C).

10.3.1.1   Fat-Soluble Vitamins

Fat-soluble vitamins are vitamins that can easily be dissolved in fat. They are, to a great extent, stored in the body, and so, do not require frequent intake (Naik, 2012). Examples are: vitamins A, D, E and K.

10.3.1.1.1   Vitamin A (Retinol)

This vitamin contains a single 6-membered ring to which is attached an 11-carbon side-chain (Figure 10.8) (Naik, 2012). Vitamin A can exist in three different active forms (retinol, retinal and retinoic acid) all of which are derived from the plant precursor molecule, β-carotene.

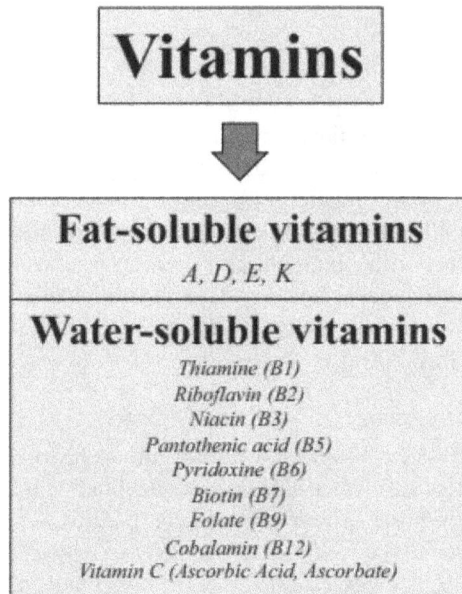

FIGURE 10.7   Classification of vitamins.

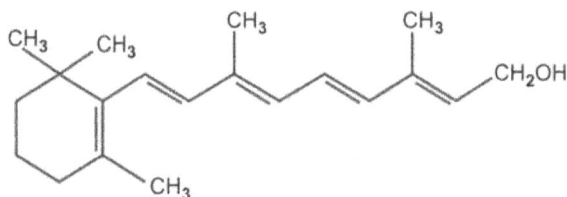

FIGURE 10.8   Structure of vitamin A.

Vitamin A supports bone growth and immune function. It is involved in cellular differentiation and physiological function of epithelial glands. It also supports the skin and partakes in the uptake of visual sharpness (Muhammad *et al.*, 2020). Deficiency of it leads to lack of rhodopsin in the retinol rod cells, visual impairment, xerophthalmia, keratomalacia, respiratory and intestinal infections. Excess of it can result into vomiting, nausea and anorexia. Important sources of vitamin A include leafy vegetables, meat, fish, green mango, egg, spinach, cabbage, cod liver oil, etc.

10.3.1.1.2   Vitamin D (Cholecalciferol)

Vitamin D could exist in several kinds (Figure 10.9). Four crystalline D vitamins are isolated, and at least ten pro-vitamins D are known (Muhammad *et al.*, 2020). However, there are primarily two prominent ones naturally produced cholecalciferol (D_3), which is gotten from animal sources in the diet, like from ultraviolent light from sunlight on 7-dehydrocholesterol (Naik, 2012). The second type is the one that is artificially produced form D_2 or ergocalciferol and it is made in the laboratory by irradiation of plant sterol, ergosterol.

The absorption and deposition of phosphorus and calcium in the intestine and bones, respectively, is greatly enhanced by vitamin D. Another crucial role of vitamin D is the modulation of transcription of cell cycle proteins that decreases and increases the cell proliferation and differentiation of a number of specialized cells in the body, which include keratinocytes, osteoclastic precursors, enterocytes, etc. Studies have shown that vitamin D also possesses antioxidant and immunomodulatory properties (Christakos *et al.*, 2015). Deficiency of vitamin D can affect development of the bone in both children and adults (Kennel *et al.* 2010). It causes rickets in children, while, in adults, it causes osteomalacia (Nair and Maseeh, 2012). The main source of vitamin D is sunlight-induced synthesis; likewise, cod liver oil, fish oil, liver and egg yolk are very good sources (Naik, 2012).

10.3.1.1.3   Vitamin E (Tocopherol)

Vitamin E is a natural antioxidant and also an anti-sterility factor that consists of eight naturally occurring tocopherols, of which A-tocopherol is the most active form (Figure 10.10) (Naik, 2012).

As earlier stated, this vitamin is a natural antioxidant that scavenges free radicals and molecular oxygen. Some of the other numerous important properties of vitamin K are that it prevents peroxidation of polyunsaturated fatty acids in cell membranes and also partakes in wound healing and immunity (Schmölz *et al.*, 2018). Deficiency of this vitamin leads to hemolytic anemia and retrolental fibroplasia (RLF), while excessive intake of it can lead to interference with the utilization of vitamins A and K, intestinal irritability, prolonged prothrombin time, etc. (Gomez-Pomar *et al.*, 2018; Moisa *et al.*, 2018). Sources of vitamin K include fat and oils – i.e. germ oil, corn oil, fish oil, eggs and lettuce (Naik, 2012).

10.3.1.1.4   Vitamin K

Vitamin K is known as an anti-hemorrhagic factor because its deficiency leads to uncontrolled hemorrhages due to a defect in blood coagulation (Figure 10.11) (Naik, 2012). There are mainly

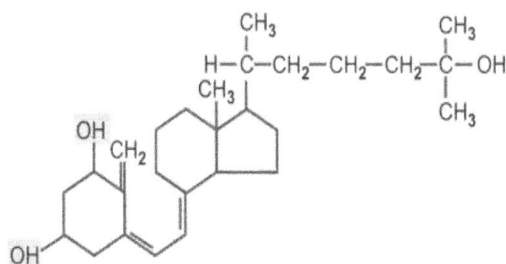

FIGURE 10.9   Structure of vitamin D.

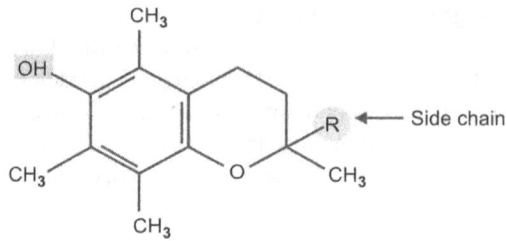

FIGURE 10.10   Structure of A-tocopherol (vitamin E).

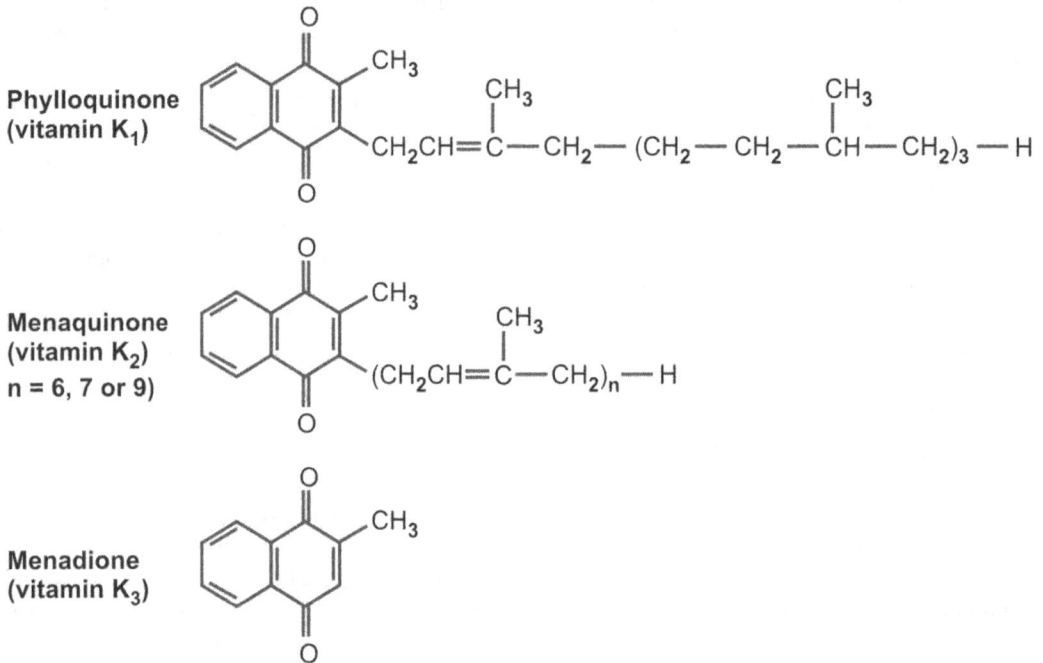

FIGURE 10.11   Vitamin K.

three classes of vitamin K, which are K_1, K_2 and K_3 (K_1 – phylloquinone and K_2 – menaquinone are naturally occurring, while K_3 – menadione is synthetic). As earlier said, the major function is the role it plays in blood coagulation by the activation of blood clotting factors produced in the liver in the inactive form (Reddy and Jialal, 2018).

Deficiency of this vitamin can lead to generalized bleeding, prolonged clotting time in adults and development of hemorrhagic disease in new borns (Reddy and Jialal, 2018). Excessive intake can lead to hyperbilirubinemia, hemolytic anemia and jaundice. Good sources of this vitamin include fresh green vegetables, lettuce, cabbage, cauliflower, spinach, tomatoes, liver, egg yolk, etc.

10.3.1.2   Water-Soluble Vitamins

10.3.1.2.1   Vitamin B_1 (Thiamine)

This vitamin consists of a pyrimidine ring attached to a thiazole ring by a methylene bridge (Figure 10.12). The active coenzyme form of this enzyme is thiamine pyrophosphate (TPP).

Vitamin B_1 plays a key role in carbohydrate metabolism, especially in hexose monophosphate shunt. It is also a very efficient neuro-protective agent (Ikeda *et al.*, 2016). Thiamine is a co-catalyst

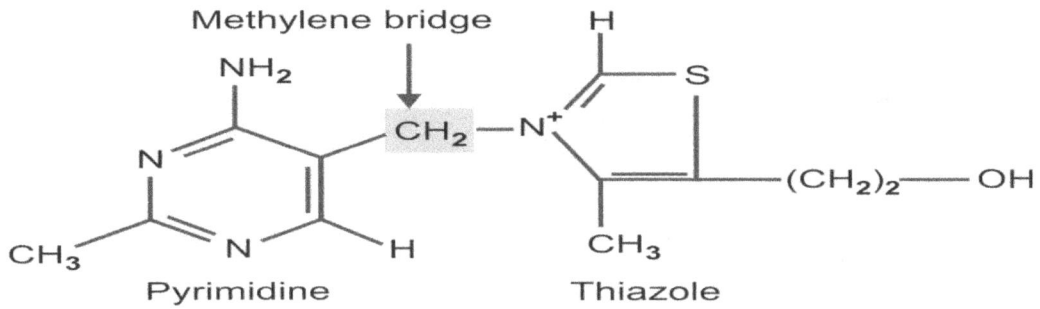

FIGURE 10.12 Thiamine.

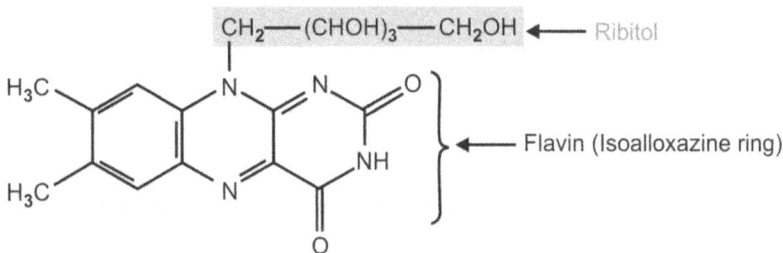

FIGURE 10.13 Riboflavin.

in sugar digestion and is necessary to the function of the heart, nerves, and muscles. (Muhammad *et al.*, 2020). Deficiency of vitamin B_1 results in a condition known as beri-beri, while its excess can lead to tachycardia, migraines and peevishness (Wiley and Gupta, 2019). Sources of this vitamin include unrefined cereals, wheat germ, nuts, lentils, green vegetables, etc.

10.3.1.2.2 Vitamin B_2 (Riboflavin)
Riboflavin is a yellow crystalline substance that consists of a isoalloxazine ring with a ribitol (sugar alcohol) side chain (Naik, 2012) (Figure 10.13).

Its derivatives FAD and $FADH_2$ are involved in oxidative-reduction reactions. Vitamin B_2 is also involved in protection against peroxidation in metabolism of xenobiotics and maintenance of mucosal epithelial and ocular tissue (Naik, 2012). Its deficiency results in ariboflavinosis (Muhammad *et al.*, 2020). Sources of vitamin B_2 include green verdant vegetables, liver, oats, milk, grain, etc.

10.3.1.2.3 Vitamin B_3 (Niacin)
Niacin is a simple derivative of pyrimidine and it is a general name for nicotinic acid and nicotinamide (Figure 10.14) (Naik, 2012).

It is a precursor of coenzymes NAD^+ and $NADH^+$ which are involved in many oxidation-reduction reactions like the oxidative pathways, reductive synthesis, etc. (Muhammad *et al.*, 2020). Deficiency results in pellagra, while high intake leads to vasodilation, flushing and liver damage (Naik, 2012). Sources of vitamin B_3 include yeast, legumes, liver, etc., while limited quantities of this vitamin can be obtained from tryptophan (Naik, 2012).

10.3.1.2.4 Vitamin B_5 (Panthothenic acid)
Pantothenic acid is a vitamin formed by combination of pantoic acid an β-alanine (Naik, 2012). It is widely distributed in food. This vitamin has components of coenzymes that participate in reactions

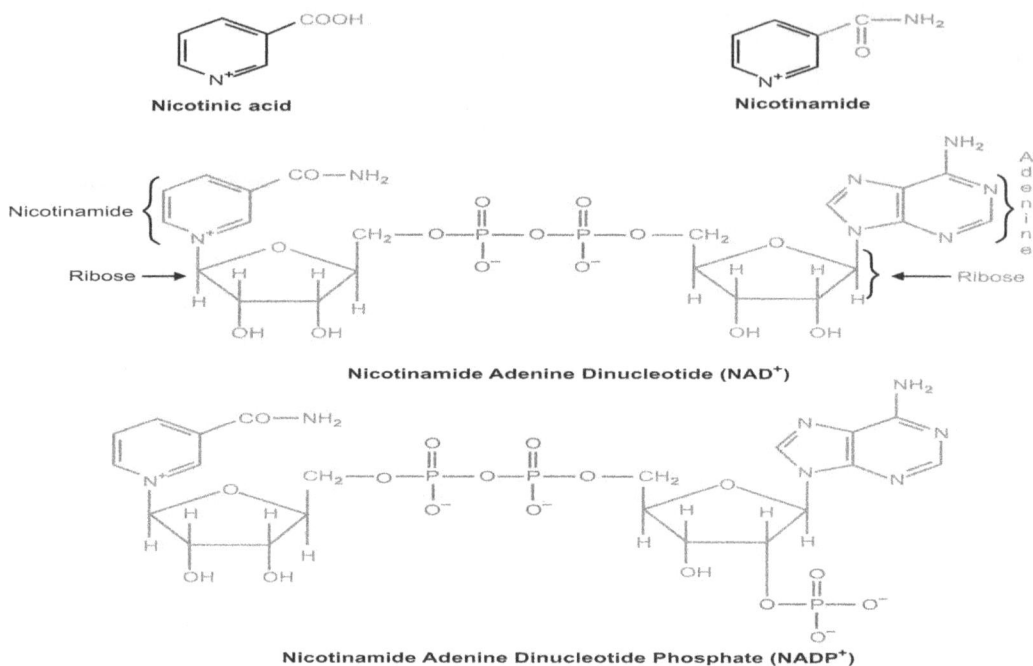

FIGURE 10.14   Structure and active coenzyme forms of niacin.

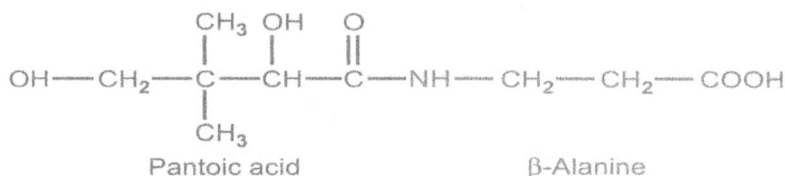

FIGURE 10.15   Pantothenic acid.

concerned with fatty acid synthesis. It also plays a key role in homonogenesis and energy production (Figure 10.15) (Muhammad *et al.*, 2020).

Deficiency of this vitamin may lead to burning feet syndrome, dermatitis, alopecia, etc. (Lykstad and Sharma, 2019). As stated earlier, its wide distribution in food allows for varieties of sources, and these include yeast, liver, wheat germs, cereals, eggs, etc.

10.3.1.2.5   *Vitamin B$_6$ (Pyridoxine)*

Three natural vitamers (different forms of the vitamin) of vitamin B$_6$ – namely, pyridoxine, pyridoxamine and pyridoxal – are known, and they can be interconverted in the body. The active form of vitamin B$_6$ is pyridoxial phosphate, and it is formed from the phosphorylation of the three forms of Vitamin B$_6$ (Figure 10.16).

The active form of this vitamin acts as coenzyme in major reactions of amino acid metabolism, and this includes transamination reactions, decarboxylation, nonoxidative deamination condensation of amino acids (Naik, 2012). This vitamin is of high therapeutic use, as it is actively involved in the treatment of autism, seizures, Down's syndrome, premenstrual tension syndrome, etc. Deficiency can lead to irritability, nervousness and depression. Sources of this vitamin include mainly plant products (for pyriodoxine), whereas, for pyridoxamine and pyridoxal, they

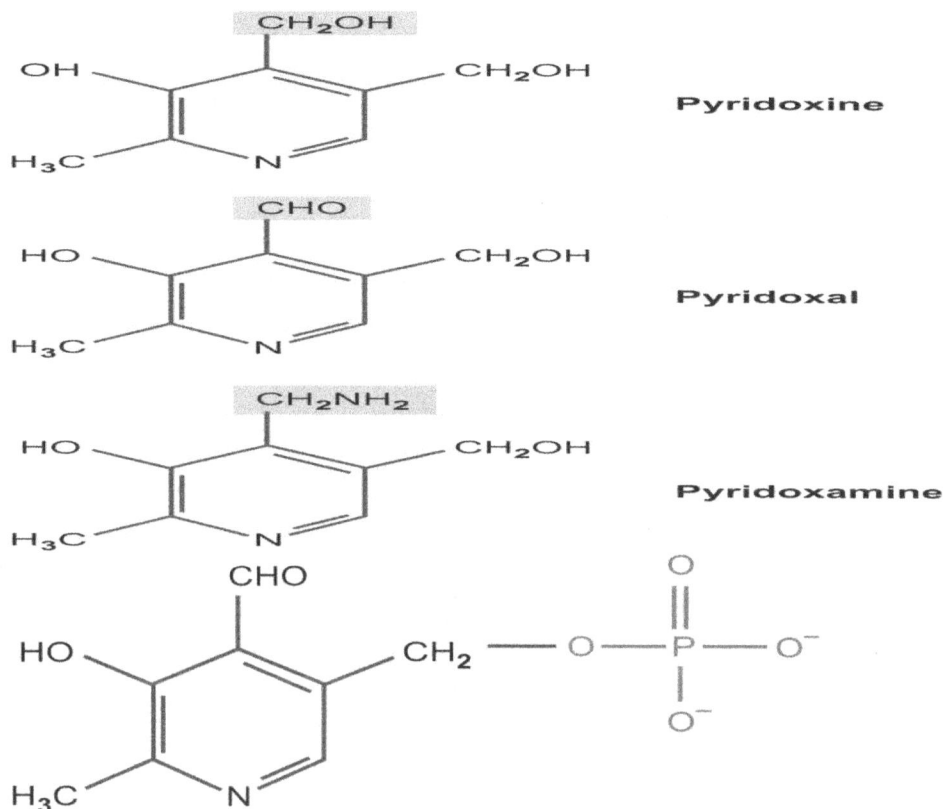

FIGURE 10.16 The three forms of pyridoxine and pyridoxal phosphate.

are animal products. However, there are excellent dietary sources, which include yeast, pulse, meat, poultry, fish, etc.

10.3.1.2.6 Vitamin B₇ (Biotin)

Biotin, formerly known as vitamin H, is an imidazole derivative that consists of a tetrahydrothiophene ring that is bound to an imidazole ring and a valeric acid side-chain (Figure 10.17). It plays a crucial role in glucose, vitamin B_{12} and folic acid utilization, metabolism of protein and synthesis of fatty acids. Although some scientists believe that there are no known effects of the deficiency and excess of biotin (Muhammad et al., 2020), it is also documented by some that biotin deficiency causes anorexia, glossitis, alopecia, depression, muscular pain, etc. Dietary sources of biotin include green beans, egg yolk, dark green vegetables, liver, kidney.

10.3.1.2.7 Vitamin B₉ (Folic acid)

Three components make up folic acids, and they are pteridine ring, p-amino benzoic acid (PABA) and L-glutamic acid (Figure 10.18) (Muhammad et al., 2020). The synthesized form of folic acid is folate, which is now converted to the active form tetrahydrofolate.

Folic acid is an essential molecule in the synthesis of nucleic acids (DNA and RNA) and also plays a key role in the metabolism of amino acids ((Lykstad and Sharma, 2019). Deficiency causes neural tube defects, megaloblastic and macrocytic anemia and hyperhomocysteinemia (Hodgetts et al., 2015). Dietary sources include green vegetables, liver, yeast, fruits.

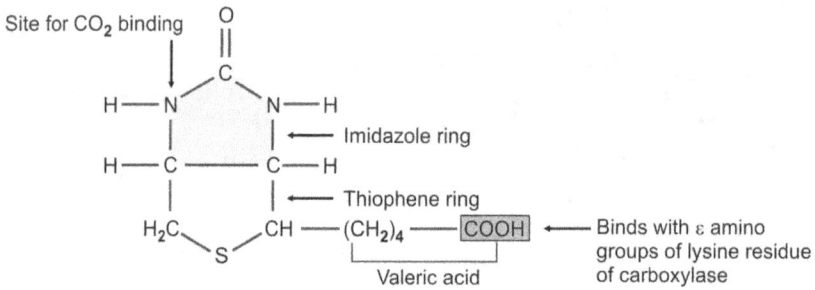

FIGURE 10.17   Biotin.

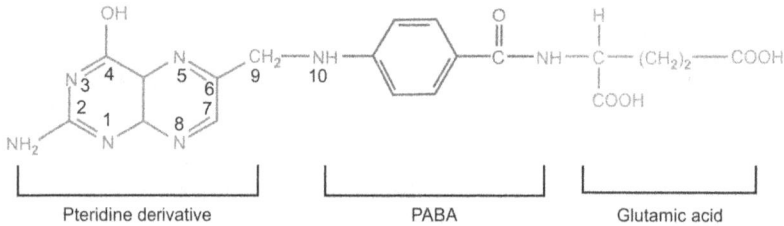

FIGURE 10.18   Folic acid.

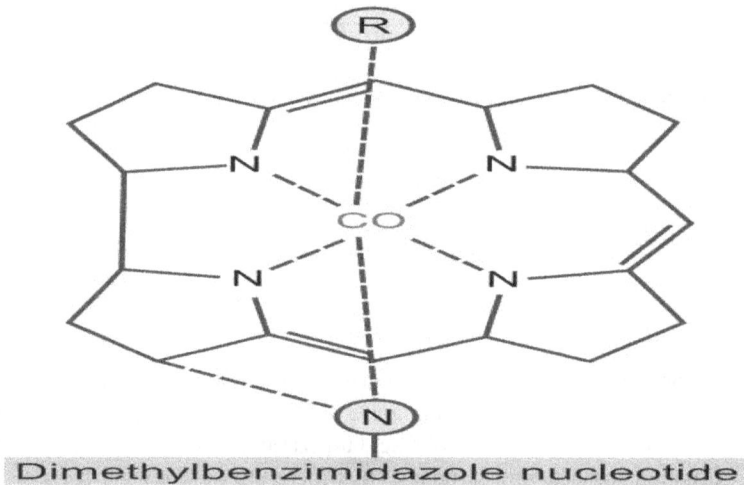

FIGURE 10.19   Cobalamin (R: either methyl or deoxyadenosyl or hydroxy group).

10.3.1.2.8   Vitamin B_{12} (Cobalamin)

Vitamin B_{12} bears a complex corrin ring (containing pyrrols similar to porphyrin), linked to a cobalt atom held in the center of the corrin ring by four coordination bonds with the nitrogen of the pyrrole groups (Naik, 2012). The remaining coordination bonds of the cobalt are linked with the nitrogen of dimethylbenzimidazole nucleotide, and the sixth bond is linked to either methyl or 5'-deoxy-adenosyl or hydroxy group to form methylcobalamin, adenosylcobalamin or hydroxycobalamin, respectively (Figure 10.19) (Naik, 2012). The active forms of cobalamin are methylcobalamin and deoxyadenosylcobalamin.

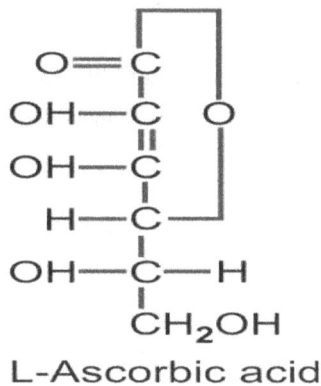

L-Ascorbic acid

FIGURE 10.20 Ascorbic acid.

They play a key role in normal production of red blood cells by the bone marrow, growth of nervous cells and metabolism of amino acids. Deficiencies can lead to pernicious and megaloblastic anemia, methylmalonic aciduria as well as neuropathy (Lykstad and Sharma 2019; Ankar and Kumar, 2019). Dietary sources are mainly animal products like meat, dairy products, fish, eggs, etc.

10.3.1.2.9 Vitamin C (Ascorbic acid)

Vitamin C is also known as ascorbic acid, and it is a six-carbon sugar derivative (Figure 10.20). Most animals can synthesize vitamin C but humans cannot due to lack of the enzyme gluconolactone oxidase, a key enzyme required for the synthesis of vitamin C. Vitamin C is a crystalline solid soluble in water (Halliwell, 2001).

Vitamin C acts as antioxidant and free oxygen radical scavenger and can be used topically in skin disorders, including those caused by photo-aging (Sorice *et al.*, 2014; Luis Gomez *et al.*, 2018). It also performs various metabolic processes, which include collagen biosynthesis, degradation of tyrosine, absorption of iron and steroid synthesis. Deficiency of vitamin C can lead to poor wound healing, abnormal bone development and osteoporosis, scurvy, spongy swollen bleeding gums, etc. Dietary sources are leafy vegetables and fruits, especially citrus fruits, strawberries, tomatoes, etc.

10.3.2 MINERALS AND HEALTH BENEFITS

Minerals plays a vital role in the human body; they are required for major physiological function and also play a role in the functions of important biomolecules present in the body. The minerals that are required for human nutrition are classified into macrominerals and microminerals based on their daily requirement.

10.3.2.1 Macrominerals

10.3.2.1.1 Sodium

Sodium is a vital cation of the extracellular fluid. It serves as a buffer for the body system. It regulates muscle and nerve irritability at the proper level. It ensures cell membrane permeability (Cogswell *et al.*, 2016). An insufficient amount of sodium in the body leads to acidosis, while its excess leads to hypertension and edema. Dietary sources include table salt, salty food, animal food and milk.

10.3.2.1.2 Potassium

Potassium is a major intracellular cation. It is also a constituent of the buffer, and it plays a key role in acid and base balance. It is essential for many enzymatic reactions (Weaver, 2013). Several

TABLE 10.1
Minerals Required in Human Nutrition

Macrominerals	Microminerals, or trace elements
Sodium	Chromium
Potassium	Cobalt
Chlorine	Copper
Calcium	Fluoride
Phosphorus	Iodine
Magnesium	Iron
Sulfur	Manganese
	Molybdenum
	Selenium
	Zinc

Source: Naik (2012).

glycolytic enzymes require potassium ions to function properly. It is required for the normal functioning of the heart and skeletal muscle fibres. It is also required in protein metabolism and transmission of nerve impulses. Deficiency of this macromineral leads to hypokalemia, cardiac disturbances and paralysis, while excess of it can lead to hyperkalemia, cardiac disturbances and paralysis (He and MacGregor, 2008). Dietary sources include whole and skimmed milk, banana, meat, tender coconut water.

10.3.2.1.3 Chloride
Chloride is a principal extracellular anion that is required for electrolyte, osmotic and acid base balance. It is required for the formation of hydrochloric acid in the gastric mucosa and for the activation of the enzyme amylase (Naik, 2012). Deficiency results in metabolic acidosis, vomiting and excessive sweating, while excessive concentration leads to dehydration and metabolic acidosis. Dietary sources of this include table salt, vegetables, milk, egg.

10.3.2.1.4 Calcium
Calcium is the most abundant mineral in the human body, and it is essential for adequate growth and bone development. It is also involved in various metabolic processes, which include release of hormones and neurotransmitters, blood coagulation, muscle contraction and cardiac activity (Hall *et al.,* 1991). Deficiency of calcium can result in rickets, osteoporosis and osteomalacia, while its excess can result in kidney stones.

10.3.2.1.5 Phosphorus
Phosphorus is an important mineral in the bones and teeth; likewise, it is an important component of ribonucleic acids; it is present in phospholipids; and it forms parts of cell membranes. Deficiency of phosphorous results into growth retardation, skeletal deformities, muscle weakness and cardiac arrhythmia, while hyperphosphatemia can result in renal failure (Arai and Sakuma, 2015).

10.3.2.1.6 Magnesium
The human body contains about 25 g of magnesium, of which about 55% of it is found in the bone. Therefore, it is an important constituent of the bone, thereby maintaining bone growth and integrity. Magnesium influences the secretion of parathyroid hormone by the parathyroid gland, and it also functions in the regulation of cardiac cycle. Deficiency diseases associated with lack of magnesium

include hypomagnesaemia and neuromuscular irritability, while symptoms due to toxicity of magnesium are hypotension, respiratory failure and cardiac disturbances (Allen and Sharma, 2019). Dietary sources are cereal, meat, milk, green leafy vegetable, banana, etc.

10.3.2.1.7 Sulfur

The major source of sulphur in the body is mainly from protein-rich foods, especially the sulphur-containing amino acids (Naik, 2012). They are therefore constituents of proteins. Likewise, they are a component of bile acid, glycans, thiamine, lipoic acid and are also involved in detoxification processes. The effect of their deficiencies and excessive intake are not known yet. Dietary sources are plant and animal proteins, eggs, cauliflower.

TABLE 10.2
Microminerals: Functions and Sources

S/N	Minerals	Functions	Sources	References
1	Iron (Fe)	Helps in the formation of heme proteins needed for the transport of oxygen to the red blood cells, flavoproteins and other enzymes.	Fe is widely distributed in organ meats, red meats (30–70% is haem iron), egg yolks; legumes; dried fruits; dark, leafy greens; iron-enriched breads and cereals; fortified cereals; fish; poultry; shellfish.	Fairweather-Tait and Hurrell (1996)
2	Copper (Cu)	Part of many enzymes including metalloenzymes; needed for red blood cell formation, connective tissues.	Foods high in copper include liver, kidney, shellfish, whole-grain cereals and nuts. Soft or acidic water passing through copper pipes can also contribute copper to the diet.	Fairweather-Tait and Hurrell (1996)
3	Zinc (Zn)	It plays main roles in cell-mediated immunity, bone formation, tissue growth, brain function, growth of the fetus and child. It also has role in pathogenesis of some dermatological disorders.	Meats, fish, poultry, oysters, leavened whole grains, vegetables.	Bagherani and Smoller (2016)
4	Iodine (I)	Growth and development, metabolism, reproduction, thyroid hormone production.	Seafood, foods grown in iodine-rich soil, iodized salt, bread, dairy products.	Fairweather-Tait and Hurrell (1996)
5	Selenium (Se)	Anti-oxidant; selenium is needed for the proper functioning of the immune system and appears to be a key nutrient in counteracting the development of virulence and inhibiting HIV progression to AIDS. It is required for sperm motility and may reduce the risk of miscarriage.	Meats, seafood, grains, cereals, seafood and meat products are the richest sources of Se and are the main contributors to the daily Se intake, whereas vegetables, fruits and beverages are generally rich in Se.	Combs (1988), Fairweather-Tait and Hurrell (1996) and Margaret (2000)
6	Chronium (Cr)	Chromium acts as an antioxidant. It also helps to decrease insulin resistance in diabetic patients.	Dietary sources of chromium include brewer's yeast, cheese, pork kidney, whole grain breads and cereals, molasses, spices and some bran cereals. Lean beef, oysters, eggs, and turkey are sources of chromium.	Anderson *et al.* (1992), Anderson (2000 and Tulasi and Rao (2014)

(Continued)

TABLE 10.2 *(Continued)*
Microminerals: Functions and Sources.

S/N	Minerals	Functions	Sources	References
7	Manganese (Mn)	It activates numerous enzymes – such as hydrolases, transferases, kinases, and decarboxylases – and is a constituent of some enzymes. Manganese also plays a role in blood clotting and hemostasis in conjunction with vitamin K.	Manganese is present in a wide variety of foods, including whole grains, clams, oysters, mussels, nuts, soybeans and other legumes, rice, leafy vegetables, coffee, tea and many spices, such as black pepper.	Watts (1990), Aschner and Aschner (2005) and Buchman (2014)
8	Fluoride (F)	It is involved in formation of bones and teeth; helps prevent dental decay and cavities.	Drinking water (either fluoridated or naturally containing fluoride), fish and most beverages, from oral toothpastes as well.	O'Mullane *et al.* (2016)
9	Molybdenum (Mo)	Functions as a cofactor for at least four enzymes: sulfite oxidase, xanthine oxidase, aldehyde oxidase and mitochondrial amidoxime reducing component.	Legumes; nuts, breads and grains; leafy greens; leafy, green vegetables; milk; liver.	Novotny (2011)

Source: Modified from www.uofmhealth.org/health-library/ta3912.

10.4 PHYTONUTRIENTS

Phytonutrients are bioactive substances found in plant-based foods that offer various health benefits to humans. They include essential nutrients like vitamins and minerals as well as antioxidants and phytochemicals. Phytochemicals, specifically, are a diverse group of plant compounds that are known to prevent chronic illnesses such as heart disease, cancer and diabetes. There are numerous phytochemicals, such as beta-carotene and lycopene, that are found in fruits and vegetables with unique structures and functions. In addition to phytochemicals, plant-based foods also contain vitamins and minerals that are crucial for good health. Incorporating plant-based foods into the diet can help reduce the risk of chronic diseases and promote overall well-being.

10.4.1 Types of Phytonutrients and Dietary Sources

10.4.1.1 Flavonoids

Flavonoids are a large and diverse class of phytochemicals that are found in fruits, vegetables and grains. Flavonoids have been linked to a range of health benefits, such as reducing the risk of cardiovascular disease, cancer and neurodegenerative diseases. One study found that flavonoids can modulate signaling pathways involved in inflammation and cancer development (Panche *et al.*, 2016; Oladele *et al.*, 2020).

10.4.1.2 Carotenoids

Carotenoids are another class of phytochemicals that are found in fruits and vegetables. They are responsible for the bright red, orange and yellow colors of many plant-based foods. Carotenoids have been linked to a range of health benefits, such as reducing the risk of cardiovascular disease and cancer. One study found that carotenoids have antioxidant and anti-inflammatory properties that may help protect against chronic diseases (Goltz and Campbell, 2012).

10.4.1.3 Phenolic Acids

Phenolic acids are a class of phytochemicals found in fruits, vegetables, whole grains and legumes. They have been shown to have antioxidant and anti-inflammatory properties and may help reduce the risk of chronic diseases such as cardiovascular disease and diabetes (Liu, 2013).

10.4.1.4 Alkaloids

Alkaloids are a diverse group of phytochemicals found in various plants, including coffee, tea and cocoa. Alkaloids have various biological effects, including acting as stimulants, analgesics and anti-inflammatory agents. One study found that caffeine, an alkaloid found in coffee, has neuroprotective effects and may reduce the risk of neurodegenerative diseases (Cao and Loewenstein, 2021).

The phytochemistry of phytonutrients is a complex area of study with potential health benefits. Consuming a diverse range of plant-based foods is important to ensure a variety of phytonutrients in diet.

10.4.2 Pharmacological and Biological Activities of Phytonutrients

10.4.2.1 Antioxidant Activities of Phytonutrients

10.4.2.1.1 Turmeric

The phytonutrients in turmeric have potent antioxidant properties. Specifically, curcumin, which is the main active ingredient in turmeric, was found to exhibit strong antioxidant activity (Oladele *et al.*, 2020, 2023).

10.4.2.1.2 Garlic

The phytonutrients in garlic, particularly allicin, were found to have significant antioxidant activity, according to a study by Agarwal and Gupta (2019). The study suggested that the antioxidant properties of garlic may be useful in preventing diseases related to oxidative stress.

10.4.2.1.3 Cinnamon

The phytonutrients in cinnamon, particularly cinnamaldehyde, were found to have strong antioxidant activity (Zare *et al.*, 2019; Oladiji and Oladele, 2023). The study also suggested that cinnamon may be a promising candidate for preventing and treating oxidative stress-related diseases.

10.4.2.1.4 Granola

According to Liu *et al.* (2020a, 2020b), granola's phytonutrients, especially polyphenols, have potent antioxidant activity. The study suggested that the antioxidant properties of granola may be beneficial in reducing oxidative stress and inflammation in the body.

10.4.2.1.5 Oregano

Eşrefoğlu *et al.* (2020) found that oregano's phytonutrients, particularly phenolic compounds, have strong antioxidant activity. The study also found that oregano extract was effective in scavenging free radicals.

10.4.2.2 Anti-inflammatory Activities of Phytonutrients

Inflammation is a natural process that the body's immune system uses to defend against foreign pathogens and injury. Excessive and prolonged inflammation can lead to various diseases, such as diabetes, cancer and cardiovascular diseases (Oladele *et al.*, 2020). Phytonutrients are bioactive compounds present in plant-based foods that have anti-inflammatory properties (Oladiji and Oladele, 2023).

Curcumin is a polyphenol that is commonly found in turmeric and has been widely researched for its anti-inflammatory effects (Oladele *et al.*, 2023). It inhibits the activation of NF-κB, a transcription factor that regulates inflammation. A study conducted by Aggarwal *et al.* (2007) showed that cur-cumin can reduce the production of pro-inflammatory cytokines such as IL-1, IL-6 and TNF-A.

Resveratrol is another polyphenol found in grapes, berries and peanuts (Oladele *et al.*, 2021). It has been shown to have anti-inflammatory properties by inhibiting the activation of NF-κB and the production of pro-inflammatory cytokines. Resveratrol also inhibits COX-2, which is a crucial enzyme involved in the inflammatory response (Chen *et al.*, 2014; Oladele *et al.*, 2022).

Quercetin, a flavonoid, is present in many fruits and vegetables (Oladele *et al.*, 2021). It has anti-inflammatory properties by inhibiting the production of pro-inflammatory cytokines such as IL-1, IL-6 and TNF-A (Kim *et al.*, 2015). Quercetin also inhibits the activation of NF-κB (Oladele *et al.*, 2021).

EGCG is a catechin that is present in green tea. It has been shown to have anti-inflammatory properties by inhibiting the production of pro-inflammatory cytokines and the activation of NF-κB (Mokra *et al.*, 2023). EGCG also inhibits the expression of COX-2.

10.4.2.2.1 Turmeric

Curcumin, which is the primary phytonutrient in turmeric, has been found to have anti-inflammatory properties in a review conducted by Gupta *et al.* (2013). The review suggests that curcumin's anti-inflammatory effects may be beneficial in preventing and treating different inflammatory diseases.

10.4.2.2.2 Garlic

The phytonutrients present in garlic, particularly allicin, were found to have potent anti-inflammatory activity in a study by Rahman *et al.* (2021). The study proposes that garlic may have therapeutic potential in the treatment of inflammatory diseases.

10.4.2.2.3 Cinnamon

In a study by Yerra *et al.* (2019), it was discovered that the phytonutrients in cinnamon, especially cinnamaldehyde, exhibit anti-inflammatory properties. The study suggests that cinnamon could have therapeutic applications in the treatment of inflammatory diseases (Oladiji and Oladele, 2023).

10.4.2.2.4 Granola

The polyphenols present in granola were found to have significant anti-inflammatory activity in a study by Liu *et al.* (2020a). The study suggests that the anti-inflammatory properties of granola may be useful in reducing inflammation and associated disorders.

10.4.2.2.5 Oregano

Carvacrol and thymol, the primary phytonutrients in oregano, were found to have potent anti-inflammatory activity in a study by Silva *et al.* (2020). The study suggests that oregano may have therapeutic potential in the treatment of inflammatory diseases due to its anti-inflammatory and antioxidant properties.

Phytonutrients like curcumin, resveratrol, quercetin and EGCG have been found to have anti-inflammatory properties. These compounds can reduce the activation of NF-κB and the production of pro-inflammatory cytokines, which play a crucial role in the inflammatory response. Consuming these phytonutrients through a balanced diet may help to prevent chronic diseases by reducing inflammation.

10.4.2.3 Antiviral Activities of Phytonutrients

Viruses are a significant cause of infectious diseases globally, and while vaccines and antiviral drugs exist, drug-resistant strains and high treatment costs have emphasized the need for alternative options. Phytonutrients are bioactive substances found in plant-based foods that have antiviral properties. Several phytonutrients such as quercetin, EGCG, curcumin and resveratrol have antiviral effects against various viruses, including influenza, hepatitis B and C, HIV and herpes simplex virus. These phytonutrients work by inhibiting viral entry, viral gene expression and viral assembly and release.

Quercetin is a flavonoid found in many fruits and vegetables and has antiviral activity against influenza, hepatitis C and HIV. EGCG is a catechin present in green tea and has antiviral effects against influenza, hepatitis B and herpes simplex virus. Curcumin, a polyphenol found in turmeric, exhibits antiviral activity against influenza, hepatitis B and herpes simplex virus. Resveratrol, a polyphenol found in grapes, berries and peanuts, shows antiviral activity against influenza, HIV and herpes simplex virus.

10.4.2.3.1 Turmeric

In a review study conducted by Oladiji and Oladele (2023), it was discovered that the phytonutrient curcumin found in turmeric has antiviral properties. The research suggests that curcumin has potential as an antiviral agent against various viruses.

10.4.2.3.2 Garlic

A review by Nantz *et al.* (2012) indicates that garlic has antiviral properties, particularly against influenza viruses. The study suggests that phytonutrients such as allicin and alliin present in garlic have the potential to treat and prevent viral infections.

10.4.2.3.3 Cinnamon

A study conducted by Khan *et al.* (2020a) found that the phytonutrient cinnamaldehyde present in cinnamon has antiviral properties against several viruses. The research suggests that cinnamon can be a potential natural antiviral agent.

10.4.2.3.4 Granola

In a study by Kim *et al.* (2018), it was discovered that oats, a primary ingredient in granola, contain phytonutrients that have antiviral properties against several viruses. The research suggests that oats' antiviral properties can help prevent and treat viral infections.

10.4.2.3.5 Oregano

Astani *et al.* (2010) conducted a study on oregano and discovered that its phytonutrients, including carvacrol and thymol, have antiviral properties against several viruses. The research suggests that oregano has potential as a natural antiviral agent.

10.4.2.4 Immunological Activities of Phytonutrients

Phytonutrients help improve immune system functioning through multiple mechanisms, such as augmenting immune cell activity and mitigating inflammation. For instance, quercetin is a phytonutrient that may improve immune function by improving immune cell function. Another phytonutrient, beta-carotene, which is converted to vitamin A in the body, plays a crucial role in immune function. Furthermore, curcumin, found in turmeric, has anti-inflammatory and antioxidant characteristics that enhance immune function.

10.4.2.4.1 Turmeric

According to research conducted by Aggarwal *et al.* (2007), the presence of curcumin in turmeric has immunomodulatory properties. The study suggests that curcumin can boost the immune system's function and response.

10.4.2.4.2 Garlic

A review by Oladiji and Oladele (2023) suggests that garlic has immunomodulatory properties. The research indicates that phytonutrients present in garlic, including allicin and alliin, can enhance the immune system's response to infections and diseases.

10.4.2.4.3 Cinnamon

Oladiji and Oladele (2023) found that cinnamon has immunomodulatory properties. The study indicates that the presence of cinnamaldehyde, a phytonutrient in cinnamon, can stimulate the immune system's function and response.

10.4.2.4.4 Granola

Delaney *et al.* (2003) found that oats, which are a primary ingredient in granola, have immunomodulatory properties. The research indicates that beta-glucans, a type of phytonutrient present in oats, can enhance the immune system's response.

10.4.2.4.5 Oregano

According to Leyva-López *et al.* (2017), oregano has immunomodulatory properties. The research indicates that phytonutrients in oregano, including carvacrol and thymol, can enhance the immune system's function and response.

10.4.2.5 Antibacterial Activities of Phytonutrients

Phytonutrients are natural compounds that occur in plants and have been linked to various health benefits, including antibacterial properties. According to research, flavonoids, phenolic acids and terpenoids are among the phytonutrients with the potential to hinder the growth of bacterial pathogens, including those that are multidrug-resistant (Khan *et al.*, 2020b).

For instance, flavonoids like quercetin and kaempferol have been proven to impede the growth of diverse bacterial strains, including *Escherichia coli, Staphylococcus aureus* and *Pseudomonas aeruginosa* (Kumar *et al.*, 2019). Additionally, phenolic acids like gallic acid and ellagic acid have demonstrated antibacterial effects against several bacterial species (Borges *et al.*, 2013). Similarly, terpenoids such as carvacrol and thymol, present in essential oils, have exhibited potent antibacterial activity against both Gram-positive and Gram-negative bacteria.

10.4.2.5.1 Turmeric

Curcumin, a phytonutrient found in turmeric, has been found to possess antibacterial properties in a study conducted by Khan *et al.* (2020b). Their research has demonstrated that curcumin can inhibit the growth of different bacterial strains, including *E. coli, S. aureus* and *P. aeruginosa*.

10.4.2.5.2 Garlic

According to Khan *et al.* (2020b) and Oladiji and Oladele (2023), garlic has been identified to possess antibacterial properties. The research suggests that phytonutrients, such as allicin and ajoene, found in garlic, can prevent the growth of different bacterial strains.

10.4.2.5.3 Cinnamon

Oladiji and Oladele (2023) have found that cinnamon has antibacterial properties. Their review suggests that cinnamaldehyde, a phytonutrient in cinnamon, has the potential to inhibit the growth of various bacterial strains, including *E. coli, S. aureus* and *P. aeruginosa*.

10.4.2.5.4 Granola

In a study by Delaney *et al.* (2003), beta-glucans, a type of phytonutrient present in oats, a primary ingredient in granola, were found to possess antibacterial properties. The research indicates that beta-glucans can prevent the growth of different bacterial strains.

10.4.2.5.5 Oregano

Oregano has been identified to possess antibacterial properties, according to a review by Leyva-López *et al.* (2017). The research suggests that carvacrol and thymol, phytonutrients in oregano, can prevent the growth of different bacterial strains.

10.4.2.6   Antifungal Activities of Phytonutrients

Phytonutrients are active compounds found in plants and are known to have various therapeutic properties, including antifungal activity. The antifungal potential of phytonutrients is due to their ability to interfere with fungal cellular machinery, leading to cell death. Recent research has shown that several types of phytonutrients, including phenolics, flavonoids and terpenoids, exhibit antifungal activity against different fungal pathogens (Mishra *et al.*, 2021; Oladele *et al.*, 2022b).

For instance, essential oils containing phenolic compounds such as eugenol and thymol have potent antifungal activity against *Candida albicans* and *Aspergillus fumigatus* (Kumar *et al.*, 2017). Flavonoids, like quercetin and kaempferol, have also been found to possess antifungal properties and can inhibit the growth of *Candida* species (Silva *et al.*, 2017). Terpenoids, including carvacrol and linalool, have been shown to be effective against several fungal pathogens, including *Candida* and *Aspergillus* species (Soliman *et al.*, 2017).

The antifungal potential of phytonutrients highlights their potential as alternative treatments for conventional antifungal agents. Moreover, the use of phytonutrients as adjunct therapy to conventional antifungal agents could be a strategy to combat antifungal resistance, which is an increasingly concerning issue.

10.5   BIOAVAILABILITY OF PHYTONUTRIENTS

Phytonutrients are natural compounds found in plants that offer various health benefits. The degree and speed at which they are absorbed into the bloodstream and reach the target tissues, known as bioavailability, determines their positive impact on health. The bioavailability of phytonutrients can be influenced by various factors, including the food matrix, processing and individual factors such as age and gut microbiota. The food matrix, which refers to the physical and chemical structure of the food, can affect the solubility, stability and absorption of phytonutrients. Processing techniques like cooking, grinding and fermentation can also alter the chemical and physical properties of phytonutrients, affecting their bioavailability. Individual factors like aging and gut microbiota composition can affect the absorption of phytonutrients. Understanding these factors is crucial in optimizing the health benefits of phytonutrients. Techniques like optimizing the food matrix, preserving the integrity of phytonutrients during processing and regulating gut microbiota can help improve their bioavailability. Proper bioavailability of phytonutrients ensures the maximum health benefits that they offer.

10.6   CONCLUSION AND FUTURE PROSPECTS

Dietary fibres and phytonutrients are important components of our diet and have various health benefits. This might be due to their structural properties and their interaction with other components of the biological system. Vitamins and minerals are micronutrients required in smaller quantities when compared with macronutrients. They are very key to normal body functioning and health status of the body. Phytonutrients are bioactive compounds found in plant-based foods that offer a range of potential health benefits. They have been linked to reduced risk of chronic diseases such as cancer, heart disease and diabetes as well as improved overall health and well-being. While more research is needed to fully understand the mechanisms of phytonutrients and their effects on the body, incorporating a variety of colorful fruits and vegetables into the diet is a simple and effective way to increase intake of these important nutrients. Future research is to focus on the mechanistic interaction of the constituents of these dietary molecules with the biomarkers known for specific health challenges.

REFERENCES

AACC (2001). Report of the dietary fibre definition committee to the Board of Directors of the American Association of Cereal Chemists. 46: 3. W-2001-0222-010.

Agarwal, K. C. and Gupta, A. (2019). Garlic and its constituents: Implication in cancer prevention and therapy. In L. G. Nagpal (Ed.), *Functional foods and human health* (pp. 143–166). Heidelberg: Springer. https://doi.org/10.1007/978-981-13-9405-8_7

Aggarwal, B. B., Sundaram, C., Malani, N. and Ichikawa, H. (2007). Curcumin: The Indian solid gold. In Aggarwal, B.B., Surh, YJ., Shishodia, S. (eds): *The molecular targets and therapeutic uses of curcumin in health and disease* (pp. 1–75). New York City: Springer US.

Allen, M. J. and Sharma, S. (2019). Magnesium. [Updated 2023 Feb 20]. In: StatPearls [Internet]. Treasure Island (FL): StatPearls Publishing; 2023 Jan-. Available from: https://www.ncbi.nlm.nih.gov/books/NBK519036/

Anderson, R. A. (2000). Chromium in the prevention and control of diabetes. *Diabetes Metab*, 26(1), 22–27.

Anderson, R. A., Bryden, N. A. and Polansky, M. M. (1992). Dietary chromium intake: Freely chosen diets, institutional diets and individual foods. *Biol Trace Elem Res*, 32, 117–121.

Ankar, A. and Kumar, A. (2019). Vitamin B12 deficiency (cobalamin) [Updated 2019 January 11]. In *StatPearls* [Internet]. Treasure Island, FL: StatPearls Publishing, January. Available from: www.ncbi.nlm.nih.gov/books/NBK441923/

Arai, H. and Sakuma, M (2015). Bone and nutrition. Bone and phosphorus intake. *Clin Calcium,* 25(7), 967–972.

Aschner, J. L. and Aschner, M. (2005). Nutritional aspects of manganese homeostasis. *Mol Asp Med,* 26, 353–362.

Astani, A., Reichling, J. and Schnitzler, P. (2010). Screening for antiviral activities of isolated compounds from essential oils. *Evidence-Based Complementary and Alternative Medicine*, 2011, 1–8. https://doi.org/10.1093/ecam/neq074

Awuchi, C. G., Igwe, V. S., Amagwula, O. I. and Echeta, C. K. (2020). Health benefits of micronutrients (vitamins and minerals) and their associated deficiency diseases. A systemic review. *International Journal of Food Sciences*, 3(1), 1–32.

Bagherani, N. and Smoller, B. R. (2016). An overview of zinc and its importance in dermatology-Part I: Importance and function of zinc in human beings. *Glob Dermatol,* 3(5), 330–336. https://doi.org/10.15761/GOD.1000185.

Borges, A., Ferreira, C., Saavedra, M. J. and Simoes, M. (2013). Antibacterial activity and mode of action of ferulic and gallic acids against pathogenic bacteria. *Microbial Drug Resistance*, 19(4), 256–265. https://doi.org/10.1089/mdr.2012.0163

Buchman, A. R. (2014). Manganese. In A. C. Ross, B. Caballero, R. J. Cousins, K. L. Tucker, and T. R. Ziegler (Eds.), *Modern nutrition in health and disease* (11th edn, pp 238–244). Baltimore: Lippincott Williams & Wilkins.

Bulló, M., Casas-Agustench, P., Amigó-Correig, P., Aranceta, J. and Salas-Salvadó, J. (2007). Inflammation, obesity and comorbidities: The role of diet. *Public Health Nutrition*, 10(10A), 1164–72.11.

Cao, C. and Loewenstein, D. A. (2021). Caffeine as a protective factor in dementia and Alzheimer's disease. *Journal of Alzheimer's Disease*, 83(3), 1003–1015. https://doi.org/10.3233/JAD-210262

Chen, C. C., Chow, M. P., Huang, W. C., Lin, Y. C., Chang, Y. J. and Flavonoids, Y. C. (2014). Flavonoids inhibit tumor necrosis factor-A-induced up-regulation of intercellular adhesion molecule-1 (ICAM-1) in respiratory epithelial cells through activator protein-1 and nuclear factor-κB: Structure–activity relationships. *Molecular Pharmacology*, 66(3), 683–693.

Christakos, S., Dhawan, P., Verstuyf, A., Verlinden, L. and Carmeliet, G. (2015). Vitamin D: Metabolism, molecular mechanism of action, and pleiotropic effects. *Physiol Rev*, 96(1), 365–408.

Clifford, J., Niebaun, K. and Bellows, L. (2015). Food and nutrition series. fact Sheet. Colorado State University Extension. No. 9: 333.

Codex Alimentarius Commission (CAC) (2005). Report of the 27th session of the codex committee on nutrition and foods for special dietary uses, Bonn, Germany 21–25 November 2005. ALINORM 06/29/26.

Cogswell, M. E., Mugavero, K., Bowman, B. A. and Frieden, T. R. (2016). Dietary sodium and cardiovascular disease risk – measurement matters. *N Engl J Med*, 375(6), 580.

Combs Jr, G. F. (1988). Selenium in foods. *Adv Food Res*, 32, 85–113.

Delaney, B., Nicolosi, R. J., Wilson, T. A., Carlson, T., Frazer, S., Zheng, G. H., Hess, R., Ostergren, K., Haworth, J. and Knutson, N. (2003). Beta-glucan fractions from barley and oats are similarly antiatherogenic in hypercholesterolemic Syrian golden hamsters. *The Journal of Nutrition*, 133(2), 468–475. https://doi.org/10.1093/jn/133.2.468. PMID: 12566485.

Devinder, D., Mona, M., Hradesh, R. and Patil, R. T. (2012). Dietary fibre in foods: A review. *J Food Sci Technol,* May–June, 49(3), 255–266. https://doi.org/10.1007/s13197-011-0365-5

Eşrefoğlu, M., Gül, M. and Öztürk, N. (2020). Antioxidant activity of Origanum vulgare L. extract: An in vitro study. *Turkish Journal of Medical Sciences*, 50(4), 1117–1122. https://doi.org/10.3906/sag-1909-171

Fairweather-Tait, S. and Hurrell, R. F. (1996). Bioavailability of minerals and trace elements: Members of EC flair concerted action no. 10: Measurements of micronutrient absorption and status. *Nutr Res Rev*, 9(1), 295–324.

Goltz, S. R. and Campbell, W. W. (2012). Carotenoids and cardiovascular health. *American Journal of Lifestyle Medicine*, 6(6), 361–371. https://doi.org/10.1177/155982761245330

Gomez-Pomar, E., Hatfield, E., Garlitz, K., Westgate, P. M. and Bada, H. S. (2018). Vitamin E in the preterm infant: A forgotten cause of Hemolytic Anemia. *Am J Perinatol*, 35(03), 305–310.

Gray, J. (2006). *Dietary fibre: Definition, analysis, physiology and health*. International Life Science Institute. Brussels Belgium: ILSI Europe Concise Monograph Series. 1–44.

Gupta, S. C., Patchva, S. and Aggarwal, B. B. (2013). Therapeutic roles of curcumin: Lessons learned from clinical trials. *The AAPS Journal*, 15(1), 195–218. https://doi.org/10.1208/s12248-012-9432-8

Hall, D., Cromwell, G. and Stahly, T. (1991). Effects of dietary calcium, phosphorus, calcium: Phosphorus ratio and vitamin K on performance, bone strength and blood clotting status of pigs. *J Anim Sci*, 69(2), 646–655.

Halliwell, B. (2001). Vitamin C and genomic stability. *Mutat Res/Fundam Mol Mech Mutagen*, 475(1), 29–35.

He, F. J. and MacGregor, G. A. (2008). Beneficial effects of potassium on human health. *Physiol Plant*, 133(4), 725–735.

Heredia, A., Jimenez, A., Fernandez-Bolanos, J., Guillen, R. and Rodriguez, R. (2002). *Fibra Alimentaria*. Madrid: Biblioteca de Ciencias, pp. 1–117.

Hipsley, E. H. (1953). Dietary "Fibre" and pregnancy toxemia. *Br Med J*, 2, 420–422.

Hodgetts, V., Morris, R., Francis, A., Gardosi, J. and Ismail, K. (2015). Effectiveness of folic acid supplementation in pregnancy on reducing the risk of small-for-gestational age neonates: A population study, systematic review and meta-analysis. *BJOG: Int J Obstet Gynaecol*, 122(4), 478–490.

Ikeda, K., Liu, X., Kida, K., Marutani, E., Hirai, S., Sakaguchi, M. et al. (2016). Thiamine as a neuroprotective agent after cardiac arrest. *Resuscitation*, 105, 138–144.

Kay, M. C. (1982). Dietary fibre. *Journal of Lipid Research*, 23, 221–235.

Kennel, K. A., Drake, M. T. and Hurley, D. L. (2010). Vitamin D deficiency in adults: When to test and how to treat. *Mayo Clin Proc*, 85(8), 752–758.

Khan, A., Khan, T., Ali, S. S., Mehmood, M. H., Khan, A. and Ahmed, F. (2020a). Cinnamaldehyde and its derivatives: Mechanisms for antiviral effect. *Journal of Medicinal Plants Research*, 14(3), 89–97. https://doi.org/10.5897/JMPR2019.6929

Khan, R., Islam, B., Akram, M., Shakil, S., Ahmad, A., Ali, S. M. and Siddiqui, M. (2020b). Antibacterial activities of phytonutrients against multidrug-resistant bacteria. *Journal of Taibah University Medical Sciences*, 15(3), 188–194. https://doi.org/10.1016/j.jtumed.2020.01.011

Kim, Y., Narayanan, S., Chang, K. O. and Inhibition, I. V. (2015). Inhibition of influenza virus replication by plant-derived isoquercetin. *Antiviral Research*, 118, 68–78.

Kim, Y., Narayanan, S., Chang, K. O. and Inhibition, V. P. (2018). Antiviral activities of cereal grains against human norovirus surrogates. *Journal of Food Science*, 83(3), 734–740. https://doi.org/10.1111/1750-3841.14036

Kumar, S., Pandey, A. K. and Pandey, A. C. (2019). Medicinal attributes of flavonoids: A review. *International Journal of Pharmaceutical Sciences and Research*, 10(5), 2298–2311. https://doi.org/10.13040/IJPSR.0975-8232.10(5).2298-11

Kumar, V., Yadav, D. K. and Ahmad, A. (2017). Antifungal activity of eugenol and thymol against fungi isolated from onychomycosis. *Brazilian Journal of Microbiology*, 48(1), 145–152. https://doi.org/10.1016/j.bjm.2016.10.002

Leyva-López, N., Gutiérrez-Grijalva, E. P., Vazquez-Olivo, G. and Heredia, J. B. (2017). Essential oils of Oregano: Biological activity beyond their antimicrobial properties. *Molecules*, 22(6), 989. doi: 10.3390/molecules22060989.

Liu, R., Xue, Y., Huang, X. and Liu, Y. (2020a). Evaluation of the antioxidant activity of granola using in vitro models. *Food Science and Technology*, 40(2), 392–397. https://doi.org/10.1590/fst.17419

Liu, R., Xue, Y., Huang, X. and Liu, Y. (2020b). In vitro anti-inflammatory activity of granola extracts. *Journal of Food Biochemistry*, 44(7), e13239. https://doi.org/10.1111/jfbc.13239

Liu, R. H. (2013). Health-promoting components of fruits and vegetables in the diet. *Advances in Nutrition*, 4(3), 384S–392S. https://doi.org/10.3945/an.112.003517

Lotternberg, A. M. P., Fan, P. L. T. and Buonacorso, V. (2010). Effects of dietary Fibre intake on inflammation in chronic diseases. *Medical Developments*, 8, 254–258.

Luis Gomez, A., Tchekalarova, J. D., Atanasova, M., da Conceição Machado, K., de Sousa Rios, M. A., Jardim, M. F. P. et al (2018). Anticonvulsant effect of anacardic acid in murine models: Putative role of GABAergic and antioxidant mechanisms. *Biomed Pharma*cother, 106, 1686–1695. https://doi. org/10.1016/j.biopha.2018.07.121.

Lykstad, J. and Sharma, S. (2019). Biochemistry, water soluble vitamins. [Updated 2019 February 16]. In *StatPearls* [Internet]. Treasure Island, FL: StatPearls Publishing, January. Available from: www.ncbi. nlm.nih.gov/books/

Margaret, P. R. (2000). The importance of selenium to human health. *Lancet*, 356(9225). https://doi. org/10.1016/S0140–6736(00)02490–9.

Mishra, A., Sharma, A. K., Kumar, S. and Saxena, A. K. (2021). Phytonutrients: Promising antifungal agents for the management of fungal infections. *Pharmacognosy Reviews*, 15(30), 66–81. https://doi.org/10.4103/ phrev.phrev_16_20

Moisa, C., Gaman, M. A., Pascu, E. G., Dragusin, O. C., Assani, A. D., Epingeac, M. E. and Gaman, A. M. (2018). The role of oxidative stress in essential thrombocythemia. *Arch Balk Med Union,* 53(1), 70–75.

Mokra, D., Joskova, M. and Mokry, J. (2023). Therapeutic effects of green tea polyphenol (–)-epigallocatechin-3-gallate (EGCG) in relation to molecular pathways controlling inflammation, oxidative stress, and apoptosis. *International Journal of Molecular Sciences*, 24(1), 340. https://doi.org/10.3390/ijms24010340

Muhammad, A., Munir, N., Daniyal, M., Egbuna, C., Găman, M.-A., Onyekere, P. F. and Olatunde, A. (2020). Vitamins and minerals: Types, sources and their functions. In C. Egbuna and G. Dable-Tupas (Eds.), *Functional foods and nutraceuticals*. New York: Springer. https://doi.org/10.1007/978-3-030-42319-3_9.

Naik, P. (2012). *Essentials of biochemistry*. New Delhi and Panama City, London: Jaypee Brothers Medical Publishers (P) Ltd.

Nair, R. and Maseeh, A. (2012). Vitamin D: The "sunshine" vitamin. *J Pharmacol Pharmacother*, 3(2), 118.

Nantz, M. P., Rowe, C. A., Muller, C. E., Creasy, R. A., Stanilka, J. M. and Percival, S. S. (2012). Supplementation with aged garlic extract improves both NK and γδ-T cell function and reduces the severity of cold and flu symptoms: A randomized, double-blind, placebo-controlled nutrition intervention. *Clinical Nutrition*, 31(3), 337–344. https://doi.org/10.1016/j.clnu.2011.11.019

Novotny, J. A. (2011). Molybdenum Nutriture in Humans. *J Evid Based Complement Alter Med,* 16(3), 164–168.

Oda, T., Aoe, S., Sanada, H. and Ayano, Y. (1993). Effects of soluble and insoluble fibre preparations isolated from oat, barley, and wheat in liver cholesterol accumulation in cholesterol-fed rats. *J Nutr Sci Vitaminol*, 39, 73–79.

Oladele, J. O., Oladele, O. T., Adewole, T. S., Oyeleke, O. M. and Oladiji AT. (2022). Phytochemicals and natural products: Efficacy in the management/treatment of neurodegenerative diseases. Chapter 10. In Ajeet Singh. (ed): *Handbook of research on advanced phytochemicals and plant-based drug discovery*. Hershey, USA, Pennsylvania: IGI Publisher Hershey. https://doi.org/10.4018/978-1-6684-5129-8.ch010

Oladele, J. O., Oladele, O. T. and Oyeleke, O. M. (2021). Possible health benefits of polyphenols in neurological complications associated with COVID-19. *Acta facultatis medicae Naissensis*, 38, 294–309.

Oladele, J. O., Oyeleke, M. O., Adewole, S. T., Ademiluyi, O. A., Olowookere, B. D. and Oladele, O. T. (2023). Ethanol extract of Curcuma longa protects against carbon tetrachloride induced oxidative stress, renal and hepatic damage in rats. *Journal of Pharmacology and Toxicology,* 18(1), 32–41. https://doi. org/10.3923/jpt.2023.32.41

Oladele, J. O., Oyeleke, M. O., Awosanya, O. O. and Oladele, T. O. (2020). Effect of *Curcuma longa* (turmeric) against potassium bromate-induced cardiac oxidative damage, hematological and lipid profile alterations in rats. *Singapore Journal of Scientific Research*, 10, 8–15.

Oladele, O. T., Aladejana, M. O., Adewole, T. S., Olowookere, B. D. and Oladele, J. O. (2022b). Phytochemicals as a antimicrobial agents: Application in infectious diseases. Chapter 11. In Ajeet Singh. (ed): *Handbook of research on advanced phytochemicals and plant-based drug discovery*. Hershey, USA, Pennsylvania: IGI Publisher Hershey, https://doi.org/10.4018/978-1-6684-5129-8.ch011

Oladiji, A. T. and Oladele, J. O. (2023). Spices as potential human disease panacea. Chapter 16. In L. Kambizi and C. Bvenura (Eds.), *Sustainable uses and prospects of medicinal plants*. London: CRC. Taylor and Francis. https://doi.org/10.1201/9781003206620-16

O'Mullane, D. M., Baez, R. J., Jones, S., Lennon, M. A., Petersen, P. E., Rugg Gunn, A. J., Whelton, H. and Whitford, G. M. (2016). Fluoride and oral health. *Community Dent Health*, 33, 69–99.

Ormsbee, M. J., Bach, C. W. and Baur, D. (2014). Pre-exercise nutrition: The role of macronutrients, modified starches and supplements on metabolism and endurance performance. *Nutrients*, 6(5), 1782–1808.

Panche, A. N., Diwan, A. D. and Chandra, S. R. (2016). Flavonoids: An overview. *Journal of Nutritional Science*, 5, e47. https://doi.org/10.1017/jns.2016.41

Rahman, M. A., Rahman, M. M., Kundu, S. K., Hossain, M. J. and Hasan, M. M. (2021). Allicin, a phytonutrient of garlic, in the management of inflammatory diseases: A review. *Phytotherapy Research*, 35(1), 1–18. https://doi.org/10.1002/ptr.6853

Reddy, P. and Jialal, I. (2018). Biochemistry, vitamin, fat soluble. [Updated 2018 November 23]. In *StatPearls* [Internet]. Treasure Island, FL: StatPearls Publishing, 2019 January. Available from: www. ncbi.nlm.nih. gov/books/NBK534869/.

Rivellese, A., Riccardi, G., Giacco, A., Pacioni, D., Genovese, S., Mattioli, P. L. and Mancini, M. (1980). Effect of dietary fibre on glucose control and serum lipoproteins in diabetic patients. *Lancet*, 2, 447–449.

Schmölz, L., Schubert, M., Kluge, S., Birringer, M., Wallert, M. and Lorkowski, S. (2018). The hepatic fate of Vitamin E. In J. A. Morales-Gonzalez (Ed.), *Vitamin E in health and disease*. IntechOpen. https://doi.org/10.5772/intechopen.79445. Available from: www.intechopen.com/books/vitamin-e-in-health-and-disease/the-hepatic-fate-of-vitamin-e.

Silva, L. N., da Silva, C. R., de Souza, T. B., Ferreira, G. F., Silva, N. C. and Dias, D. F. (2017). Antifungal activity of flavonoids and their potential application in the development of new antifungal agents. *Frontiers in Microbiology*, 8, 125. https://doi.org/10.3389/fmicb.2017.00125

Silva, M. M., da Silva, M. S., Souza, M. A., de Souza, C. R., de Almeida, T. S., dos Santos, M. H., . . . Costa, E. A. (2020). Oregano (Origanum vulgare L.) essential oil and its main phytonutrients exhibit anti-inflammatory and antioxidant properties. *Food Research International*, 137, 109703. https://doi. org/10.1016/j.foodres.2020.109703

Soliman, S. S. M., Almahdy, D. A. and El-Keblawy, A. A. (2017). Antifungal activity of some plant extracts against fungal strains isolated from poultry farms in Egypt. *Journal of Applied Pharmaceutical Science*, 7(1), 181–187. https://doi.org/10.7324/JAPS.2017.70125

Sorice, A., Guerriero, E., Capone, F., Colonna, G., Castello, G. and Costantini, S. (2014). Ascorbic acid: Its role in immune system and chronic inflammation diseases. *Mini Rev Med Chem*, 14(5), 444–452.

Takahashi, H., Yang, S. I., Hayashi, C., Kim, M., Yamanaka, J. and Yamamoto, T. (1993). Effect of partially hydrolyzed guar gum on fecal output in human volunteers. *Nutr Res*, 13, 649–657.

Tulasi, G. and Rao, K. J. (2014). Essentiality of chromium for human health and dietary nutrition. *J Entomol Zoolgy Stud*, 2(1), 107–108.

Tungland, B. C. and Meyer, D. (2002). Nondigestible oligo and polysaccharides (dietary fibre): Their physiology and role in human health and food. *Compr Rev Food Sci Food Saf*, 1, 73–92.

Velioglu, Y. S., Mazza, G., Gao, L. and Oomah, B. D. (1998): Antioxidant activity and total phenolics in selected fruits; vegetables; and grain products. *Journal of Agricultural and Food Chemistry*, 46, 4113–4117.

Watts, D. L. (1990). The nutritional relationships of manganese. *J Orthomolecular Med*, 5(4), 219–222.

Weaver, C. M. (2013). Potassium and health. *Adv Nutr*, 4(3), 368S–377S.

Wellen, K. and Hotamisligil, G. S. (2005). Inflammation, stress, and diabetes. *J Clin Invest.*, 115(5), 1111–1119.

Wiley, K. D. and Gupta, M. (2019). Vitamin B1 thiamine deficiency (beriberi) [Updated 2019 January 2]. In *StatPearls* [Internet]. Treasure Island, FL: StatPearls Publishing, January. Available from: www.ncbi. nlm.nih.gov/books/NBK537204/

Xu, H., Barnes, G. T., Yang, Q., Tan, G., Yang, D. and Chou, C. J. (2003). Chronic inflammation in fat plays a crucial role in the development of obesity-related insulin resistance. *J Clin Invest.*, 112(12), 1821–1830.

Yerra, V. G., Kalvala, A. K., Kumar, A. and Ismail, A. (2019). Cinnamaldehyde and its derivatives, a novel class of antihyperglycemic agents with anti-inflammatory and antioxidant properties. *Current Medicinal Chemistry*, 26(11), 1993–2003. https://doi.org/10.2174/0929867325666180515144241

Zare, R., Hajiaghaee, R., Mohammadi, M., Sadeghi, M. and Akbari, H. (2019). Antioxidant activity and total phenolic content of cinnamon extracts obtained from different accessions. *Journal of Food Measurement and Characterization*, 13(4), 2928–2934.

11 Nutrition and Mental Health

*Fatima Alaba Ibrahim, Taoheed Olawale Bello,
Idowu Yetunde Fakolujo, Johnson Olaleye
Oladele, and Adenike Temidayo Oladiji*

11.1 INTRODUCTION

Nutrition is the scientific study of foods, eating habits, nutrient composition, nutritional status, and individual and population health and disease (ADA, 2006; Ajayi et al., 2021). Nutrition is the field of science that encompasses a wide range of information, including data from the basic sciences, behavioral economics, and other disciplines. Nutritional research and knowledge are continually evolving, but implementing new findings into clinical practice or incorporating them into public policy takes time. Even if the research findings are promising, new research findings are difficult to adopt into clinical practice (ADA, 2006; Ajayi et al., 2021).

Nutrients are nutritional components that the body needs in the correct amounts to grow, reproduce, and live a normal, healthy life. Nutrients include carbohydrates, water, lipids, proteins, vitamins, and minerals (Mudambi and Rajagopal, 2007; Ajayi et al., 2021). Each group contains a diverse range of nutrients, such as carbs, water, lipids, proteins, vitamins, and minerals. As a result, food delivers over 40 basic nutrients that are used to make thousands of compounds necessary for life and physical fitness (Mudambi and Rajagopal, 2007). Nutrition is determined by the types of foods consumed by the body and the efficiency with which the body processes those foods. It also suggests that such nutrients are used in the body in such a way that one's physical and mental health is preserved at the maximum degree possible throughout one's life (Mudambi and Rajagopal, 2007).

According to Saxena et al. (2007), the vast majority of nations devote less than 1% of their health expenditures to mental health, resulting in a treatment difference of greater than 75% in many lower- and medium-income nations (Saxena et al., 2007; WHO, 2011).

Behavioral and mental-health disorders (e.g., depression, nervousness, substance misuse, aggressiveness, attention-deficit and behavioral problems, and post-traumatic stress) are the major causes of adjustment problems in adolescents and young people (Gore et al., 2011). Mental health issues are frequently regarded as a lesser concern in developing and low-income countries; nevertheless, even high-income countries have de-prioritized mental health and devoted substantially fewer supplies to mental health compared to physical health.

As a result, it's critical to address this increasing trend of mental illnesses, which will lower people's well-being, increase mortality and impairment due to mental disease, and possibly worsen the underlying health sickness (Alexopoulos, 2005). Mental problems can also increase rates of suicide, cause economic damage (absenteeism from work), and impair general family functioning if not treated properly. Furthermore, mental illness raises the risk of complications of physical illnesses like heart disease, endocrine diseases, respiratory problems, and a variety of others. As a result, mental illness has far-reaching consequences for both the person and society as a whole (Aucoin et al., 2018).

Many epidemiologies are being undertaken in order to reveal changeable risk factors for the prevention of mental illness; one such key element has been identified as dietary considerations. Different dietary habits, foods, and nutrients have also been suggested as having an impact on the start, maintenance, and magnitude of mental problems (Benton et al., 1995). Numerous biological and epidemiological researches have shown the role of diet and nutrition in the prevention and treatment of mental illnesses.

DOI: 10.1201/9781003361497-13

11.2   THE IMPACT OF NUTRITION ON MENTAL HEALTH

Omega-3, -6, and other necessary fatty acids, which are mostly received from external sources and support the healthy growth of brain neurons, make up the majority of the fat in the human brain (Bilici et al., 2004).

Diets that are Western include meat pies, processed meats, pie, chips, hamburgers, white bread, sweetener, flavored milk drinks, beer; traditional: vegetables, fruit, meat, fish, whole-grain foods; and modern: fruits, vegetables, fish, tofu, beans, nuts, dairy, red wine (Bourre, 2004). Major research on diet and mental health is compiled in Table 11.1.

TABLE 11.1
Major Research on Diet and Mental Health

Psychiatric Illness	References	Nutrition understudy	Major Highlight
Distress	Penckofer et al., 2010; Maurizi, 1990; Eritsland, 2000; Mohandas and Rajmohan, 2007 and	Vitamin D rich diet Adjuvant treatment with omega-3 fatty acids Zinc and selenium Vitamins and minerals (folate, vitamin B12)	Reduced risk of depression lowered chance of mood disorders like depression decreased chance of depression decreased chance of depression
An emotional disorder of the bipolar schizophrenia spectrum	Stoll et al., 1999	Omega-3 fatty acids	superior in social, occupational, and also other domains as well as intellect.
	Aucoin et al., 2018	Improper eating practices using processed sugars and fats; adhering to a low-fibre diet; and including omega-3 and omega-6 fatty acids, vegetables, fruit, and particular minerals and vitamins	The incidence of metabolic syndrome is increased by medications.
Developmental disorder	Humphries et al. (2004)	Unhealthy diet	A secondary learning impairment brought on by inadequate diet.
Eating store attention, eating store	Hilbert et al. (2017)	Unhealthy diet	Lower reaction to treatment
Hyperactivity deficiency disorders (ADHD)	Sinn (2008)	Iron, zinc, and magnesium deficiency	ADHD is a threatening factor
Addiction	Cook et al. (1998)	Lack of some of these vitamins and minerals, or malnourishment	Increases the risk of anemic, neurological issues (including Wernicke's encephalopathy, cognitive deficits, impaired vision, and Korsakoff's psychosis in alcoholics), and other problems.
Mental decline	Valls-Pedret et al. (2012, 2015)	Glucose management is aided by polyphenols, the Mediterranean diet, and dietary supplements like olive oil and almonds.	Both young adults and the elderly experience cognitive deterioration.

Source: Kumar et al., 2020.

11.2.1 DEPRESSION

In those who have poor eating habits and are overweight, obesity, depression, and nutritional variables have all been associated with an increase in depressed symptomatology. Additionally, it has been found that women who eat foods high in vitamin D have a reduced risk of developing depression (Bourre, 2004). Studies have also demonstrated the efficacy of omega-3 fatty acids as an additional treatment for major depressive illness (Bourre, 2006). Numerous studies have confirmed this finding and found that omega-3 fatty acid also reduce inflammation, suggesting they may be helpful in the production of neurotransmitters (Brown et al., 1990). It has been demonstrated that a low-fat diet has the ability to depress mood; alterations in dietary fat consumption can impair focus and cause fatigue, while a high-protein diet boosts alertness.

In the onset and management of depression, minerals and vitamins (such as folate and vitamin B12) are also crucial (Bruinsman and Taren, 2009). One of the most typical neuropsychiatric signs of folate insufficiency is depression (Buydens-Branchey et al., 2003). Depressed people have levels that are over 25% lower than those of their healthy counterparts. Depression has been associated with low levels of selenium and zinc. A diet strong in sugar, processed flour, and saturated/trans fatty acids and poor in antioxidants and fibre-rich foods may make depression more frequent, according to a study (Curtis and Patel, 2008). Nutrition, a body's natural defense system, and the proper running of the nervous system are fully accountable for an individual 's mental well-being, according to research in the fields of psychoneuroimmunology and chemical routes. Twenty researchers are beginning to accept diet and nutrition as significant factor in the prevention of mental illnesses (Alexopoulos, 2005).

Forgetfulness is a critical challenge in many mental conditions; it can be enhanced by eating memory-boosting foods like berries (which have flavonoids), nuts, and seedlings (omega-3 fatty acid widely known as alpha-linolenic acid). Caffeine boosts memory by increasing concentration and alertness (Grotzkyj-Giorgi, 2009). Our mental health has a significant impact on our physical health. Numerous studies have discovered a connection between the two. Depression and other psychiatric conditions can aggravate or cause a wide range of medical situations, which include insomnia, cardiovascular disease, gastrointestinal disorders, metabolic disease, and fatigue. As the saying goes, "Let meal be thy medicine-Hippocrates." When there is a psychiatric imbalance, such as depression and other mood disorders, acting quickly can improve well-being.

11.2.2 MANIC-DEPRESSIVE DISORDER (MDD)

In a study of manic-depression patients, omega-3 fatty acids were linked to overall course of the illness. In studies comparing the response of omega-3 fatty acids, anticonvulsants (lithium carbonate), and a placebo (olive oil), sick people on omega-3 fatty acids had a much higher rate of remission compared to the placebo group. Other areas where the omega-3 fatty acid group surpassed the others included intelligence, social interaction, and occupational achievement (Humphries et al., 2009).

11.2.3 PSYCHOSIS SUSCEPTIBILITY SYNDROME (PSS)

Nutrition is essential in patients with psychopathy because it improves general health and reduces antipsychotic medication after-effects such as metabolic syndrome. Unhealthy dietary habits have been linked to the use of finely tuned carbohydrates and fat, a low-fibre diet, omega-3 and omega-6 fatty acids, veggies, fruit, and particular vitamins and minerals (folic acid, selenium, vitamins B_{12}, vitamin B_6, ascorbic acid, and zinc) (Khanna et al., 2019). According to studies, patients with severe psychosis have faulty eating patterns and a deficient meal organization, such as eating heavy meals in the night and omitting breakfast (Lian et al., 2019).

Schizophrenic patients have extremely high levels of glycated hemoglobin and insulin and also a relatively wider waist circumference and higher value for diastolic blood pressure than their healthy counterparts. As a result, these findings corroborate the benefits of a balanced dietary pattern and general well-being as part of schizophrenia therapy, lowering the condition's overall burden (Mohandas and Rajmohan, 2007).

11.2.4 COGNITIVE DISABILITIES (DD)

In terms of cognitive/intellectual disorders, a systematic dietary review found that deficient nutrition (e.g., anemia) is a potential risk for the source of secondary learning problems, exacerbating the existing illness (Owen and Corfe, 2017).

11.2.5 ANOREXIA NERVOSA (AN)

Correct nutrition-value knowledge of a specific item aids in an improved treatment response in individuals suffering from anorexia nervosa (eating disorders). In these patients, a nutritional remedy, in addition to pharmacological treatment, is vital (Popa, 2012).

11.2.6 ATTENTION-DEFICIT DISORDER (ADD)

Microelement deficiencies levels such as magnesium, iron, and zinc have been found to aggravate hyperactivity and attention difficulties in ADD children. Thus far, omega-3 polyunsaturated fatty acids (PUFA) have provided the most powerful evidence of a dietary contribution (Rocks et al., 2014).

11.2.7 SUBSTANCE DEPENDENCE (SD)

Substance dependence disorders, particularly alcoholism, are influenced by nutrition. Malnourishment (protein-calorie malnutrition) is an indicator of chance of living in patients with alcohol hepatic disease in patients co-occurring with alcoholism (ALD). Furthermore, a deficiency of vitamins and minerals such as folic acid, retinol, pyridoxine, and vitamin B_1 actually adds to malnourishment, raising the risk of anemic conditions and neurological complications (developmental delays, nyctalopia [night blindness], Wernicke's disease, and Korsakoff's syndrome) (Roick et al., 2007).

11.2.8 COGNITIVE DECLINE

Nutritional deficiencies can intensify cognitive decline. Inadequate diet causes vascular defects, which are commonly linked to senile dementia and other cognitive disorders. Poor glucose control has been connected to cognitive dysfunctions, even in younger people (Sarris, 2019). Diet not only benefits the elderly, but it also reduces the risk of cognitive impairment in adults. Additionally, some study has focused on the impact of polyphenols and supplements from the Mediterranean diet, which include olive oil and nuts, in enhancing cognitive performance in both young adults and the old (Sarris, 2019).

11.3 PREDISPOSING FACTORS FOR MENTAL HEALTH ISSUES

The link between a healthy diet and mental wellness includes brain growth. A number of disparities, such as the increase in threatening factors linked to the intake of fast foods and additives, mental well-being, and socio-economic issues including poverty, alcoholism, and obesity can all influence the development of mental health disorders. It has been established that both of these disparities and malnutrition are intricately related.

11.3.1 PROCESSED FOODS AND FOOD ADDITIVES

Inadequate dietary habits in children and teenagers are linked to worse mental health, including increased consumption of saturated fat, processed carbohydrates, and fast foods. O'Neil and associates (2014) and Beyer and Payne (2016) found that manic depression patients have a nutritional pattern that is of worse quality and higher in glucose, lipids, and starches (Beyer and Payne, 2016).

Depression rates growing concurrently with those of conventional diets rich in polyunsaturated fatty acids were also being deserted in favor of more packaged foods, according to research on how people in the Artic and sub-Artic regions were modifying their diets (McGrath-Hanna et al., 2003).

11.3.2 DEFICIT PHYSICAL HEALTH

A number of major physical health problems, including myocardial ischemia, several malignancies, osteoporosis, and dental ailments, have been related to changes in food production methods, such as processing, the use of supplements, and industrial farming (Ferro and James, 2001).

11.3.3 POVERTY

Nutrition and mental health are significantly impacted by poverty. The complicated and cumulative consequences of poverty and mental health issues on nutrition quality are influenced by a variety of factors, including revenue, comprehension and capability, food accessibility and standard, as well as time, wellness, and comfort. The standard of a person's, a household's, and a community's nutrition varies according to socioeconomic status. Energy-dense, nutrient-poor meals are more frequently consumed by persons with lower socioeconomic standing and less financial means, while higher-quality diets are linked to greater affluence (PHE, 2013).

Food preferences are influenced by socioeconomic status and household earnings, which is a factor that is getting more and more significant as household earnings drops.

Comparatively lower portions of fruits and vegetables are consumed in statutory aid households than in non-benefit households. Malnourished patients were brought to hospitals at a rate of more than 5,400 in 2012, although 347,000 people were served by food banks during the same year (BMJ, 2013). It is important to look into how nutritional difficulties affect these groups' mental health conditions.

11.3.4 OBESITY

A complex association exists between obesity and mental health issues. According to a review of longitudinal studies published in 2010, there is a bidirectional association between depression and obesity, with those who are obese having a 55% higher lifetime risk of acquiring the condition, while those who are sad have a 58% higher lifetime risk (Luppino et al., 2010).

Although poor nutrition can lead to obesity, other demographic characteristics, including the degree of obesity, socioeconomic position, educational levels, sex, age, and ethnic background, may affect area/extent of the link between obesity and mental health (Luppino et al., 2010).

11.3.5 ALCOHOL

Alcohol and mental wellbeing have a complex relationship. In addition to being a contributing factor to excessive alcohol use, mental health problems can also be the result of it. In short, alcohol is a depressant that can quickly worsen mood. Alcohol alters sleep patterns, which may result in less energy. Alcohol can produce mood swings by depressing the central nervous system. Some people use it as a way to suppress their feelings and keep from dealing with uncomfortable situations. Additionally, drinking alcohol is connected to altered eating habits, nutritional inadequacies, and disturbed sleep patterns. Although the effects of dietary changes brought on by alcohol consumption on mental health are not fully understood, studies have indicated that vitamin B is crucial in avoiding dementia brought on by alcohol (Korsakoff psychosis) (Tolmunen et al., 2004).

11.4   NUTRITIONAL PROTECTIVE FACTORS FOR MENTAL HEALTH

The brain can sustain healthy neurotransmitter activity with the aid of a diet high in polysaccharides, vital lipids, proteins, vitamins, minerals, and water. It has been demonstrated to defend the brain from the consequences of oxidants, which have been demonstrated to have a detrimental influence on mental and emotional well-being. Throughout the lifetime, there is proof of nutrition's protective abilities.

From an early age, good eating has been connected to academic success. A number of studies have confirmed that giving kids breakfast improves their academic performance (Meyers et al., 1989). Numerous studies that have been published have demonstrated that children who are under-nourished behave poorly at school, with claims of decreased fighting, absences, and increased concentration when nourishing foods are offered (Murphy et al., 1998).

A diet rich in omega-3 and omega-6 fatty acid and lower in saturated fatty acids appears to prevent the deterioration of memory and other cognitive issues as we age (Gómez-Pinilla, 2008). Fruits and vegetables and vitamins, minerals, and acids make up the two divisions.

11.4.1   FRUITS AND VEGETABLES

High levels of mental health have been associated with eating vegetables. The eating of fruits and vegetables by an individual, together with smoking, was found to be the behavioral risk factor most frequently linked to both poor and excellent mental health in both genders (Stranges et al., 2014).

11.4.2   MINERALS, VITAMINS AND ACIDS

Micronutrients such as vitamins and minerals play a range of significant roles, including supporting amino acids in turning into neurotransmitters and helping vital fatty acids enter the brain.

Due to the fact that they can transform carbohydrates into simple sugars, fatty acids into healthy nerve cells, and amino acids into neurotransmitters, they play a significant role in defending mental well-being.

Numerous mental health problems have been connected to micronutrient deficits. Research findings have demonstrated that increased intake of these fatty acids can assist in controlling manic-depressive illness. For example, unbalanced dietary intakes of essential fatty acids have been connected to a variety of psychiatric problems, including depression and problems with attention and memory problems (Beyer and Payne, 2016).

According to research, these fatty acids are linked to greater mental well-being, even after accounting for other variables (such as revenue, age, and eating habits) as well as a lower chance of cognitive deficits in midlife (Kalmijn et al., 2004).

11.5   MOLECULAR MECHANISM IMPACT OF NUTRITION ON MENTAL HEALTH

A balanced nutrition pattern can influence mental health and wellness via inflammation and oxidative stress, neuroplasticity, microbiota gut-brain axis, mitochondrial dysfunction, and microbiome immune-modifying mechanisms as well as epigenetic changes (Marx et al., 2017). Dietary profile influences not only brain composition, formation, and purpose but also endogenous hormones,

TABLE 11.2

List of Essential Vitamins and Minerals as well as Their Effects and Sources

Nutrients	Effect of nutrients deficiency	Sources of food
Thiamine (vit.B$_1$)	Inability to concentrate and pay attention	Vegetables and whole grains
Niacin (vit.B$_3$)	Depression	Wholegrains Vegetables
Panthothenic acid (vit.B$_5$)	Poor memory and stress are both caused by deficiency in vitamin B$_5$.	Wholegrains and vegetables
Pyridoxine (vit.B$_6$)	Irritability, poor memory, stress, and depression are all symptoms of vitamin B$_6$ deficiency.	Bananas and wholegrains
Cobalamin (vit.B$_{12}$)	Confusion, poor memory, and psychosis are all symptoms of vitamin B$_{12}$ deficiency.	Meat, fish, dairy products, and eggs are all examples of animal products
Ascorbic acid (vit.C) deficiency	Depression.	Fruits and vegetables
The mineral folic acid	Anxiety, depression, and psychosis.	Vegetables with green leaves
Magnesium	Irritability, insomnia, and sadness from magnesium.	Nuts and seeds as well as green leafy vegetables
Selenium	Irritability to selenium and sadness.	Whole meal, liver, fish, sunflower spore, Brazil nuts, clove, and baker's yeast
Zinc	Manifestations of zinc deficiency include uncertainty, untaught state, sadness, appetite loss, and a lack of desire.	Oysters, seafood, nuts, and seeds

Source: Holford (2003).

peptides, chemical messenger, and microbiota-gut-brain axis, which, in turn, plays an important role in anxiety and inflammatory modulation and cognitive ability retention (Adan et al., 2019).

Several pathways are implicated in mental health and can be regulated by diet (Berk et al., 2013 and Moylan et al., 2014). Despite being described as specific pathways, it is possible that these biochemical mechanisms overlap synergistically and interconnect with one another.

11.5.1 Inflammation and Oxidative Stress

Inflammation, defined as the presence of pro-inflammatory cytokines and acute phase response, is connected to the growth of manic depression, dementia, and de novo depression (Berk et al., 2013 and Fernandes et al., 2016). Despite the absence of clinical symptoms, oxidative stress and impaired antioxidant properties have been linked to a variety of non-communicable diseases, including mental illness (Cunningham, 2013). The genesis of this inflammation are multidimensional and include a variety of lifestyle factors such as psychological stress, smoking, fatness, insomnia, and most importantly, inadequate diet (Berk et al., 2013). With reference to mental illness, there is developing body of investigation probing the viable dialogue between pathological changes in sleep patterns (Clark and Vissel, 2014), stress (Lee and Giuliani, 2019), and mental disorders (Salim et al., 2012) and inflammatory diseases that require a rise in inflammatory cytokines in order to be liberated.

Several studies have also found transforming growth factor β1 (TGF-β1) to play a significant function in regulating gut microbiota (Bauche and Marie, 2017), and its deficiency can perform a crucial role in the physiopathology of mental instability both in stress and Alzheimer's disease (AD) (Caraci et al., 2018). It has been reported by different researchers that a deficiency in the role of inflammatory cytokines to reduce inflammation, which include TGF-β1, can lead to the origin of mental instability. TGF-β1 production and liberation from intestinal epithelial cell interference can occur from gut imbalance-reliant alterations of butyrate (Martin-Gallausiaux et al., 2018).

Sleep disturbance is hypothesized to affect inflammatory state, activating microglia in the central nervous system (Irwin et al., 2016), decreasing neuron plasticity and hippocampus ontogenesis, changing chemical transmitter synthesis, and gene copy, detecting epigenetic alterations that lead to short-term and long-term imbalances of neuronal role and behavior (Irwin et al., 2016). Thus, stress and mental disorders have been linked with elevated inflammatory status and disturbance in brain usefulness and may be connected to insomnia. Recently, investigations have shown a bifacial connection between mental illness, swelling, and oxidative pressure. Insomnia, stress, and worry may therefore be related with elevated degree of IL-6 and CRP (Tayefi et al., 2017). Dietary patterns and food intake, for example, can influence the expression of inflammatory biomarkers, which, one by one, affect inflammation. Several nutritional factors have been proposed to influence inflammatory reactions via pro- or anti-inflammatory cytokine production and control of the nuclear factor kappa-light-chain-enhancer of activated B cells (NF-kB) biochemical cascade (Minihane et al., 2015). Plant-based foods, which including vegetables, fruits, leafy greens, lentils, and whole cereals, have been shown to have neuroprotection and anti-inflammatory impacts because of their significant vitamin and phytochemicals content (Irwin et al., 2016). Similarly, monounsaturated fatty acid (MUFA) obtained from olive oil as well as certain polyunsaturated fatty acid (PUFA) from fish, such as omega-3 fatty acid, have anti-inflammatory outcomes, which enhance cognitive performance (Irwin et al., 2016).

Foods high in calories, artificial sweeteners, hydrogenated oils, and additives, on the other hand, may influence the production of pro-inflammatory cytokines, worsening both the inflammatory factor and cognitive abilities (Irwin et al., 2016). Similarly, rich glycemic foods and packaged meat intake have been linked to the synthesis of inflammatory biomarkers (Alisson-Silva et al., 2016). Finally, the previously mentioned phenyl-valerolactones, which are derived from gut microbiota transformation of flavan-3-ols, may exert neuroprotective effects in secondary preventative measures for AD via an anti-inflammatory mechanism, as they have been found to reduce glial overactivation in amyloid-oligomer-treated mice (Ruotolo et al., 2020).

11.5.2 Neuroplasticity

Neurogenesis, especially in the hippocampus, is linked to studying, recollection, and emotional control, whereas altered neurogenesis is linked to mental illness (Zainuddin and Thuret21). Brain-derived neurotrophic factor (BDNF) and other neurotrophins (such as bcl-2 and vascular endothelial growth factor) are thought to be involved in hippocampal neurogenesis (Fernandes et al., 2014, 2015). Currently, clinical research on the effect of diet on this pathway is limited; however, preliminary data confirms the importance of nutrition in boosting BDNF levels. For example, in people with schizophrenia, a 4-week nutritional intercession to increase the intake of fruit and vegetables that have high carotenoid content (eight servings daily) led to higher serum levels of BDNF compared to the control group (Guimaraes et al., 2008). Furthermore, an epidemiological study of older adults found a link between inadequate diet and decreased hippocampal volume (Jacka et al., 2015). Nutrients such as n-3 fatty acids (Kawakita et al., 2006), polyphenols (Williams et al., 2008), l-theanine, and vitamin E, in addition to having antioxidant and anti-inflammatory properties, can also stimulate neurogenesis, whereas foods that are high in calories, refined sugar, and fat impair this process (Molteni et al., 2002; Zainuddin and Thuret, 2012;Martire et al., 2014).

11.5.3 Microbiota Gut-Brain Axis

The composition of the intestinal microbiota in healthy adults is generally steady over time, with Firmicutes (including Enterococcus genus, Clostridium, and Lactobacillous) and Bacteroidetes (i.e., Bacteroides genus) dominating the gut microbiome (Cenit et al., 2017). Pathogenic conditions may result from changes in the gut microbiome characterized by an abundance of facultative anaerobes (*Escherichia coli*), pro-inflammatory *Ruminococcus*, or nonbacterial microbes (Hills et al., 2019). As a result, the diversity and balance of gut microbiota strains are significant determinant of overall body wellness (Fava et al., 2018). Furthermore, the type, quality, and origin of food influence the structure and feature of the gut microbiota (Dawson et al., 2016). Fibre, prebiotics, and probiotics have been found to modify the gut microbiota (Makki et al., 2018 and Houghton et al., 2018). Healthy eating habits, such as the Mediterranean diet and other plant-rich diets, have been linked to increased microbiota diversity (St-Onge and Zuraikat, 2019). Although preliminary, some research has suggested a link between gut microbiota composition and depressed mood and reaction to chronic stress (Dash et al., 2015).

The current focus of research is on the exchange of signals affected by gut microbiota that are discovered and transduced in details from the gut to the nervous system via inflammatory, endocrine, and neural mechanisms (Osadchiy et al., 2019). The production of molecules such as SCFAs, secondary bile acids, and tryptophan metabolites (O'Mahony et al., 2015) – as well as folate and GABA (Tuohy et al., 2015) – by the gut microbiota has been demonstrated to significantly impact neurotransmitter metabolism, with implications for enteric and central nervous system function. The signal can be spread by interacting with enteroendocrine cells (EECs) and enterochromaffins cells (ECCs), which can induce central responses (for example, by controlling serotonin release) via long-distance neural signaling via sensory nerve fibres that extend into intestinal villi (Gershon, 2013).

The intestinal microbiota influence the modulation of gut peptides, which are part of the complicated pathway that characterizes the gut-brain axis (Lach et al., 2018). The neuropeptide Y, which is abundant in the brain (including the nucleus of the solitary tract, hypothalamus, and amygdala) and is highly controlled by peripheral signaling, has the capacity to control GABA release (Martin et al., 2018). Another mechanism may rely on hormone-like, glucagon-like peptide-1, an incretin hormone involved in the modulation of the HPA axis and overall stress response as well as in lowering after-meal blood glucose via augmentation of gastric inhibitory peptide release and obstruction of glucagon secretion (Zietek and Rath, 2016). Cholecystokinin (CKK) is a peptide that is formally called pancreazymin that can regulate gastric emptying, gallbladder contraction, pancreatic enzyme liberation, and appetite suppression. It has been shown to play a role in anxious behavior at the central-nervous-system level by activating CCK2 receptors in limbic regions (Ballaz, 2017). Serum ghrelin, known for its adipogenic effects and role in stress response (i.e., triggering motivation for rewards), has been linked to changes in certain gut bacteria strains, such as being negatively correlated with commensal *Bifidobacterium* and *Lactobacillus* strains, and proportionate with *Bacteroides/Prevotella* species (Morris et al., 2018). When subjected to chronic stress, corticotropin-releasing factor (CRF) plays a vital role in response to stressful situations by arbitrating the neural control of adrenocorticotropin release from pituitary corticotropes, which, in turn, control cortisol production acutely but may result to the formation of stress-related disorders (i.e., anxiety and depression) (Fox and Lowry, 2013). The CRF system, as well, impacts some gastrointestinal functions, such as motility and permeability (Galley and Bailey, 2014). Interestingly, animal experiments revealed that increased CRF was associated with changes in the intestinal microbial community (i.e., a decrease in *Lactobacillus*) as well as an inverse relationship between CRF receptor signaling (i.e., corticotropin-releasing factor mediated activation of the hypothalamic – pituitary – adrenal) and altering the gut microbiota (Chatoo et al., 2018).

One of the most intriguing links between brain and gut microbiota is the latter's rearrangement of the structure of (poly)phenols (Del-Rio et al., 2013), resulting in the release into the bloodstream of smaller compounds that are putatively active at the nervous system level. Among these, the chemical reorganization of flavan-3-ols, one of the most common flavonoid subclasses, has received a lot of attention (Mena et al., 2019). The main flavan-3-ol colonic metabolites – namely, phenyl-valerolactones – have recently been discovered to be capable of crossing the blood-brain barrier and being accessible to neuronal cells (Angelino et al., 2019), where they might efficiently impede with amyloid-oligomer assembly, depicting a potential novel therapeutic agent to prevent Aβ aggregation and Aβ-induced neurodegeneration in Alzheimer's disease (AD) (Ruotolo et al., 2020). Moreover, some other small colonic metabolites are the subject of similar research, as they have been shown to have anti-inflammatory activity at the neuronal level (Carregosa et al., 2020). In terms of human intervention studies, a recent trial found that acute supplementation with a grape and Western blueberry high in polyphenol extract enhanced cognitive performance, with a significant impact on specific brain function such as working memory and attentiveness (Philip et al., 2019).

An impaired intestinal microbiota, distinguished by a limited number of different species and a predominance of harmful bacterial species over the others (so-called "dysbiosis"), results in increased permeability of the intestinal mucosa ("leaky gut"), among indirect mechanisms. This clinical condition allows some bacterial components to pass through as lipopolysaccharides (LPS), which bind to circulating monocytes and macrophages and stimulate the production of cytokines (TNF-a, IL-1, IL-6), resulting in a rise in the inflammatory state (Irwin et al., 2016). SCFAs may have anti-inflammatory properties by binding to G-protein receptors found in a variety of cells, including sensory fibres, EECs, gliocytes in the brain, and adipocytes, which suppress a neuro-inflammatory response – i.e., against LPS inflammatory responses in microglia (Sherwin et al., 2016). Furthermore, there is proof to support anti-inflammatory action via neuroglia activation (Kaczmarczyk et al., 2012). Furthermore, gut chemical transmitters, which include serotonin, have been found to possess both pro-inflammatory effects and anti-inflammatory activities, thereby regulating inflammatory and immune reactions (Khan and Ghia, 2010).

11.5.4 MITOCHONDRIAL DYSFUNCTION

Decreased mitochondrial power generation, size, and distribution have been linked to depression, mental illness, and bipolar disorder (Morris et al., 2017; Morris and Berk, 2015). These changes could be attributed to decreased antioxidant activities and a pro-inflammatory cytokine-mediated rise in mitochondrial-derived oxygen and nitrogen-free radicals, implying that inflammation and oxidative stress are to blame for mitochondrial impairment (Morris and Berk, 2015). In animal models, nutrition and functional compounds such as coenzyme Q10, lipoic acid, carnitine, creatine, resveratrol, NAC, and some antidepressants increase mitochondrial respiratory function (Wright et al., 2015; Maes et al., 2012 and Dean et al., 2015).

11.5.5 MICROBIOME MECHANISM IN MENTAL HEALTH

Diet is known to have an impact on the microbiome and can either control or dysregulate it. When the ratio of "probiotic" and "pathogenic" bacteria is off, diseases might arise. A respiratory disorder, obesity, metabolic syndrome, diabetes, emotional and intellectual problems, spastic colon, and others are examples of conditions where the constitution and interconnections of microorganisms, the gut lining, and the immune response go wrong.

Numerous tasks are carried out by healthy gut bacteria, such as the digestion of polysaccharides, the creation of short chain fatty acids, vitamins, and other nutrients. Additionally, they help to detoxify the body, defend against microbes, strengthen the immune system, and regulate the nervous system (ZinAcker and Linseth, 2018).

In terms of mental health, the gut has 90% of 5-hydroxytryptamine receptors (5-HT receptors). Therefore, it is not unexpected that gastrointestinal issues are the most frequent adverse reactions to antidepressants like sertraline or fluoxetine. Frequent complaints from patients include diarrhea, dry mouth, and, in exceptional cases, nausea. These reactions usually leave after 1 to 2 weeks, if not shortly. Prescription antibiotics can also cause gut dysbiosis. Antibiotics have a negative impact on the good bacteria in the gut. One remedy is to consume meals high in probiotics or take a probiotic to shield healthy gut flora (ZinAcker and Linseth, 2018).

Recently, ZinAcker and Linseth examined the Western diet, the relationship between the microbiota and the host, and its impact on metabolic disorders (ZinAcker and Linseth, 2018). They claim that the microbiome (or gut environment) is affected by what we consume and that the Western diet, which is comprised of highly processed foods, has an effect on it. As a result, the gut becomes inflamed, which leads to disorder-related symptoms. The authors explore the effects that these food preservatives have on inflammation in the body and how they may influence disease, even though we already know that processed meals are poor nutritional substitutes for natural fruits and veggies.

Fast foods and obesity, diabetes, and coronary artery disease have been connected in numerous studies. This study examined the idea that diet-microbiome-host interactions during food processing affect inflammatory processes in the body (and consequently, illnesses). Without fully analyzing their effects on the microbiota, the food industry has gradually increased the amount of food preservatives. The results of this study suggest that removing processed foods from our nutrition might reduce the likelihood of developing disorders linked to inflammation.

The withdrawal features that individuals go through when they quit eating packaged meals were the subject of a University of Michigan study (Schulte et al., 2018). The study examined data showing that, in some individuals, food addiction (e.g., consuming highly processed meals) might result in addictive disorder, including withdrawal symptoms. By modifying self-report measurements of drug withdrawal symptoms, the Heavily Packaged Food Withdrawal Scale (ProWS) was created. The researchers think that this scale has the potential to be a reliable psychometric instrument for next studies on human withdrawal from heavily packaged foods (Schulte et al., 2018).

11.5.5.1 Prebiotics and Probiotics

Consuming both prebiotic and probiotic foods establishes microbial equilibrium. Prebiotics are soluble fibres that help feed the probiotics, or good bacteria, in our stomach. The large intestine already contains probiotics. The probiotics will function better the more prebiotics they consume. Examples of prebiotic foods include bulb onions, garden leeks, sparage, edible bananas, sunchoke, chicory root, clove, and dandelion greens (ZinAcker and Linseth, 2018).

Fermented foods that contain these microorganisms such as sauerkraut, dairy with live cultures, cucumbers, kefir, kimchi, kombucha, and soybean paste are examples of "encourage your patients to carefully read labels and steer clear of extra sugar and preservatives." For instance, pickles and dairy may have refined sugar or food coloring. A healthy substitute for sugar is plain yogurt or kefir with berries and cinnamon (ZinAcker and Linseth, 2018).

A recent study suggests that consuming a balanced diet, like the Mediterranean diet, and staying away from foods that cause inflammation may help prevent depression (Lassale et al., 2018). The most convincing evidence came from the Mediterranean diet, which places an emphasis on eating whole grains, fish, and poultry at least twice a week, along with beans, legumes, fruits and vegetables (spinach, kale, salad rocket, "cos" lettuce), dry drupes (almonds, walnuts), broccoli, cabbage, healthy fats (olive and canola oil), and reducing meat (Schulte et al., 2018).

11.6 CELLULAR ASPECT OF NUTRITION AND MENTAL HEALTH

There is little or no awareness of the link between nutrition and depression, whereas there is much awareness of the link between nutritional deficiencies and physical illness. Depression is commonly thought to be solely biochemical or emotionally based. On the contrary, nutrition can influence the onset, severity, and duration of depression. Many of the easily noticeable food patterns that occur prior to depression are also found during depression. These may include a lack of appetite, skipping meals, and a predominance of sweet foods (Shaheen and Vieira, 2008).

The general population's food consumption pattern in many developing and developed countries reflects that they are frequently deficient in many nutrients, particularly important vitamins, minerals, and omega-3 fatty acids (Shaheen and Vieira, 2008). The severity of insufficiency in these nutrients is a prominent part of the nutrition of people with mental disorders. Daily supplements of vital nutrients have been shown in studies to be beneficial in easing patients' symptoms (Shaheen et al., 2008). The classes of foods and how it affects mental health are given in the sections that follow.

11.6.1 CARBOHYDRATES AND MENTAL HEALTH

Carbohydrates occur naturally as polysaccharides that play a vital role in an organism's structure and function. Scientists are growingly interested in the impact of carbohydrates on overall well-being and disorders (Gopinath et al., 2016). The ability of carbohydrate-rich foods to raise blood glucose levels is referred to as their "glycaemic index (GI)," which varies between foods and serves as a criterion of carbohydrate quality. Dietary glycemic load (GL) is the sum of the glycemic index and total carbohydrate content of a given amount of food (Gopinath et al., 2016). Many studies have found that GI has a significant correlation with psychological distress and mental disorders, whereas GL has a negative correlation.

Dietary carbohydrates raise serum insulin levels, which increase tryptophan (a precursor to serotonin) uptake in the brain (Pellegrin et al., 1998). As a result, carbohydrate-rich foods are expected to reduce the occurrence of depression (Murakami et al., 2010). Sweet foods have an immediate and short-term effect on emotions. However, a high intake of low GI foods such as fruits, vegetables, and whole grains is recommended to maintain mental health (Rao et al., 2008).

11.6.2 PROTEINS AND MENTAL HEALTH

Amino acids are the building blocks of proteins. These amino acids influence brain function because they are precursors to neurotransmitters that impact emotions and behaviors. Tyrosine isa precursor to dopamine, and tryptophan is a precursor to serotonin. A lack of these amino acids can result in decreased production of the corresponding neurotransmitters, which can lead to poor mental health and depression. Excessive consumption of these amino acids may also result in mental illnesses and brain injury (Rao et al., 2008). Tryptophan influences neural processing in brain neurocircuits that control mood (Kroes et al., 2014). It has been discovered that reducing tryptophan has a greater influence on mood disruption than increasing carbohydrate intake Shepherd and Raats (2006). However, because tryptophan competes with large neutral amino acid (LNAA) for transport from the blood to the brain, any disparity caused by this mechanism can be alleviated by increasing the tryptophan/LNAA (large neutral amino acid) ratio Kroes and colleagues (2014).

11.6.3 ESSENTIAL FATTY ACIDS AND MENTAL HEALTH

11.6.3.1 Omega-3 Fatty Acids

Lipid content (fats) comprise of a major part of the brain. Brain lipids, which are made up of fatty acids, are structural components of membranes. Grey matter is thought to contain 50% polyunsaturated fatty acids (about 33% of which belong to the omega-3 family), which are obtained through diet. The omega-3 fatty acids (specifically, alpha-linolenic acid [ALA]) participate in the effect of dietary nutrients on the formation and function of the brain, which was the initial confirmation. A lack of omega-3 fatty acids may raise the likelihood of developing mental illnesses such as anxiety, distress, cognitive decline, manic depression, hyperactivity disorder, psychosis, and autism spectrum disorder. According to some research results, lowering plasma cholesterol through diet and prescription drugs increases depressive episodes. The amount and proportion of omega-6 and omega-3 fatty acids that influence serum lipids and change the biochemical and biophysical properties of cellular membrane are important factors to consider (Stoll et al., 1999).

Polar phospholipids, spingolipids, and cholesterol are functional and structural outer layer constituents in brain cells, which is a lipid-rich organ. The brain's glycerophospholipids contain a high proportion of PUFA obtained from essential fatty acids (EFAs), linoleic acid, and linolenic acid. DHA, derived from the omega-3 fatty acids linolenic acid, arachidonic acid (AA), and docosatetraenoic acid, derived from the omega-6 fatty acid linoleic acid, are the most abundant PUFA in the brain. Experiments have shown that diets low in omega-3 PUFA cause significant disruptions in neural function (Sinclair et al., 2007). Eicosapentaenoic acid (EPA) and docosa-hexaenoic acid (DHA) are linked to the maintenance of psychological disorders, and their deficits may contribute to the pathophysiology of psychological illnesses if other contributing factors such as genetic makeup and stressors are present (Lange, 2020; McNamara, 2009). It has been proposed that consuming enough long-chain polyunsaturated acids (PUFAs), particularly DHA, may help to prevent the development of depression. DHA and EPA reduce inflammation by controlling the magnitude and duration of the inflammatory response. They provide depression resistance and anti-depressant effects via anti-inflammatory mechanisms (McNamara, 2009). DHA (22: 6n-3) accounts for approximately 15% (the most abundant) of total fatty acids. DHA must be obtained through diet because mammals do not produce it (Levant, 2013). Intake of EPA between 1.5g to 2g has an effect on patients' depressive symptoms (Lakhan and Vieira, 2008).

11.6.4 Micronutrients

Productions of some neurotransmitters are achieved with the help of Vitamins B_6 and B_{12}. Supplementing with vitamin B_{12} protects the myelin sheath of the axon while also improving mental cognition and intellectual capacity (Rao et al., 2008). Benton et al., 1995 discovered that a year of excessive vitamin supplementation enhanced behaviors and feelings in all test groups. Vitamins B_1, B_2, and B_6 were mainly responsible for these advancements.

Vitamin E, also known as alpha-tocopherol, is a component of cell membranes. It is in charge of neurological processes as well as growing the regularity of lipid packaging. Lipid peroxidation can be hindered by acting as an antioxidant and anti-inflammatory, and it piles up in places where free radical generation is high, such as mitochondrial membranes (Rizvi et al., 2014). It regulates immune response, and a lack of it can impair both inborn and specific immunity (Lewis et al., 2019), significantly raise pregnancy risks, and cause neurological anomalies (Traber, 2014).

Folic acid, or folate, also known as water-soluble vitamin B_9, is converted into the bioavailable form L-methyl folate. The production of serotonin, noradrenaline, and dopamine can be regulated by L-methyl folate, which has a significant impact on mental cognition and function (Leahy, 2017). Folate deficiency is characterized by depressive symptoms. According to research, patients with depression have a 25% lower blood folic acid concentration compared to healthy people (Rao et al., 2008). Vitamin B_9 deficit is caused by insufficient food intake and can result in neural tube anomalies in fetuses and neurological diseases in adults (Polavarapu & Hasbani, 2017).

Magnesium is involved in cell energy metabolism, neurotransmission, nerve conduction study, and plasma membrane stability. It has anti-inflammatory properties as well as the ability to liberate pro-inflammatory molecules (Nielsen, 2018). Magnesium deficiency occurs as a result of poor dietary habits, liquor, illegal substances, and gastrointestinal malabsorption (Polavarapu and Hasbani, 2017).

Iodine performs a key role in mental illness and is supplied by the thyroid hormone to ensure the energy metabolism of the cerebrum. During the pregnancy period, the nutritional reduction of iodine induces serious cerebral impairment, eventually resulting to cretinism (Bourre, 2006).

Iron is required for oxygenation and energy production in the cerebral parenchyma (via cyto-chrome oxidase) as well as the production of neurotransmitters and myelin. Children with hyperactivity disorder have iron deficiency. Iron concentrations in the umbilical artery are critical during fetal development and in relation to child IQ; infantile anemia, with related iron deficiency, is associated with disruption in cognitive function development (Bourre, 2006). Iron is required for oxygenation and energy production in the cerebral parenchyma (via cytochrome oxidase) as well as the production of neurotransmitters and myelin.

Zinc, for example, is involved in the gustation process. At least five studies have found that people with clinical depression have lower zinc levels (Levenson, 2006). Furthermore, intervention studies show that oral zinc can affect the efficacy of antidepressant treatment. Zinc also shields brain cells from the potential damage caused by free radicals.

Several studies have revealed that a child's full genetic potential for physical and mental development may be jeopardized due to a deficiency (even subclinical) of micronutrients. When children and adolescents with poor nutritional status are exposed to changes in mental and behavioral functions, dietary measures can help to correct them, but only to a certain extent. It has been discovered that the nutrient composition of a diet and meal pattern can have either positive or negative, instant or long-term, effects. Deficiencies in antioxidant activity and nutrients (micro-elements, vitamins, and non-essential micronutrients such as polyphenols) in the diet during aging may precipitate neurological diseases due to a failure of the defensive measure against free radicals (Nowak and Szewczyk, 2005).

11.7 NUTRIENTS FOR THE PREVENTION AND TREATMENT OF MENTAL HEALTH PROBLEMS

In particular for individuals at risk or residing in underdeveloped areas, there is strong evidence that a better diet can result in healthy cognitive development and a decreased risk of mental illness. Growth monitoring and supplemental feeding are two of the most effective intervention methods. These strategies integrate nutritional interventions such as food fortification, nutrient supplementation, and functional foods.

The nutrients that impact the central nervous system (CNS) and are most likely to be low in levels necessary for proper brain function are those that are most significant in clinical psychiatric treatment. Nutritional needs are affected by a variety of factors, including dietary inadequacies, malabsorption, stress, disease, age, brain injury, and genetic polymorphisms. Under conditions of oxidative stress, oxygen deficiency, inflammation, or mitochondrial insufficiency, larger quantities of nutrients may be needed to maintain cell function and restoration as well as to prevent cumulative damage.

Iodine is also crucial for preventing learning problems as well as physical and intellectual disability (WHO, 2002c). Children receive enough iodine, thanks to iodine supplementation programs that iodize salt or water. Seventy percent of homes worldwide now use table salt (iodized salt) as a consequence of global initiatives, including those backed by UNICEF. Indirectly, this also prevents the iodine deficit that affects 91 million babies (UNICEF, 2002) and indirectly averts mental and physical health issues.

11.7.1 FOOD FORTIFICATION

To ensure that all necessary trace nutrients are obtained, food fortification adds nutriments (i.e., vitamins and minerals). The procedure of adding fortifiers (essential micro-elements and vitamins) to food during processing is called as food fortification. These additional nutriments are helpful to the food because the general health policy focus is to decrease the number of individuals in a populace who have nutritional deficiencies. Since the late 1990s, folate, often known as vitamin B_9, has been added to flours, cereal crops, and other food grain products. It is a good illustration of the advantages of nutrient fortification. In order to lower the chance of neural tube defects in children, such as spina bifida, diets abundant in folic acid are advised for women who are or aspiring to become pregnant. Other nutrients are added to foods and supplements as well, and for the most part, this fortification is considered advantageous (ADA, 2006).

11.7.2 DIETARY SUPPLEMENTS

Nutrient supplements, which are usually pills containing various nutrients, make it easy for users to get all of the key nutrients (i.e., vitamins and minerals) they need each day. It must be recognized that a supplement may still not comprise all of the vital nutrients required. Specific age groups are targeted by certain supplement formulations (e.g., adolescent, adult female, pregnant women, adult male, and older adults). In the future, nutrient supplements may be developed to meet the demands of specific people, especially those with genetically linked nutrient deficiencies.

11.7.3 NUTRITIOUS FOODS

Nutritious foods or functional foods are food ingredients that may provide health benefits or reduce the risks of chronic conditions. Because of the quantitatively substantial amount of a specific nutrient or phytoconstituents contained in one serving of the meal, the Food and Drug Administration (FDA) of the United States allows numerous specific food products to be regarded as nutritious food or functional foods. A nutritious food, or functional food, is one that contains a biologically active ingredient (nutrient or phytoconstituent) that has substantial health benefits beyond its basic nutritional function, particularly for improving health and reducing the risk of developing disease. The health benefit of the particular nutrient or ingredient of interest must be supported by published research (ADA, 2006).

The focus is on the health benefits of specific foods. A health claim for a nutritious or a functional food, which includes fortified foods, is generally made on the food's tag or carton. The term "functional food" does not, in general, refer to preservatives, supplements, or herb-tea. Functional foods include swamp blueberry, cranberry juice, love apple, spinach, brussels sprouts, garlic, soya, green tea, seafoods, nuts, and granola. Red wine is also considered a functional food. Epidemiological data have shown that these food products have human health benefits, such as a decrease in cardiovascular disease. Examples of "super" functional foods include blueberries and other vegetables (ADA, 2003).

Functional foods can be an extremely good way to meet everyday nutrient requirements. A food-based technique to meet nutritional requirements, rather than depending on supplements or herbal products, which are not truly foods, is important for healthy food habits. Nutritionally rich foods and plant-based foods that are also high in phytochemicals aid body functions effectively.

11.8 NUTRITIONAL PSYCHIATRY

Nutritional psychiatry is becoming a viable medical intervention option for people suffering from worry and misery. Nutritional psychiatrists, as opposed to regular psychiatrists, integrate food into their overall treatment plans (Sarris et al., 2015). Nutritional psychiatry prefers nutrient-rich foods high in vital nutrients, minerals, phytochemicals, dietary fibre, pro- and prebiotics, and protein over nutritionally "empty" calories (such as sugar). These modifications are intended to reduce brain inflammation, improve serotonin and dopamine regulation, and impact a variety of other mood-enhancing responses.

In addition to allopathic medications, some people seek alternative medicine, such as dietary and lifestyle interventions, to enhance their mood and anxiety. While such alternative medicine may be beneficial for mild to moderate depression and nervousness, they are unlikely to improve with suicidal ideation or a behavioral emergency (Marx et al., 2017).

11.9 CONCLUSION

The emergence of mental health is increasing rapidly, but growing evidence suggests a strong link between a poor diet and the worsening of mood disorders such as anxiety and depression as well as other neuropsychiatric conditions. A diet substantial in fruits, vegetables, and protein low in processed and fatty foods, can help to maintain physical and mental well-being. Food fortification, nutrient supplements, and functional foods should be studied further as mood-altering and cognitive-skill agents in both clinical and healthy populations. Priority must also be given to the new research area of nutritional psychiatry, which examines the capacity of nutrition in mental health.

REFERENCES

Adan, R.A.H., Vander-Beek, E.M., Buitelaar, J.K., Cryan, J.F., Hebebrand, J. and Higgs, S. (2019). Nutritional psychiatry: Towards improving mental health by what you eat. Eur Neuropsychopharmacol. 29:1321–1332.

Ajayi, E.I.O., Molehin, O.R., Adefegha S.A., Fakayode, A.E., Oladele, J.O. and Adewumi, S.O. (2021). Nutritional regulation of metabesity. In Nutrition, Food and Diet in Ageing and Longevity. Healthy Ageing and Longevity. 14. https://doi.org/10.1007/978-3-030-83017-

Alexopoulos, G.S. (2005). Depression in the elderly. Lancet. 365:1961–1970.

Alisson-Silva, F., Kawanishi, K. and Varki, A. (2016). Human risk of diseases associated with red meat intake: Analysis of current theories and proposed role for metabolic incorporation of a non-human sialic acid. Mol Asp Med. 51:16–30.

American Dietetic Association. (2003). Position of the American Dietetic Association and Dietitians of Canada. Vegetarian diets. J Acad Nutr Diet. 103:748–765.

American Dietetic Association. (2006). Position of the American Dietetic Association: Food and nutrition misinformation. J Acad NutrDiet. 106:601–607.

Angelino, D., Carregosa, D., Domenech-Coca, C., Savi, M., Figueira, I., Brindani, N., Jang, S., Lakshman, S., Molokin, A. and Urban, J.F. (2019). 5-(Hydroxyphenyl)-γ-valerolactone-sulfate, a key microbial metabolite of Flavan-3-ols, is able to reach the brain: Evidence from different in silico, In Vitro and In Vivo experimental models. Nutrients. 11.

Aucoin, M., LaChance, L. and Cooley, K. (2018). Diet and psychosis: A scoping review. Neuropsychobiology. 10:1–23.

Ballaz, S. (2017). The unappreciated roles of the cholecystokinin receptor CCK(1) in brain functioning. Rev Neurosci. 28:573–585.

Bauche, D. and Marie, J.C. (2017). Transforming growth factor β: A master regulator of the gut microbiota and immune cell interactions. Clin Transl Immunol. 6:e136.

Benton, D., Haller, J. and Fordy, J. (1995). Vitamin supplementation for 1 year improves mood. Neuropsychobiology. 32(2):98–105.

Berk, M., Williams, L.J. and Jacka, F.N. (2013). Depression is an inflammatory disease, but where does the inflammation come from? BMC Med. 11:200.

Beyer, J. and Payne, M.E. (2016). Nutrition and bipolar depression. Psychiatric Clin North Am. 39(1):75–86.

Bilici, M., Yıldırım, F. and Kandil, S. (2004). Double-blind, placebo-controlled study of zinc sulfate in the treatment of attention deficit hyperactivity disorder. Prog Neuro-Psychopharmacol Biol Psychiatry. 28(1):181–190.

Bourre, J. (2004). The role of nutritional factors on the structure and functioning of the brain: An update on dietary requirements. Rev Neurol (Paris). 160(8–9):767–792.

Bourre, J. (2006). Effects of nutrients (in food) on the structure and function of the nervous system: Update on dietary requirements for brain. Part 1: Micronutrients. J Nutr Health Aging. 10(5):377–385.

Brown, R., Blum, K. and Trachtenberg, M. (1990). Neurodynamics of relapse prevention: A neuronutrient approach to outpatient DUI offenders. J Psychoact Drugs. 22(2):173–187.

British Medical Journal. (2013). The rise of food poverty in the UK. BMJ. 347:f7157.

Bruinsma, K. and Taren, D. (2009). Dieting, essential fatty acid intake, and depression. Nutr Rev. 58(4):98–108.

Buydens-Branchey, L., Branchey, M. and McMakin, D. (2003). Polyunsaturated fatty acid status and relapse vulnerability in cocaine addicts. Psychiatry Res. 120(1):29–35.

Caraci, F., Spampinato S.F., Morgese M.G., Tascedda F., Salluzzo M.G., Giambirtone M.C., Caruso G., Munafo A., Torrisi S.A. and Leggio, G.M. (2018). Neurobiological links between depression and AD: The role of TGF-β1 signaling as a new pharmacological target. Pharmacol Res. 130:374–384.

Carregosa, D., Carecho, R., Figueira I. and Santos, C.N. (2020). Low-molecular weight metabolites from polyphenols as effectors for attenuating neuroinflammation. J Agric Food Chem. 68:1790–1807.

Cenit, M.C., Sanz, Y. and Codoner-Franch, P. (2017). Influence of gut microbiota on neuropsychiatric disorders. World J Gastroenterol. 23:5486–5498.

Chatoo, M., Li, Y., Ma, Z., Coote, J., Du, J. and Chen, X. (2018). Involvement of corticotropin-releasing factor and receptors in immune cells in irritable bowel syndrome. Front Endocrinol. 9:21.

Clark, I.A. and Vissel, B. (2014) Inflammation-Sleep interface in brain disease: TNF, insulin, orexin. J Neuroinflamm. 11:51.

Cook, C., Hallwood, P. and Thomson, A. B. (1998). vitamin deficiency and neuropsychiatric syndromes in alcohol misuse. Alcohol. 33(4):317–336.

Cunningham, C. (2013). Microglia and neurodegeneration: The role of systemic inflammation. Glia. 61:71–90.

Curtis, L. and Patel, K. (2008). Nutritional and environmental approaches to preventing and treating autism and attention deficit hyperactivity disorder (ADHD): A review. J Altern Complement Med. 14(1):79–85.

Dash, S., Clarke, G., Berk, M. and Jacka, F.N. (2015). The gut microbiome and diet in psychiatry: Focus on depression. Curr Opin Psychiatry. 28:1–6.

Dawson, S.L., Dash, S.R. and Jacka, F.N. (2016). The importance of diet and gut health to the treatment and prevention of mental disorders. Int Rev Neurobiol. 131:325–346.

Dean, O.M., Turner, A. and Malhi, G.S. (2015) Design and rationale of a 16-week adjunctive randomized placebo-controlled trial of mitochondrial agents for the treatment of bipolar depression. Rev Bras Psiquiatr. 37:3–12.

Del-Rio, D., Rodriguez-Mateos, A., Spencer, J.P., Tognolini, M., Borges, G. and Crozier, A. (2013). Dietary (poly)phenolics in human health: Structures, bioavailability, and evidence of protective effects against chronic diseases. Antioxid. Redox Signal. 18:1818–1892.

Eritsland, J. (2000). Safety considerations of polyunsaturated fatty acids. The American Journal of Clin Nutr. 71(1):1975–2015.

Fava, F., Rizzetto, L. and Tuohy, K.M. (2018). Gut microbiota and health: Connecting actors across the metabolic system. Proc Nutr Soc. 2018:1–12.

Fernandes, B.S., Berk, M. and Turck, C.W. (2014) Decreased peripheral brain-derived neurotrophic factor levels are a biomarker of disease activity in major psychiatric disorders: A comparative meta-analysis. Mol Psychiatry. 19:750–751.

Fernandes, B.S., Molendijk, M.L. and Kohler, C.A. (2015) Peripheral brain-derived neurotrophic factor (BDNF) as a biomarker in bipolar disorder: A meta-analysis of 52 studies. BMC Med. 13:289.

Fernandes, B.S, Steiner, J. and Molendijk, M.L. (2016). C-reactive protein concentrations across the mood spectrum in bipolar disorder: A systematic review and meta-analysis. Lancet Psychiatry. 3:1147–1156.

Ferr-Luzzi, A. and James, W.P.T. (2001). European diet and public health: The continuing challenge. Public Health Nutr. 4(2A):275–292.

Fox, J.H. and Lowry, C.A. (2013). Corticotropin-Releasing factor-related peptides, serotonergic systems, and emotional behavior. Front Neurosci. 7:169.

Galley, J.D. and Bailey, M.T. (2014). Impact of stressor exposure on the interplay between commensal microbiota and host inflammation. Gut Microbes. 5:390–396.

Gershon, M.D. (2013). 5-Hydroxytryptamine (serotonin) in the gastrointestinal tract. Curr Opin Endocrinol Diabetes Obes. 20:14–21.

Gómez-Pinilla, F. (2008). Brain foods: The effects of nutrients on brain function. Nat Rev Neurosci. Jul; 9(7):568–578.

Gopinath, B., Flood, V.M., Kifley, A., Louie, J.C. and Mitchell, P. (2016). Association between carbohydrate nutrition and successful aging over 10 years. J Gerontol Ser A, Biol Sci Med Sci. 71(10):1335–1340.

Gore, F.M., Bloem, P.J., Patton, G.C., Ferguson, J., Joseph, V., Coffey, C., Sawyer, S.M. and Mathers, C.D. (2011). Global burden of disease in young people aged 10–24 years: A systematic analysis. The Lancet. 377(9783):2093–2102.

Grotzkyj-Giorgi, M. (2009). Nutrition and addiction – can dietary changes assist with recovery? Drugs Alcohol Today. 9(2):24–28.

Guimaraes, L.R., Jacka, F.N. and Gama, C.S. (2008) Serum levels of brain-derived neurotrophic factor in schizophrenia on a hypocaloric diet. Prog Neuropsychopharmacol Biol Psychiatry. 32:1595–1598.

Hilbert, A., Hoek, H. and Schmidt, R. (2017). Evidence-based clinical guidelines for eating disorders. Curr Opin Psychiatr. 30(6):423–437.

Hills, R.D., Jr., Pontefract, B.A., Mishcon, H.R., Black, C.A., Sutton, S.C. and Theberge, C.R. (2019). Gut microbiome: Profound implications for diet and disease. Nutrients. 11.

Holford, P. (2003). Optimum Nutrition for the Mind. London: Piatkus.

Houghton, D., Hardy, T., Stewart, C., Errington, L., Day, C.P., Trenell, M.I. and Avery, L. (2018). Systematic review assessing the effectiveness of dietary intervention on gut microbiota in adults with type 2 diabetes. Diabetologia. 61:1700–1711.

Humphries, K., Traci, M. and Seekins, T. (2004). A preliminary assessment of the nutrition and food-system environment of adults with intellectual disabilities living in supported arrangements in the community. Ecol Food Nutr. 43(6):517–532.

Humphries, K., Traci, M. and Seekins, T. (2009). Nutrition and adults with intellectual or developmental disabilities: Systematic literature review results. Intellect Dev Disabil. 47(3):163–185.

Irwin, M.R., Olmstead R. and Carroll, J.E. (2016). Sleep disturbance, sleep duration, and inflammation: A systematic review and meta-analysis of cohort studies and experimental sleep deprivation. Biol Psychiatry. 80:40–52.

Jacka, F.N., Cherbuin, N. and Anstey, K.J. (2015) Western diet is associated with a smaller hippocampus: A longitudinal investigation. BMC Med. 13:215.

Kaczmarczyk, M.M., Miller, M.J. and Freund, G.G. (2012). The health benefits of dietary fibre: Beyond the usual suspects of type 2 diabetes mellitus, cardiovascular disease and colon cancer. Metabolism. 61:1058–1066.

Kalmijn, S., Van-Boxtel, M.P., Ocke, M., Verschuren, W.M., Kromhout, D. and Launer, L.J. (2004). Dietary intake of fatty acids and fish in relation to cognitive performance at middle age. Neurology. 62(2):275–280.

Kawakita, E., Hashimoto, M. and Shido, O. (2006). Docosahexaenoic acid promotes neurogenesis in vitro and in vivo. Neuroscience. 139:991–997.

Khan, W.I. and Ghia, J.E. (2010). Gut hormones: Emerging role in immune activation and inflammation. Clin Exp Immunol. 161:19–27.

Khanna, P, Chattu, V.K. and Aeri, B. (2019). Nutritional aspects of depression in adolescents – A systematic review. Int J Prev Med. 10:42.

Kroes, M.C.W., Wingen, G.A., Wittwer, J., Mohajeri, M.H., Kloek, J. and Fernández, G. (2014). Food can lift mood by affecting mood-regulating neurocircuits via a serotonergic mechanism. Neuro Image, 84, 825–832.

Kumar, K., Bansal, K. and Mina, S. (2020). Role of nutrition in mental well-being. Int J Curr Res Rev. 12.

Lach, G., Schellekens, H., Dinan, T.G. and Cryan, J.F. (2018). Anxiety, depression, and the microbiome: A role for gut peptides. Neurotherapeutics. 15:36–59.

Lakhan, S.E. and Vieira, K.F. (2008). Nutritional therapies for mental disorders. Nutr J. 7:2.

Lange, K.W. (2020). Omega 3 fatty acids and mental health. Global Health J. 4(1):18–30.

Lassale, C., Batty, G.D. and Baghdadli, A. (2018). Healthy dietary indices and risk of depression outcomes; a systematic review and meta-analysis of observational studies. Mol Psychiatry. September 26, E-pub ahead of print.

Leahy, L.G. (2017). Vitamin B supplementation: What's the right choice for your patients? J Psychosoc Serv Mental Health Serv. 55(7):7–11.

Lee, C.H. and Giuliani, F. (2019). The role of inflammation in depression and fatigue. Front. Immunol. 10:1696.

Levant, B. (2013). N-3(omega-3)polyunsaturated Fatty acids in the pathophysiology and treatment of depression: Pre-clinical evidence. CNS and Neurological Disorders – Drug Targets | Bentham Science. 12(4):450–459.

Levenson, C.W. (2006). Zinc, the new antidepressant? Nutr Rev. 6:39–42.

Lewis, E.D., Meydani, S.N., Wu, D. (2019). Regulatory role of vitamin E in the immune system and inflammation. IUBMB Life. 71: 487–494.

Lian, B., Forsberg, S. and Fitzpatrick, K. (2019). Adolescent anorexia: Guiding principles and skills for the dietetic support of family-based treatment. J Acad of Nutr Diet. 119(1):17–25.

Luppino, F.S., de –Wit, L.M., Bouvy, P.F., Stijnen, T., Cuijpers, P. and Penninx, B.W.J.H. (2010). Overweight, obesity, and depression: A systematic review and meta-analysis of longitudinal studies. Archive Gen Psychiatr. 67(3):220–229.

Maes, M., Fisar, Z. and Medina, M. (2012) New drug targets in depression: Inflammatory, cell-mediated immune, oxidative and nitrosative stress, mitochondrial, antioxidant, and neuroprogressive pathways. And new drug candidates – Nrf2 activators and GSK-3 inhibitors. Inflammopharmacology. 20:127–150.

Makki, K., Deehan, E.C., Walter, J. and Backhed, F. (2018). The impact of dietary fibre on gut microbiota in host health and disease. Cell Host Microbe. 23:705–715.

Martin, C.R., Osadchiy, V., Kalani, A. and Mayer, E.A. (2018). The brain-gut-microbiomeaxis. Cell Mol Gastroenterol Hepatol. 6:133–148.

Martin-Gallausiaux, C., Beguet-Crespel, F., Marinelli L., Jamet A., Ledue F., Blottiere H.M. and Lapaque, N. (2018). Butyrate produced by gut commensal bacteria activates TGF-beta1 expression through the transcription factor SP1 in human intestinal epithelial cells. Sci Rep. 8:9742.

Martire, S.I., Maniam, J. and South, T. (2014) Extended exposure to a palatable cafeteria diet alters gene expression in brain regions implicated in reward, and withdrawal from this diet alters gene expression in brain regions associated with stress. Behav Brain Res. 265:132–141.

Marx, W., Moseley, G., Berk, M. and Jacka, F. (2017). Nutritional psychiatry: The present state of the evidence. Proc Nutr Soc 76:427–436.

Maurizi, C. (1990). The therapeutic potential for tryptophan and melatonin: Possible roles in depression, sleep, Alzheimer's disease and abnormal aging. Med Hypotheses. 31(3):233–242.

McGrath-Hanna, N.K., Greene, D.M., Tavernier, R.J. and Bult-I, A. (2003). Diet and mental health in the Arctic: Is diet an important risk factor for mental health in circumpolar peoples? – a review. Int J Circumpolar Health. 62(3):228–241.

McNamara, R.K. (2009). Evaluationof docosahexaenoic acid deficiency as a preventable risk factor for recurrent affective disorders: Current status, future directions, and dietary recommendations. Prostaglandins Leukot. Essent. Fatty Acids. 81(2–3):223–231.

Mena, P., Bresciani, L., Brindani, N., Ludwig, I.A., Pereira-Caro, G., Angelino, D., Llorach, R., Calani, L., Brighenti, F. and Clifford, M.N. (2019). Phenyl-γ-valerolactones and phenylvaleric acids, the main colonic metabolites of flavan-3-ols: Synthesis, analysis, bioavailability, and bioactivity. Nat. Prod. Rep. 36:714–752.

Meyers, A.F., Sampson, A.E., Weitzman, M., Rogers, B.L. and Kayne, H. (1989). School breakfast program and school performance. Am J Dis Child. 143(10):1234–1239.

Minihane, A.M., Vinoy, S., Russell, W.R., Baka, A., Roche, H.M., Tuohy, K.M., Teeling, J.L., Blaak, E.E., Fenech, M., Vauzour, D., McArdle, H.J., Kremer, B.H., Sterkman, L., Vafeiadou, K., Benedetti, M.M., Williams, C.M. and Calder, P.C. (2015). Low-grade inflammation, diet composition and health: Current research evidence and its translation. Br J Nutr. 114(7):999–1012.

Mohandas, E. and Rajmohan, V. (2007). Lithium use in special populations. Indian J Psychiatry. 49(3): 211.

Molteni, R., Barnard, R.J. and Ying, Z. (2002). A high-fat, refined sugar diet reduces hippocampal brain-derived neurotrophic factor, neuronal plasticity, and learning. Neuroscience. 112:803–814.

Morris, G. and Berk, M. (2015). The many roads to mitochondrial dysfunction in neuroimmune and neuropsychiatric disorders. BMC Med. 13:68.C

Morris, G., Walder, K. and McGee, S.L. (2017). A model of the mitochondrial basis of bipolar disorder. Neurosci Biobehav Rev. 74(Pt A):1–20.

Morris, L.S., Voon, V. and Leggio, L. (2018). Stress, motivation, and the gut-brain axis: A focus on the ghrelin system and alcohol use disorder. Alcohol Clin Exp Res. 42.

Moylan, S., Berk, M. and Dean, O.M. (2014) Oxidative and nitrosative stress in depression: Why so much stress? Neurosci Biobehav Rev. 45:46–62.

Mudambi, S.R. and Rajagopal, M.V. (2007). Fundamental of Foods, Nutrition and Diet Therapy. 5th Edition. New Delhi, India: New Age International Publisher Limited. ISBN (13): 978-81-224-2972-5.

Murakami, K., Miyake, Y., Sasaki, S., Tanaka, K., Fukushima, W., Kiyohara, C., Tsuboi, Y., Yamada, T., Oeda, T., Miki, T., Kawamura, N., Sakae, N., Fukuyama, H., Hirota, Y., Nagai, M. (2010). Dietary glycemic index is inversely associated with the risk of Parkinson's disease: A case–control study in Japan. Nutrition. 26:515–521.

Murphy, J.M., Pagano, M.E., Nachmani, J., Sperling, P., Kane, S. and Kleinman, R.E. (1998). The relationship of school breakfast to psychosocial and academic functioning: Cross-sectional and longitudinal observations in an inner-city school sample. Arch Pediatr Adolesc Med 152(9):899–907

Nielsen, F.H. (2018). Magnesium deficiency and increased inflammation: Current perspectives. J Inflamm Res. 11: 25–34.

Nowak, G. and Szewczyk, A. (2005). Zinc and depression, An update. Pharmacol Rep. 57:713–718.

O'Mahony, S.M., Clarke, G., Borre, Y.E., Dinan, T.G. and Cryan, J.F. (2015). Serotonin, tryptophan metabolism and the brain-gut-microbiome axis. Behav. Brain Res. 277:32–48.

O'Neil, A., Quirk, S.E., Housden, S., Brennan, S.L., Williams, L.J., Pasco, J.A. and Jacka, F.N. (2014). Relationship between diet and mental health in children and adolescents: A systematic review. Am J Public Health. 104(10):e31–e42.

Osadchiy, V., Martin, C.R. and Mayer, E.A. (2019). The gut-brain axis and the microbiome: Mechanisms and clinical implications. Clin. Gastroenterol. Hepatol. 17:322–332.

Owen, L. and Corfe, B. (2017). The role of diet and nutrition on mental health and wellbeing. Proc Nutr Soc. 76:425–426.

Pellegrin, K.L., O'Neil, P.M. and Stellfson, E.J. (1998). Average daily nutrient intake and mood among obese women. Nutr Res. 18:1103–1112.

Penckofer, S., Kouba, J. and Byrn, M. (2010). Vitamin D and depression: Where is all the sunshine? Issues Ment Health Nurs. 31(6):385–393.

Philip, P., Sagaspe, P., Taillard J., Mandon C., Constans J., Pourtau L., Pouchieu C., Angelino D., Mena, P. and Martini, D. (2019). Acute intake of a grape and blueberry polyphenol-rich extract ameliorates cognitive performance in healthy young adults during a sustained cognitive effort. Antioxidants. 8.

Polavarapu, A. and Hasbani, D. (2017). Neurological complications of nutritional disease. Seminars in Pediatric Neurol. 24:70–80.

Popa, T. (2012). Nutrition and depression at the forefront of progress. J Med Life. 5(4):414–419.

Public Health England. (2013). Social and Economic Inequalities in Diet and Physical Activity. London: Public Health England.

Rao, T.S.S., Asha, M.R., Ramesh, B.N. and Rao, K.S.J. (2008). Understanding nutrition, depression and mental illnesses. Indian J Psychiatry. 50(2):77–82.

Rizvi, S., Raza, S. T., Ahmed, F., Ahmad, A., Abbas, S. and Mahdi, F. (2014). The role of vitamin E in human health and some diseases. Sultan Qaboos University Med J. 14(2):e157–e165.

Rocks, T, Pelly, F. and Wilkinson, P. (2014). Nutrition therapy during initiation of refeeding in underweight children and adolescent in patients with anorexia nervosa: A systematic review of the evidence. J Acad Nutr and Diet. 114(6):897–907.

Roick, C., Fritz-Wieacker, A. and Matschinger, H. (2007). Health habits of patients with schizophrenia. Soc Psychiatry Psychiatr Epidemiol. 42(4):268–276.

Ruotolo, R., Minato, I., La Vitola, P., Artioli, L. and Curti, C., Franceschi, V., Brindani N., Amidani, D., Colombo, L. and Salmona, M. (2020). Flavonoid-Derived human phenyl-gamma-valerolactone metabolites selectively detoxify amyloid-β oligomers and prevent memory impairment in a mouse model of Alzheimer's disease. Mol Nutr Food Res. 64:e1900890.

Salim, S., Chugh, G. and Asghar, M. (2012). Inflammation in anxiety. Adv Protein Chem Struct Biol. 88:1–25.

Sarris, J. (2019). Nutritional psychiatry: From concept to the clinic. Drugs. 79:929–934.

Sarris, J., Logan, A.C. and Akbaraly, T.N. (2015). Nutritional medicine as main stream in psychiatry. Lancet Psychiatr. 2:271–274.

Saxena, S. G., Thornicroft, M., Knapp, and Whiteford, H. (2007). Resources for mental health: Scarcity, inequity and inefficiency. The Lancet. 370:878–889.

Schulte, E.M., Smeal, J.K., Lewis, J. and Gearhardt, A.N. (2018). Development of the highly processed food withdrawal scale. Appetite. 131:148–154.

Shaheen, Lakhan, S.E. and Vieira, K.F. (2008). Nutritional therapies for mental disorders. Nutr Jr. 2008;7:2.

Shepherd, R. and Raats, M. (2006). The Psychology of Food Choice. Oxfordshire, London, UK: CABI.

Sherwin, E., Sandhu, K.V., Dinan, T.G. and Cryan, J.F. (2016). May the force be with you: The light and dark sides of the microbiota-gut-brain axis in neuropsychiatry. CNS Drugs. 30:1019–1041.

Sinclair, A.J., Begg, D., Mathai, M. and Weisinger, R.S. (2007). Omega-3 fatty acids and the brain: Review of studies in depression. Asia Pac J Clin Nutr. 16:391–397.

Sinn, N. (2008). Nutritional and dietary influences on attention deficit hyperactivity disorder. Nutr Rev. 66(10):558–568.

Stoll, A.L., Severus, W.E, Freeman, M.P., Rueter, S., Zboyan, H.A, Diamond E. (1999). Omega 3 fatty acids in bipolar disorder: A preliminary double-blind, placebo-controlled trial. Arch Gen Psychiatry. 56:407–412.

St-Onge, M.P. and Zuraikat, F.M. (2019). Reciprocal roles of sleep and diet in cardiovascular health: A review of recent evidence and a potential mechanism. Curr Atheroscler Rep. 21:11.

Stranges, S., Samaraweera, P.C., Taggart, F., Kandala, N.B. and Stewart-Brown, S. (2014). Major health-related behaviours and mental well-being in the general population: The Health Survey for England. BMJ Open. 4(9):e005878

Tayefi, M., Shafiee, M., Kazemi-Bajestani, S.M.R., Esmaeili, H., Darroudi, S., Khakpouri, S., Mohammadi, M., Ghaneifar, Z., Azarpajouh, M.R. and Moohebati, M. (2017).Depression and anxiety both associate with serum level of hs-CRP: A gender-stratified analysis in a population-based study. Psychoneuroendocrinology. 81:63–69.

Tolmunen, T., Hintikka, J., Ruusunen, A., Voutilainen, S., Tanskanen, A., Valkonen, V.P., Viinamaki, H., Kaplan, G.A. and Salonen, J.T. (2004). Dietary folate and the risk of depression in Finnish middle-aged men. A prospective follow-up study. Psychother Psychosom. 73(6):334–339.

Traber, M.G. (2014). Vitamin E inadequacy in humans: Causes and consequences. Adv Nutr. 5(5):503–514.

Tuohy, K.M., Venuti, P., Cuva S., Furlanello, C., Gasperotti, M., Mancini, A., Ceppa, F., Cavalieri, D., De-Filippo, C. and Vrhovsek, U. (2015). Diet and the Gut Microbiota – How the Gut: Brain Axis Impacts on Autism. Amsterdam, The Netherlands: Elsevier Inc.

UNICEF (2002). UNICEF Annual Report 2002. New York: UNICEF.

Valls-Pedret, C., Lamuela-Raventós, R.M., Medina-Remón, A., Quintana, M., Corella, D., Pintó, X., Martínez-González, M.Á., Estruch, R. and Ros, E. (2012). Polyphenol-rich foods in the Mediterranean diet are associated with better cognitive function in elderly subjects at high cardiovascular risk. J Alzheimer's Dis. 29(4):773–782.

Valls-Pedret, C., Sala-Vila, A., Serra-Mir, M., Corella, D., de la Torre, R., Martínez-González, M.Á., Martínez-Lapiscina, E.H., Fitó, M., Pérez-Heras, A., Salas-Salvadó, J., Estruch, R. and Ros, E. (2015). Mediterranean diet and age-related cognitive decline: A randomized clinical trial. JAMA Int Med. 175(7):1094–1103.

WHO (1999). A Critical Link: Interventions for Physical Growth and Child Development. Geneva: World Health Organization.

WHO (2002c). The World Health Report 2002: Reducing Risks, Promoting Healthy Life Style. Geneva: World Health Organization.

Williams, C.M., Mohsen, M.A. and Vauzour, D. (2008) Blueberry-induced changes in spatial working memory correlate with changes in hippocampal CREB phosphorylation and brain-derived neurotrophic factor (BDNF) levels. Free Radic Biol Med. 45:295–305.

Wright, D.J., Renoir, T. and Smith, Z.M. (2015) N-Acetylcysteine improves mitochondrial function and ameliorates behavioral deficits in the R6/1 mouse model of Huntington's disease. Transl Psychiatry. 5:e492.

Zainuddin, M.S. and Thuret, S. (2012). Nutrition, adult hippocampal neurogenesis and mental health. Br Med Bull. 103:89–114.

Zietek, T. and Rath, E. (2016). Inflammation meets metabolic disease: Gut feeling mediated byGLP-1. Front Immunol. 7:154.

ZinAcker, M. and Lindseth, I.A. (2018). The Western diet-microbiome-host interaction and its role in metabolic disease. Nutrients. 10:pii:E365.

12 Nutrition and Fitness

Idowu Yetunde Fakolujo, Oluwafisayo Modupe
Gbadeyan, Fatima Alaba Ibrahim, Johnson Olaleye
Oladele, and Adenike Temidayo Oladiji

12.1 INTRODUCTION

It is common knowledge that the choice of food and drink consumed by humans (nutrition) has a great effect on their general well-being, quality of life and health status. Proper nutrition prevents sickness and diseases, brings about improvement of health and optimizes physical, cognitive and emotional capabilities (WHO, 2003; Arija *et al.*, 2006; Rodriguez *et al.*, 2009). Scientists discovered in the eighteenth century that particular meals (nutrients) regulate body function, restore health, guard against sickness and determine people's responses to environmental changes. In order to prevent deficiency diseases and, later, chronic non-communicable diseases, nutrition research at this time was driven by a paradigm or medical model that described the chemical structures and properties of nutrients found in foods as well as their biochemical reactions, physiological functions and human needs. When it became clear that the knowledge gathered did not enable mankind to address the worldwide issues of food insecurity and hunger, the study of nutrition evolved from a medical or pathological paradigm to a more psychosocial, behavioural one in the 1980s. As a result, nutrition was described as a fundamental human right that not only contributes to but also results in human development.

Fitness is defined as the quality or state of being fit and healthy. Fitness is described as a triangle with three sides: Physical fitness, mental fitness and emotional fitness. These three types of fitness are made up of different elements and domains that are responsible for bringing an excellent quality of health and well-being. There are different nutritional and fitness requirements to achieving a healthy living or existence in different types of individuals. These requirements are based on several factors such as gender, age, body composition and health status. Focus on adherence to the recommended intake of nutritional needs of the body alone is not enough to guarantee a perfectly healthy status. To ensure a good quality of life, free of disease and sickness, with a long life span and increased productivity, there must be a healthy balance between adhering to the recommended nutritional requirements and physical, mental and emotional fitness.

12.2 NUTRITION

Nutrition is the study of food and nutrients and how they affect our health. Both nutrition and food intake have a significant impact on health. Therefore, the single most crucial element that defines the health and fitness of an individual is their diet. A broader definition of nutrition explains it as the study of foods, the chemicals they contain, the nutrients they contain and the bodily processes they affect, including digestion, absorption, metabolism and excretion.

Human nutrition has a lot to do with the availability and supply of essential nutrients from foods critical to aid good health and human life as a whole. Poor nutrition in the form of under- or over-supply of nutrients from sources of food can cause bodily diseases that are deficiency related in humans. Examples of such diseases includes anaemia, stunted growth, beri-beri, scurvy and cretinism, amongst others (Ellie *et al.*, 2013). Overnutrition leads to diseases like cardiovascular disease, obesity (Wright *et al.*, 2007), diabetes and osteoporosis. Undernutrition may result in muscle

DOI: 10.1201/9781003361497-14

wasting, in acute conditions, protein energy malnutrition and marasmus and kwashiorkor in children with chronic malnutrition (Ellie *et al.*, 2013).

12.2.1   FOOD AND NUTRIENTS

Food is any solid or liquid which, when ingested, undergoes digestion, and is assimilated in the body, supplies the body with essential nutrients and keeps it healthy. It is a basic prerequisite for living. Benefits of nutrition conferred by food are supplying the macro- and micronutrients to aid the process of healing of injury, protecting the body against disease and fuelling immediate bio-energetic, emotional and spiritual requirements (Montain *et al.*, 2010).

Nutrients are chemical constituents of food that are required in sufficient amounts by the body to grow, reproduce and live a normal and healthy life. Various nutrient types are needed to maintain a healthy body. These nutrients include carbohydrates, proteins, fats, minerals, vitamins, water and fibre. Most foods contain more than one nutrient; for example, milk has proteins, fats, etc. Each and every nutrient has its own function, but for optimal activity, different nutrients must act together in accord.

The body uses nutrients for body building, to generate fluids such as blood, repair tissues, provide energy so that the body can stay alive and warm while moving and growing, protect the body from sickness and aid chemical processes. Nutrients can be classified according to their chemical composition as macronutrients and micronutrients on the basis of the required quantity to be consumed daily (Bhavani *et al.*, 2020).

Macronutrients are nutrients that are required in large amounts by the human body and are categorized as carbohydrates, proteins and lipids. They produce energy for normal functioning of the body (Bhavani *et al.*, 2020).

12.2.1.1   Carbohydrates

Carbohydrates occur in foods such as sugars, starches and fibre and are a major source of energy in the diet. Carbohydrates, such as starch or sugar, supply 4 calories per gram of the nutrient.

12.2.1.1.1   Functions of Carbohydrates in Human Body

Carbohydrates are a needed source of energy that is readily available for proper cell functions and physical activities. The energy needs of the brain and the central nervous system depends greatly on the continuous availability of glucose (carbohydrate) as supplied from the blood. Glycogen (> 300 g), stored as body fuel reserve in the liver and muscles, is maintained with frequent, consistent carbohydrate consumption to prevent the degradation of protein and fat tissue. Lactose is a source of galactose, which is required for development of the brain. It promotes calcium and phosphorus absorption, which aids bone formation and preservation. Lactose is converted to lactic acid within the intestine as a result of the presence and action of the bacteria (lactobacilli). Some B-complex vitamins are synthesized by lactobacilli.

Carbohydrates are major elements of some compounds that enhance infection resistance and are also needed for nerve tissues, heart valves, cartilage, bone and skin growth and preservation. They are also required for complete fat metabolism. Diets low in carbohydrates can result in loss of electrolytes (particularly sodium and potassium) and water from tissues through urination, leading to incidental dehydration.

12.2.1.2   Proteins

Proteins are the basic building blocks of our bodies as well as the main solid matter in muscles, blood, bones, teeth, skin, nails and hair. Amino acids are the building blocks of proteins; when amino acids are combined in different ways, they form thousands of distinct proteins in the body. Proteins also supply the body with energy; each gram of protein contains 4 calories.

12.2.1.2.1   Functions of Proteins in Human Body
Proteins in the body have several functions that range from body building, maintenance of tissues, regulating body processes, serving as enzymes, hormones and antibody precursors and transportation of nutrients.

12.2.1.2.1.1   Body Building or Building of New Tissues   Every cell need protein to function. Amino acids are required for the development of new cells, and proteins give them. The amount of protein required at different stages of life varies, depending on the rate of growth.

12.2.1.2.1.2   Maintenance of Tissues   Protein is required to maintain and repair aged tissues throughout one's life. Proteins in bodily tissues are constantly broken down and replaced by new protein; they do not remain static.

12.2.1.2.1.3   Regulatory Functions   Proteins in bodily fluids such as blood aid in the regulation of physiological functions. The key oxygen carrier in red blood cells, haemoglobin, is a protein and iron complex that enables the smooth running of the respiratory cycle. Plasma proteins have an impact on the exchange of water between tissue cells and the surrounding fluids as well as the body's water balance. Carbon dioxide formed in the body combines with blood proteins and is excreted by exhaling.

12.2.1.2.1.4   Proteins as Precursors of Hormones, Antibodies and Enzymes   Hormones secreted by various glands that regulate and coordinate body processes and activities are proteins in nature. Since they act as catalysts for digestion and other metabolic processes in the tissues, all enzymes are proteins by nature. Proteins have a role in the immune system of the body that involves formation of antibodies and white blood cells that protects the body from infections and disorders. A tiny amount of protein (or amino acids) is necessary for the creation of hormones, antibodies and enzymes.

12.2.1.2.1.5   Transport of Nutrients   The ideal nutrient carriers across the cell membranes – proteins, phospholipids, triglycerides, fat-soluble vitamins and cholesterol – are all transported by proteins called lipoproteins across the cell.

12.2.1.3   Fats
The human body needs fats to function. Fat is an integral component of all of the body's cells and tissues. Fats belongs to a class of chemicals called the lipids, providing about 10–30% of the total energy requirements of the body. A concentrated supply of energy is found in oils and fats, providing 9 calories per gram. The main building blocks of fats are fatty acids, and there are about 20 types of fatty acids found in foods and body tissues.

12.2.1.3.1   Types of Fatty Acids
Saturated and unsaturated fatty acids are the two different types of fatty acids.

12.2.1.3.1.1   Saturated Fatty Acid   A single bond connects each of the carbon atoms that make up saturated fatty acids. Saturated fats are unhealthy fats.

12.2.1.3.1.2   Unsaturated Fatty Acids   Fatty acids with one or more double bonds in their structure are referred to as unsaturated fatty acids. While polyunsaturated fatty acids (PUFA) have two or more double bonds, monounsaturated fatty acids (MUFA) only have one. Saturated fats are considered healthier than unsaturated fats; they are easily digestible and have better health benefits.

12.2.1.3.2   Functions of Fats in the Human Body

Dietary fats are sourced from two different types of vital nutrients: i. essential fatty acids (EFA) – these are fats that the body cannot produce on its own and must be obtained from food; and ii. non-essential fatty acids that help transport and absorb fat-soluble vitamins (such as vitamins A, D, E and K) as well as their precursors.

Cholesterol, a lipid that is produced in the liver, is used to make important hormones and bile acids. Fats make up the fatty heart of cell walls and help in transferring of nutritional components across cell membranes.

Adipose tissue is the term for the fat that is stored in different parts of the body. A cushion of this tissue, resembling a web, supports and shields the vital organs in the body. Fats provide padding for several vital organs. The fat coating protects the nerve fibres and helps with nerve impulse relay.

Fat is a poor heat conductor; therefore, having a layer beneath the skin helps to maintain body heat and regulate body temperature. Fats also improve the flavour, palatability and satiety factor of foods. Satisfaction is provided due to the slower rate of fat digestion compared to that of carbohydrates.

The fat located around joints in the body serves to a lubricate and allows smooth movement of the joints.

12.2.1.4   Micronutrients

Vitamins and minerals are needed in small quantities for a human body and are classified as micronutrients.

12.2.1.4.1   Vitamins

Organic compounds known as vitamins are found in trace levels in food. They are essential for life and growth. While vitamins do not contain calories, they are crucial to the metabolic processes that convert carbohydrates, lipids, and proteins into energy. They may work alone or in tandem with other substances. Since each vitamin serves a distinct purpose in the body, they cannot be substituted for one another. Vitamins can be found in food already formed or in an active state or they can exist as a precursor compound that can be transformed into an active state in the body; for example, carotenes are present in plant foods which are converted to vitamin A or retinol in the body.

12.2.1.4.2   Classes of Vitamins

Based on their solubility, there are two classes of vitamins:

12.2.1.4.2.1   Fat Soluble Vitamins   These are vitamins that get dissolved in fat. Vitamin A, D, E and K.

12.2.1.4.2.2   Water Soluble Vitamins   These vitamins dissolve in water and are not significantly stored by the body.; they include the B-group vitamins and vitamin C.

12.2.1.4.3   Minerals

There are at least 25 mineral elements like iron, calcium, phosphorous and zinc that occur in our food; 16 of these are regarded as essential to life and must be present in the diet. The essential minerals which are needed in minute quantities are referred to as trace elements; like vitamins, only small amounts of these minerals are needed to accomplish a great deal of functions in human body. Minerals do not supply calories. Unlike vitamins, they are not destroyed by heat, so cooking does not affect the mineral content in food. In burnt food, the ash that remains is the food's mineral content. Minerals are part of the cells, red blood cells, bones, teeth, nails and muscle structure. Minerals regulate chemical processes in the body, including maintenance of water levels within and outside of cells, keeping a regular heartbeat, aiding normal nerves response, allowing clotting of blood in wounds and regulating energy release from food.

12.2.1.4.3.1   Types of Minerals   There are basically two types of minerals: Major minerals and trace minerals.

12.2.1.4.3.1.1   Major Minerals   They are essential minerals that the body needs in large amounts for the proper function of metabolic activities. Examples of major minerals are chlorine, calcium, sodium, phosphorus, potassium, magnesium and sulphur.

12.2.1.4.3.1.2   Trace Minerals   They are minerals required by the body in minute quantities. Examples of Trace minerals: iron, iodine, zinc, copper, chromium, fluoride, molybdenum, manganese and selenium.

Among the trace minerals, iron is a crucial component necessary for the creation of haemoglobin in red blood cells and is crucial for the delivery of oxygen.

12.2.1.5   Water

Approximately 60% of the human body is made up of water. It is essential to almost all biological processes. On an ordinary day at sea level, the body loses roughly 2 to 2.5 litres of water, with 20% of that water being restored by the water in food. 80% of the water lost can be replaced by drinking water (plain) and other liquids. An average adult needs 2.2 to 3.0 litres of water per day (9–12 cups). Due to increased elevation, increased temperature, decreased humidity, increased exertion and inappropriate clothing, daily fluid requirements can more than double. Even while merely relaxing in the comfort of air conditioning, there are still significant water losses. The best beverage choice is safe water at all times.

12.3   NUTRITIONAL NEEDS

In general, the brain's regulating centres, hunger and satiety all play a role in human feeding. Numerous neurological, chemical and temperature cues can influence the centres and change feeding behaviour. Good nutrition must take into account the needs of people of all ages, with different levels of activity and individual differences.

Individual energy needs are influenced by physical activity, body size and composition, age and climate.

12.3.1   Physical Activities

The energy required by the body to fuel the participation in several physical activities such as hard labour, aerobic activities and dancing is higher when compared to that consumed while sleeping, sitting down and not performing any physical exercise.

12.3.2   Age

Nutritional requirements of infants and children is higher compared to that of adults and the aged. This is because, at this stage, the body require more energy to aid their growth to maturity. People who are older participate in activities that use less energy than children do. The recommended daily calorie requirements of individuals:

   a) Infants (1–3 years) requires about 1,000 calories/day.
   b) Children (5–8 years) requires about 1,500–1,800 calories/day.
   c) Older Children (10–12) years requires about 2,000 calories/day.
   d) Calorie requirements for adults and adolescents vary according to their level of physical activity. 13–20 years requires 2,800 calories/day (less active) – 3,500 calories/day (very active).
      • Adults – office, heavy and very heavy workers require 2,300 calories/day, 2,700 calories/day and up to 4,000 calories/day respectively.

The daily calorie requirement must be increased for pregnant women by 150 calories for the first trimester and 350 calories for the second and third trimesters. For breastfeeding mothers, the daily need must be raised by 800 calories.

12.3.3 CLIMATE

Extremely cold and hot climate restricts outdoor activities. The lesser the activities involved in, the lesser the energy requirement of the body.

12.4 FITNESS

Fitness is the state of being physically healthy and fit or having the quality of being qualified to carry out a specific task or role. Fitness can also refer to the state of a person's health and well-being as well as their capacity to carry out daily activities, sports and jobs without any restrictions (Bashari, 2018).

Greg Glassman described fitness in the CrossFit journal as a greater ability to work across a range of modal domains and time frames. Fitness is the mastery of a variety of fitness attributes such as endurance, strength, speed, balance, power and coordination as well as the ability to increase the amount of work accomplished with any of these domains in a given amount of time.

12.4.1 CLASSIFICATION OF FITNESS

Fitness can be described as a triangle with three points: physical fitness, emotional fitness and mental fitness. These three are critical components of general fitness.

12.4.1.1 Physical Fitness

Physical fitness is described by the Centers for Disease Control and Prevention (CDC) as having enough energy to engage in leisure activities and respond to crises as well as the ability to perform daily tasks with vigour and alertness, without undue exhaustion.

Achieving physical fitness typically requires proper nutrition (Tremblay *et al.*, 2010), moderate-vigorous exercise (De Groot and Fagerström, 2011) and enough rest (Malina, 2010). The obvious conclusion that human fitness and health increase when inactive people begin to exercise is supported by several scientific investigations. Low levels of physical activity are more typical in industrialized, third-world countries, but they are also becoming prevalent in developing countries too.

Prior to the Industrial Revolution, fitness was once understood to be the capacity to finish the day's work without being overly worn out. However, physical fitness is now understood to be a measure of the body's ability to function effectively and efficiently in work and leisure activities, to be healthy, to fight hypokinetic disorders and to handle emergency situations as a result of automation and changes in lifestyle. Due to the fact that mechanization and industrialization have decreased the levels of occupational physical activity, there is a need to complement occupational physical activity levels accompanied by additional regular physical exercises with an intent to enhance health and fitness.

The Department of Health and Human Services of the United States (USDHHS) released Physical Exercise Guidelines for Americans in 2018 to give people aged 3 and older science-based guidance on how to maintain their health by engaging in regular exercise. According to these recommendations, people should walk around more and sit less throughout the day to improve their mental, emotional and physical health (USDHHS, 2018). For considerable health benefits, adults should perform 75 to 150 minutes of vigorous aerobic activity, 150 to 300 minutes of moderate aerobic exercise or an equivalent combination of both, spread throughout the week. The suggestion that exercise should be carried out in at least 10-minute periods has been subtracted because recent studies indicate that any degree of physical activity, regardless of duration, can contribute to the health advantages (USDHHS, 2018). A weekly rate of more than 300 minutes (5 hours) of moderate-intensity exercise may result in additional health advantages. It was also recommended that adults should engage in muscle-strengthening exercises that require moderate to high levels of intensity for 2 or more days a week and involve all major muscle groups, as these activities have extra health benefits (USDHHS, 2018).

12.4.1.1.1 Components of Physical Fitness

With an increase in the activity levels, aerobic capacity, coordination, flexibility, muscular strength and endurance and body composition are just a few of the fitness indices that all increase. Perhaps more significantly, human health indicators also increase. The elements of fitness vary greatly depending on the source. Common elements include:

12.4.1.1.2 Muscular Endurance Activity

Activities that require muscular endurance, often known as aerobic exercise, help to increase breathing and pulse rates. These activities assist with performing daily tasks as well as maintaining one's health and fitness. Exercises that increase endurance are of great benefit to the heart, lungs and circulatory system. Additionally, they have the ability to delay or perhaps completely prevent a number of conditions that are frequent in the elderly, including as diabetes, breast and colon cancer, heart disease and others. Exercises that promote muscle endurance include brisk walking or jogging, yard work (mowing, raking), dancing, swimming, biking, climbing stairs or hills and playing tennis or basketball.

The number of repetitions of a certain exercise a person can do is often used to measure their muscular endurance. Push-ups and sit-ups are frequently used as exams.

12.4.1.1.3 Muscular Strength

Some elderly people utilize weights to bolster their strength. They begin by utilizing light weights, gradually increasing them. Others employ resistance bands, which are stretchy elastic bands with different strengths. The process of using weight to build muscle strength is known as "strength training" or "resistance training." Strong muscles make it easier to perform everyday duties like getting out of a chair, climbing stairs and carrying groceries. They also assist a person in keeping their independence. Maintaining healthy muscles can help with balance, reduce falls and other fall-related injuries. The amount of weight that can be moved in relation to repetitions is often used to measure muscular strength. Exercises like the bench press and squats that work several joints and muscle groups are commonly used. Strength workouts include lifting weights, holding a tennis ball, overhead arm curls, arm curls, wall push-ups, lifting one's own body weight and using a resistance band.

12.4.1.1.4 Cardiorespiratory Endurance

Cardiorespiratory endurance is mostly assessed by observing how long or quickly a person can perform a task and how this impacts physiological variables like heart rate and oxygen consumption.

12.4.1.1.5 Muscular Power

How much force an activity can generate serves as a common benchmark for muscular power. To measure muscle force, biomechanists frequently employ sophisticated equipment.

12.4.1.1.6 Flexibility

Flexibility can be increased through stretching. Moving more freely will make it simpler to look over the shoulder when reversing a car or reach down to lace shoes. The back of leg stretch, back stretch, ankle stretch and inner thigh stretch are all flexibility exercises.

The extent to which a muscle group or joint can be moved is the standard method for determining flexibility. The shoulders and hamstrings are typically tested.

12.4.1.1.7   Balance

How long a particular position can be held, with or without any form of activity, is normally how balance is measured. Balance can be assessed using uncomplicated exercises like standing on one leg. Standing on an unstable object and trying to catch a ball is an example of a more challenging balance test.

12.4.1.1.8   Body Composition

Simply put, body composition is the ratio of body fat to other tissues, including muscle, bone and skin. It is assessed utilizing a range of procedures and tools, which includes simple examinations such as using callipers or mathematical formulae, which are common and affordable. Advanced testing is far more expensive and far less common, including underwater weighing.

Strength and endurance are frequently the criteria used to evaluate fitness. However, combining health and athleticism with the other factors provides a more comprehensive picture of overall fitness.

12.4.1.1.9   Speed

How quickly a person can move from one spot to another is a common way to measure speed. Frequently, speed is measured using the 40-yard dash.

12.4.1.2   Mental Fitness

This is accomplished through mental exercise, much like with physical fitness. With exercises that preserve strong mental and emotional wellness, it is fitness for mental health.

While it is true that the brain weakens with age, there is evidence from neuroscience that the human brain can be trained to become even stronger, healthier and more physically active at any age, improving the overall mental fitness of a person.

12.4.1.2.1   Components of Mental Fitness

Four essential elements make up mental fitness. A person's mental health is impacted by these fundamental beliefs. Paying close attention to these facets of a person's life will significantly enhance their state of health, performance at work and overall productivity. They include psychological elements such as self-acceptance, self-esteem and resilience that aid in controlling strong emotions, social elements involving social networks and companionship, financial elements involving being in control of one's finances that lessen stress and physical elements that lower the risk of chronic illnesses developing in the body and enhance brain health.

12.4.1.2.2   Mental Fitness Improvement Skill

There are different exercises used in improving mental fitness divided into three different skills to work on:

a) Regulating strong feelings and thoughts as and when they come.
b) Identifying the processes that lead to challenging emotions and bad moods.
c) Establishing new patterns to replace the ones that are detrimental to your well-being.

Finding relatively individualized tactics that work well for each person is a part of enhancing mental fitness. Individual strategies that are most effective for each person should be employed. Ways to improve mental fitness include reading, meditation, breathing exercises, playing mental games amongst others.

12.4.1.3   Emotional Fitness

Emotional fitness is defined as the state in which the mind is able to focus on creative and constructive task while avoiding negative thoughts. According to Benneth (2019), emotional fitness is a state of being emotionally healthy, having awareness and having the capacity to manage a variety of feelings, both positive and negative. Increasing one's resilience, reducing stress and maintaining a healthy work-life balance are all aspects of emotional fitness. Emotional wellness entails maintaining equilibrium, happiness and ease. It is also being able to communicate your feelings and not bury them (Benneth, 2019). Success in all area of life depends on how emotionally fit a person is. Negative feelings like anger, worry, sadness and discomfort can make it difficult to succeed and sap the energy required for everyday tasks and activities of an individual (Envick and Martinez, 2010).

12.4.1.3.1   Elements of Emotional Fitness

There are several elements of emotional fitness: Mindfulness, gratitude, optimism and connection. Others include managing clutter and establishing useful daily routines, functioning in a way that is consistent with personal beliefs, developing resilience through learning strategies to deal with and recover from stress (Smith *et al.*, 2018) and expressing oneself artistically or adding greater beauty to existence through nature, music or the arts (Stuckey *et al.*, 2010).

12.4.1.3.2   Gratitude

Gratitude, which goes hand in hand with optimism, is a powerful catalyst of emotional fitness which warrants special attention. It requires mindful appreciation of the positive aspects of life, such as loved ones, favourite locations and priceless items as well as immaterial things like convictions, opportunities and experiences.

A good way to improve emotional fitness using gratitude is by frequently writing in a journal about things that an individual is grateful for.

12.4.1.3.3   Mindfulness

Mindfulness is an act of being fully aware of the present moment in a non-judgmental way. This does not suggest that there are no distractions; rather, it means making a conscious effort to pay close attention to thoughts as they arise as well as to emotions and sensations, without becoming overwhelmed by them. Numerous studies have connected mindfulness to emotional well-being. It can be fostered through visualization and focused exercises as well as straightforward strategies like concentration on breathing (Good *et al.*, 2016).

12.4.1.3.4   Connection

Connection, as it relates to emotional wellness, is a feeling of connection or belonging to something. One type of connection that can take many various forms and has advantages is social interactions. A closest friend at work, which boosts job happiness by 50%, improves the likelihood of having a good emotional fitness level (Riordan and Christine, 2013), having more "weak" social connections, such as frequent interactions with friends at work, the store or in a classroom (Sandstrom *et al.*, 2014). Participating in more than one social group has been linked to greater satisfaction about life (Wakefield *et al.*, 2017). Feeling a connection to a location, a pet or a cause also may be advantageous to being emotionally fit. Though individual needs differ, some sort of connection helps most people flourish.

12.4.1.3.5   Optimism

Optimism refers to the ability of an individual to having a positive perspective on the present and future (Gallagher *et al.*, 2013). Research confirms that certain actions such as acting with compassion, recognizing and exploiting personal assets and envisioning a prosperous future increases optimism, and ultimately, overall happiness, which brings about emotional fitness (Seligman *et al.*, 2005).

12.4.1.3.6   Achieving Emotional Fitness

Emotional fitness activities, while not a substitute for professional mental healthcare, may be an answer for anyone ready to go from getting through the day to making the most of it. People increasingly expect these as standard wellness programme offerings, equal with fitness and nutrition activities.

Similar to physical fitness/exercise, various emotional fitness activities are best suited to various persons at various times. Unfortunately, high-quality programme options that encourage participants to test-drive various activities and delve into whatever works best for them is lacking. Many currently available programmes are specialized (dealing with just one element of emotional fitness) rather than personalized. An efficient and effective emotional fitness programme should be one that is specially tailored to meet with the emotional needs of the participant and not restricted or exclusive.

12.5   BENEFITS OF NUTRITION AND FITNESS

12.5.1   BENEFITS OF NUTRITION

It is an open secret that a healthy weight can be maintained with good nutrition and physical activity. However, the benefits of good nutrition are not limited to weight. Good nutrition can aid in lowering cholesterol levels and high blood pressure, increase energy levels, lessen the risk of some forms of cancer, osteoporosis, diabetes, heart disease and stroke. Good nutrition improves the ability of the body to fight infection and to recover from illness or injury. It also improves the mental well-being of an individual.

12.5.2   BENEFITS OF FITNESS

Physical activity has been found in studies to enhance mental health and well-being (Callaghan, 2004). This improvement is brought about by an increase in brain blood-flow, which enables hormonal secretion, the reduction of stress hormones (such as cortisol and adrenaline) in the body and the activation of the body's natural painkillers and mood boosters. Exercise not only causes the release of these feel-good chemicals, but it also reduces anxiety and boosts self-confidence.

Physical activity clearly has been found to ameliorate three of the most prevalent chronic degenerative diseases in developed countries, both in terms of severity and outcome (hypertension, coronary heart disease and non-insulin-dependent diabetes mellitus). Virtually all chronic diseases, including but not limited to stroke, peripheral artery disease, coronary heart disease, chronic obstructive pulmonary disease, osteoporosis and some types of cancer, are positively impacted by increased levels of physical activity (Alberts and Hess, 2005).

Physical activity has been linked to the alleviation of depression and anxiety symptoms (Callaghan, 2004) and has also been shown, in schizophrenic patients, to improve their quality of life and decrease the effects of schizophrenia (Vancampfort et al., 2012).

Physical fitness is effective at reducing the signs of sadness and anxiety, having a favourable effect on mental health and bringing about a number of other advantages, as these trends get better with regular physical activity (Sharma et al., 2006). A person who is physically fit will be happier and more productive both in and outside of the gym (Envrick and Martinez, 2010).

The brain's neuronal networks are strengthened by mental workouts, which results in a more grounded reasoning process and improved emotion management and decision-making. The likelihood that negative feelings and thoughts may arise increases with their feeding.

Mental fitness is emotionally beneficial as well, through supporting someone in breaking bad habits and assisting them in feeling happier feelings more frequently. Although this makes it simple to fall into negative cycles, the brain may be rewired to support good thoughts and emotions. The sensation of resilience and confidence is energized and triggered by strengthening mental fitness. It's normal to feel sad and worried, but by improving mental fitness, it will be less likely that these emotions will progress to melancholy and anxiety.

12.6   CONCLUSION

Eating the proper amounts of a wide variety of foods promotes nutrition balance. This gives the body the protein, sugars, fats, vitamins and minerals it needs to function properly. Proper dietary intake, hydration and exercise are essential for optimum health. The number of calories required to maintain a given weight of an individual varies depending on height and weight, in addition to gender, age and physical and mental activity. Good nutrition and fitness improve social skills by bringing about increase the opportunity for social interaction. Being physically, mentally and emotionally fit generally improves one's self-esteem and mental alertness, reducing fatigue (Sharma *et al.*, 2006). Good nutrition and fitness go hand-in-hand in achieving a healthy lifestyle. An individual who feeds well, has a positive view on life, a strong resilience to infection and exhibits a number of other healthy traits like an extended, active and vigorous lifespan is one who has mastered a healthy balance of nutrition and all-round fitness. A healthy individual is one who is well-nourished, physically fit, mentally alert and emotionally stable.

REFERENCES

Alberts, D. S. and Hess, L. M. (2005). *Fundamentals of Cancer Prevention*. Berlin: Springer.

Arija, V., Esparo, G., Fernandez-Ballart, J., Murphy, M. M., Biarnes, E. and Canals, J. (2006). Nutritional Status and Performance in Test of Verbal and Nonverbal Intelligence in 6-Year-old Children. *Intelligence*; 34: 141–149.

Bashari, H. (2018). Pediatrics, Nutrition & Primary Healthcare Nursing. *Pediatrics & Therapeutics Journal*; 8: 48.

Benneth, N. (2019) Emotional Fitness for University Students. *Open Access Government*; 1: 1.

Bhavani, R. V., Gopinath, R., Nithya, D. J., Raju, S. and Sakthi Velan, A. (2020). Good Nutrition – A Handbook for Trainers. *MSSRF*; 85: 1–58.

Callaghan, P. (2004). Exercise: A Neglected Intervention in Mental Health Care? *Journal of Psychiatric and Mental Health Nursing*; 11(4): 476–483.

De Groot, G. C. and Fagerström, L. (2011). Older Adults' Motivating Factors and Barriers to Exercise to Prevent Falls. *Scandinavian Journal of Occupational Therapy*; 18(2): 153–160.

Envick, B. R. and Martinez, R. (2010). The Positive Impact of Physical Fitness on Emotional Fitness. *The Crosfit Journal*. Prescott, AZ 86305, USA. 1–6.

Fair, S. E. (2010). *Wellness and Physical Therapy*. MA: Jones and Bartlett Publisher, 176–179.

Gallagher, M. W., Lopez, S. J., Pressman, S. D. (2013). Optimism Is Universal: Exploring the Presence and Benefits of Optimism in a Representative Sample of the World. *Journal of Personality*; 81(5): 429–440. https://doi.org/10.1111/jopy.12026

Good, Darren J., et al. (2016). Contemplating Mindfulness at Work: An Integrative Review. *Journal of Management*; 42(1): 114–142.

Malina, R. (2010). Physical Activity and Health of Youth. *Constanta: Ovidius University Annals, Series Physical Education and Sport/Science, Movement and Health*; 10(2): 271–277.

Montain, S. J., Carvey, C. E. and Stephens, M. B. (2010). Nutritional Fitness. *Military Medicine*; 175(8): 65.

Riordan, C. M. (2013). We All Need Friends at Work. *Harvard Business Review*. 1: 1–2.

Rodriguez, N. R., DiMarco N. M., Langley, S., et al (2009). Nutrition and Athletic Performance. *Medicine & Science in Sports & Exercise*, 41: 709–731.

Sandstrom, G. M. and Dunn, E. W. (2014). Social Interactions and Well-Being: The Surprising Power of Weak Ties. *Personality and Social Psychology Bulletin*; 40(7): 910–922.

Seligman, M. E. P., et al. (2005). Positive Psychology Progress: Empirical Validation of Interventions. *American Psychologist;* 60(5): 410.

Sharma, A., Madaan, V. and Petty, F. D. (2006). Exercise for Mental Health. *Primary Care Companion to the Journal of Clinical Psychiatry*; 8(2): 106.

Smith, B. et al. (2018). Improvements in Resilience, Stress, and Somatic Symptoms Following Online Resilience Training: A Dose-Response Effect. *Journal of Occupational and Environmental Medicine*; 60(1): 1.

Stuckey, Heather L. and Nobel, J. (2010). The Connection Between Art, Healing, and Public Health: A Review of Current Literature. *American Journal of Public Health;* 100(2).

Tremblay, M. S., Colley, R. C., Saunders, T. J., Healy, G. N. and Owen, N. (2010). Physiological and Health Implications of a Sedentary Lifestyle. *Applied Physiology, Nutrition, and Metabolism;* 35(6): 725–740.

U.S. Department of Health and Human Services (USDHHS) (2018). *Physical Activity Guidelines for Americans*, 2nd edition. Washington, DC: U.S. Department of Health and Human Services; 1–118.

Vancampfort, D., Knapen, J., Probst, M., Scheewe, T., Remans S. and De Hert, M. (2012). A Systematic Review of Correlates of Physical Activity in Patients with Schizophrenia. *Acta Psychiatrica Scandinavica*; 125: 352–362. doi: 10.1111/j.1600-0447.2011.01814.x.

Wakefield, Helen, J. R., et al. (2017). The Relationship Between Group Identification and Satisfaction With Life in a Cross-Cultural Community Sample. *Journal of Happiness Studies*; 18(3): 785–807.

Whitney, E. and Rolfes, S. R. (2013). *Understanding Nutrition* (13th ed.). Wadsworth, Cengage Learning. 667–670. Belmont, CA 94002-3098.

World Health Organization (2003). Diet, Nutrition and the Prevention of Chronic Diseases–Report of a Joint WHO/FAO Expert Consultation. *WHO Technical Report Series No. 916, Geneva, World Health Organization, 2003*.

Wright, M. E., Chang, S., Schatzkin, A., Albanes, D., Kipnis, V., Mouw, T., Hurwitz, P., Hollenbeck, A. and Leitzmann, M. F. (2007). Prospective Study of Adiposity and Weight Change in Relation to Prostate Cancer Incidence and Mortality. *Cancer;* 109(4): 675–684.

13 Nutrition and Cancer

Omowumi O. Adewale, Ebenezer I. O. Ajayi, Johnson Olaleye Oladele, and Adenike Temidayo Oladiji

13.1 INTRODUCTION

Although cancer is multifactorial, the role that the dietary factor plays in the etiology of cancer cannot be overemphasized; it contributes to 30–35% of all cancer cases worldwide(1, 2). The foremost role that nutrition plays in cancer is becoming evident as research advances.

According to statistics from the World Cancer Research Fund and the American Institute for Cancer Research, approximately 30–40% of all cancer cases can be prevented through the adoption of appropriate diets rich in essential nutrients, regular physical activity, and maintaining a healthy body weight(3).

The link between dietary factors and cancer development was first demonstrated in the 1940s through a pioneering study conducted with mice. This study revealed that, when certain dietary factors were restricted, there was a significant decrease in the occurrence of cancer(4). Food is generally composed of chemical substances that are largely harmless and usually desirable for the survival and growth of all organisms. However, the preservation and processing of food by various methods previous to consumption affect its chemical composition as well as its nutritional value and carcinogenic potential(5). Exposure to diets processed through various means has led to an increase in the occurrence of several cancers. The understanding of various factors to which nutrition can be subjected and how these affect carcinogenetic incidences could provide a means of how the global cancer menace can be tackled. This chapter discusses various aspects relating to the role nutrition plays in cancer incidence, including but not limited to anti-cancer properties and mechanisms of nutrients, effects of GMOs, functional foods and nutraceuticals in cancer, and the prospects of the nutrition and cancer relationship.

13.2 OVERVIEW OF CANCER

Cancer is a group of diseases characterized by the uncontrolled growth and proliferation of abnormal cells. It is typically derived from a single abnormal cell, which has misplaced the normal management mechanisms and, as a result, is capable of multiplying continuously, invading close tissues, migrating to sites distant from the original site, and promoting the growth of new blood vessels (a process known as angiogenesis), from which they derive nutrients. Cancerous (malignant) cells can increase from any tissue within the body; the process by which this occurs is known as carcinogenesis. Carcinogenesis is a process with more than one stage, including transformation and mutation to genetic elements that normalize the usual function of the cell, including the processes that control cell proliferation(6).

13.2.1 STAGES OF CARCINOGENESIS

Stages involved in carcinogenesis have been identified to be: initiation, promotion, progression, and metastasis (Figure 13.1).

i. Initiation stage: this includes modification, variation, or mutation of genes rising naturally or induced by contact with an oncogenic agent. Genetic changes could end in the dysregulation of biochemical signalling pathways related to cellular propagation, existence, and variation, which can be controlled by a sum of influences, involving the degree and kind of carcinogenic metabolism and the reaction of the function of DNA repair.

ii. Promotion stage: this is well-thought-out to be a comparatively long and reversible process wherein actively multiplying pre-neoplastic cells amass. During this period, the process can be changed by chemo-preventive agents that eventually affect growth rates.

iii. Progression Stage: this is the ultimate stage of neoplastic transformation; here, genetic and phenotypic changes with cell propagation occur. At this stage, there is a rapid and significant increase in the size of the tumor. Additionally, cancer cells at this stage may undergo further mutations that enhance their ability to invade nearby tissues and potentially spread to distant parts of the body through metastasis.

iv. Metastasis: at this stage, there is the spread of cancer cells from the original site to different body parts via the bloodstream or the lymph system(7, 8).

If the spread of most cancer cells is not managed, it could bring about loss of life(9). The majority of cancers result from several external factors, including chemical materials, tobacco, infectious organisms, and radiation in addition to some internal elements such as immune conditions, inherited mutations, random mutations, and hormones(9). Cancer makes up the most causes of morbidity and mortality the world over, with an estimation of 14.1 million new cases and about 8.2 million deaths within the year 2012. Remarkably, in the next two decades, the wide variety of most cancer incidences is expected to push upward by about 70%(10).

13.2.2 COMMON CHARACTERISTICS OF MANY CANCERS

Many characteristics are common to cancer these include:

i. Anomalous cell signaling resulting in unregulated cell growth.
ii. Suppression of apoptosis or natural cell death.
iii. Invasion of surrounding tissues and facilitation of cancer spread (metastasis).
iv. Induction of angiogenesis, promoting increased blood supply to the tumor (Figure 13.1).

13.2.2.1 Abnormal Signal Transduction Leading to Uncontrolled Cell Proliferation

Normal cells require signals usually delivered by ligands to stimulate their growth and inhibit their growth when it is adequate. The signals or ligands can take the form of growth factors, inhibitors, extracellular matrix components, or cell adhesion molecules. These signals are conveyed into the cells by specific proteins located on the cell membrane surface, known as receptors(11). The ligand binds to its specific receptors; these receptors usually have three domains: the extracellular ligand-binding domain, the transmembrane domain, and the intracellular domain. The binding of the ligand signal to the receptor activates it, then the signal is transferred through the transmembrane

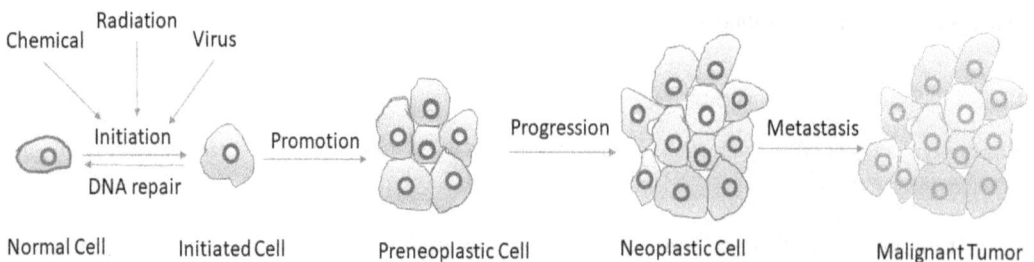

FIGURE 13.1   Multistep carcinogenesis(7).

domain, which transfers it to the receptor tyrosine kinase, which initiates a cascade of signals to the nucleus through phosphorylation. The result of this is cell proliferation or growth inhibition(12). Malignant cells produce their own growth signals, allowing them to divide, with decreased reliance on external growth stimulation. Certain cells have the remarkable ability to produce their own growth factors, essentially stimulating their own growth. This process is known as autocrine stimulation. For instance, glioblastoma cells are known to express platelet-derived growth factor (PDGF)(13); sarcoma expresses tumor growth factor (TGF-a) as well as epidermal growth factor receptor (EGFR)(14). In normal cells, the production of cell surface receptors is carefully regulated through cellular control of gene expression and protein translation. This intricate regulatory mechanism ensures the proper functioning and balance of receptor proteins on the cell surface. However, in tumor cells, this organized regulation is disrupted by mutations in genes encoding for the receptors; as a consequence, an excessive number of gene copies are produced, resulting in gene amplification. This phenomenon leads to an increased transcription and production of receptors on the tumor cell surface. This, in turn, triggers the tumor cells into the growth phase by the binding of ligands to the receptors. The overexpression of growth factor receptors can lead to ligand-independent signaling, where the receptors become active, even in the absence of stimulating molecules(15). Additionally, structural changes to receptors can also cause ligand-independent activation – e.g., truncated EGFRs that are devoid of intracellular domains are constitutively active. EGFR, also known as human epidermal receptor-1 (HER-1), belongs to the sub-family of type-1 receptor tyrosine kinases. These receptors are primarily found on the membranes of normal epithelial cells from the skin, breast, colon, lungs, etc. This receptor and its corresponding ligands play a crucial role in governing cell proliferation, differentiation, and survival. In tumors originating from the colon, rectum, head, and neck, etc., there is typically an elevated expression of this receptor.

Signal transduction is a phenomenon by which the binding of a specific ligand to its receptor elicits a conformational change in the receptor that transmits the specific signal to the intracellular membrane of the cell, thereby propagating the signal specific to that receptor in the cell. The conformational change on the receptor activates the receptor tyrosine kinase, which initiates a signaling pathway specific to the receptor. The initiation of the signal transduction pathway activates an intricate series of processes in the cytoplasm or fluid intracellular space. This cascade eventually extends to the cell nucleus, where the transcription of genes responsible for regulating cell cycle progression is induced, leading to cell progression. The Ras/raf-Mitogen activated protein, or MAP kinase pathway, is one of the major signaling cascades implicated in cancers; another is the Phosphoinositide-3-kinase (PI3K/akt MTOR) pathway(16). These two pathways are interconnected with each other and with various other signaling pathways within the cell. Many disruptions or impairments of the normal regulatory mechanisms in these pathways have been identified in all types of human cancers. Once the signals reach the nucleus, transcription factors are activated to transcribe genes that are translated into proteins such as growth factors that allow the cells to proliferate. The results of any growth factor receptor signal transduction pathway are tumor DNA replication and cell division(12). As a result, there is an exponential growth potential of tumor cells. The tumor begins to increase in size on the tissue level. Many components of signal transduction pathways are potential targets of many anticancer therapies. Components of these include: receptors, ligands, intracellular second messengers, and nuclear transcription factors that transcribe tumor genes.

13.2.2.2 Loss of Programmed Cell Death or Apoptosis

Apoptosis is one of the ways by which organisms limit the growth or replication of cells. The absence of apoptosis results in loss of control of cell growth and tissue homeostasis. Loss of apoptosis is one of the crucial mechanisms behind cancer. Genetic changes within cancer cells lead to not only enhanced cell proliferation but also diminished apoptosis. Consequently, malignant tissues exhibit a combination of increased cell growth and reduced cell death. Apoptosis occurs in normal cells to remove the damaged cell and maintained a constant number of cells in regenerating tissues, and it is a vital process in embryogenesis(17). In an average human adult, 50–70 billion cells undergo apoptosis per day. Apoptosis is characterized by changes including cell shrinkage, mitochondrial cytochrome-c release, cell DNA fragmentation into multiples of 180 base pairs, and ultimate breakage of cells into small, apoptotic bodies, which are taken up by neighboring cells through phagocytosis. There are two mechanisms by which apoptosis is initiated; these are:

i. Through death receptors or extrinsic pathways; this is triggered by activation of members of the tumor necrosis receptor superfamily.
ii. Through mitochondrial or intrinsic pathway, which is triggered by DNA damage.

Ultimately, both pathways culminate in the activation of caspases, which engage with inhibitors of apoptosis proteins (IAPs) and the BCL-2 protein family. These individual components possess either pro- or anti-apoptotic characteristics(17). Numerous malignant cells exhibit resistance to apoptosis attributed to the heightened expression of several anti-apoptotic proteins. For instance, Survivin, an IAP present in numerous cancers, has been linked to unfavorable outcomes. Overexpression of BCL-2 is observed in B-cell lymphomas, often due to gene translocation. Conversely, in certain gastrointestinal tumors and leukemias, deactivating mutations of pro-apoptotic molecules like Bax have been identified. Anticancer therapies have been devised to target anti-apoptotic molecules. For instance, strategies involve utilizing short DNA segments that complement BCL-2 RNA or designing antisense oligonucleotides to curtail the translation of these apoptotic proteins(18).

13.2.2.3 Tissue Invasion and Metastasis Promoting the Spread of Cancer

Cancer cells exhibit a direct extension and penetration into adjacent tissues, a phenomenon termed "invasion." The amalgamation of abnormal cell proliferation and sustained tumor growth contributes to the disruption of tissue barriers, enabling the tumor to infiltrate neighboring tissue. This local invasion constitutes the initial phase of secondary tumor formation or metastasis. Metastasis refers to the capability of cancer cells to infiltrate lymphatic and blood vessels, traverse these conduits, and establish invasion in healthy tissues in different parts of the body. Metastasis is derived from the Greek word *methistanai*, which means "to migrate to another area." Metastasis occurs through the "metastatic cascade," which occurs in an ordered and predictable manner(19–21). The ability of cancer cells to migrate from a primary site of disease is linked to mutations in genes that control the production of proteins that anchor cells to their surroundings. Cancer cells can escape the primary tumor site because of decreased synthesis of chemicals that naturally bind them to neighbor cells as well as aberrant creation of enzymes capable of destroying cell-tissue interactions(19–21).

13.2.2.4 Angiogenesis Leading to Enhanced Blood Supplies of Tumor

Angiogenesis is a pivotal process that supports the sustenance and advancement of tumors. Tumor angiogenesis denotes the capacity of a tumor to trigger the development of novel blood vessels(22). This key stage in tumor progression facilitates tumor growth, local infiltration, and the spread to distant sites by ensuring the supply of oxygen, nutrients, and factors essential for survival. It also fosters the generation of growth factors that aid tumor cells and serves as the foundation for tumor cell nourishment. Among the key elements of angiogenesis, vascular endothelial growth factor (VEGF) stands out as the most significant. This factor spurs the proliferation and movement of endothelial cells(23). Additional angiogenesis regulators, such as EGFL-7 and A5β1-integrin, also play roles in the facilitation of new blood vessel creation. This process is facilitated by interactions with the extracellular matrix. The involvement of endothelial cell interactions, EGFL-7, and A5β1-integrin expression has been observed in developing vessels, including those within tumors(24).

13.3 ROLE OF NUTRIENTS IN CARCINOGENESIS

Even though cancer is caused by several influences, the role that diet plays in the process of carcinogenesis is widely reported; it contributes between 30–35% of all cancer cases worldwide(1, 2).

Indeed, nutrition has emerged as a prominent modifiable factor in the context of chronic diseases, with scientific evidence substantiating the notion that dietary modifications exert substantial impacts, both favorable and unfavorable, on overall health(25). On the positive front, research has demonstrated that a significant proportion of all cancer cases can be potentially averted by consuming diets rich in essential nutrients(3). On the other hand, it is also possible for a diet to comprise carcinogens and mutagens, which may increase the risk of cancer development, predominantly in genetically vulnerable individuals(25). Altogether, diet is considered to be a blend of defensive, carcinogenic, and mutagenic mediators; the majority of these are modified by metabolizing enzymes(25) to produce their eventual effects (whether positive or negative as far as carcinogenesis is concerned). Epidemiological studies specified nutritional factors are the most auspicious area to investigate in order to obtain tangible results for the menace of cancer(26, 27). There is evidence that relates specific nutrients/substances in the diet to their impacts on specific tumor development/reversion or some other results on cancer at a specific site in the body(28).

13.3.1 ROLE OF NUTRIENTS IN THE SUPPRESSION OF CARCINOGENESIS

Naturally, humans possess a variety of protective mechanisms to protect against mutagens and carcinogens, and these comprise constant flaking of the skin surface layers as well as those of the colon, intestines, cornea, and of the stomach(29). Protection against oxygen radicals and lipid peroxidation is regarded as a pivotal defense mechanism, given that these agents play a crucial role in inducing DNA damage(30). The primary sources of endogenous oxygen radicals are identified as hydrogen peroxide and superoxide, which are generated as metabolic byproducts. Additionally, the oxygen radical burst resulting from phagocytosis in a response to viral or bacterial infections as well as inflammatory reactions contributes to the production of oxygen radicals(31). Various environmental factors also contribute to the generation of oxygen radicals. However, cells are safeguarded from oxidative harm by several enzymes, including superoxide dismutase, glutathione transferases, DT-diaphorase, and glutathione peroxidase(32). Furthermore, various small molecules present in the diet play role in the antioxidative mechanisms and therefore appear to be anticarcinogens. Studies suggest diets including fibre-rich cereals, vegetables, and fruits are rich in these small molecules and that a general increase in consumption of these foods could drastically suppress the process of carcinogenesis(33, 34). Some of these small molecules are discussed in the following sections.

13.3.1.1 Glutathione

Glutathione is a dipeptide formed from two amino acids – glutamate and cysteine (Figure 13.2). It is a potent molecule available in food and one of the main antioxidants present in the soluble portion of cells and an antimutagen. The amount of glutathione is suggested to be influenced by dietary sulphur-containing amino acids(35). Brussels sprouts, broccoli, cauliflower, and other cruciferous vegetables have been known to be rich sources of glutathione. Diets rich in kale, mustard greens, garlic, onions, shallots, poultry, and fish are also known to induce the production of glutathione(36).

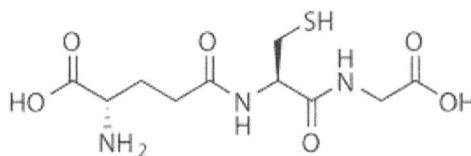

FIGURE 13.2 Glutathione.

13.3.1.2 Ascorbic Acid

Dietary ascorbic acid is another critical antioxidant; it is a water-soluble vitamin (Figure 13.3). It is presents in food such as citrus fruit (oranges and orange juice), black currants, peppers, broccoli, strawberries, potatoes, brussels sprouts, and so on. It was revealed to possess anticarcinogenic effects in rodents that were exposed to nitrite, benzo[a]pyrene, and ultraviolet radiation(37, 38). There are several evidences of the cytotoxic outcome of ascorbic acid on cancer cells, either singly or in combination with established cytotoxic drugs in vitro(39–42). Many studies also have recommended involvement of vitamin C in the treatment of progressive cancers(43) (Hoffer et al., 2015) as well as pancreatic cancer(44, 45). The mechanism of vitamin C's anticarcinogenic action has been suspected to be the formation of significant levels of hydrogen peroxide via autoxidation of normal ascorbic acid concentrations and activation of 2-oxoglutarate-dependent dioxygenase enzymes (2-OGDDs) family, which requires ascorbic acid as a cofactor.

13.3.1.3 Vitamin E (Tocopherol)

This molecule is considered a major radical snare for oxygen radicals in lipids(46) and has been useful medically against various oxidatively related illnesses(47). Tocopherols amend damage and carcinogenicity induced by daunomycin, Adriamycin, and quinones in the heart. These substances have been reported to be carcinogenic, mutagenic, cardiotoxic, and their mechanism of toxicity was reported to be through free radical generation defensive roles of vitamin E against DNA damage induced by radiation, and mutation and carcinogenesis induced by dimethylhydrazine were also reported(48). Tocopherols cause significant endurance in rats subjected to heavy exercise that normally leads to extensive oxidative damage to tissues (Figure 13.4).

13.3.1.4 Edible Plants With Their In-built Phytochemicals

Edible plants possessing phytochemicals substances including: phenols, have been described to impede carcinogenesis or mutagenesis in animal experiments(49). Most of these substances seem to impede carcinogenesis by enhancing certain metabolic enzymes like cytochrome P-450(50).

13.3.1.5 β-Carotene

β-Carotene belongs to the group of carotenoids containing isoprene units(51). It functions as a dietary antioxidant, shielding fats and lipid membranes from oxidation caused by free radicals.

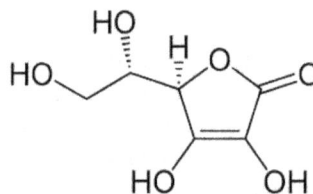

FIGURE 13.3 Ascorbic acid.

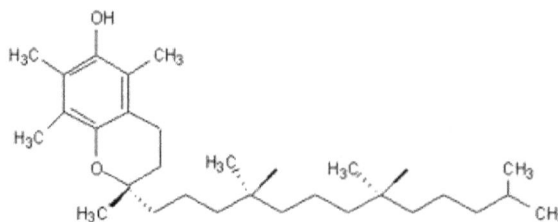

FIGURE 13.4 Vitamin E.

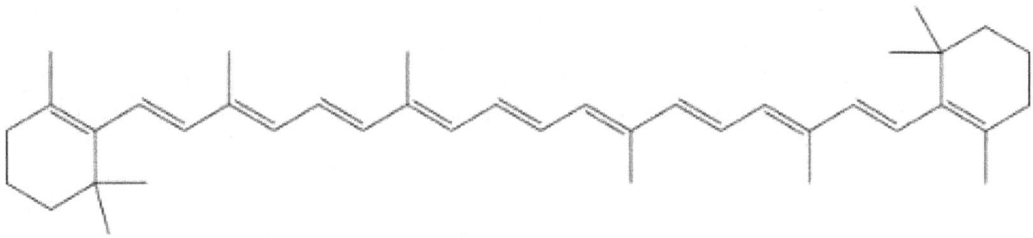

FIGURE 13.5 β-Carotene.

Carotenoids, in general, serve as scavengers for free radicals and are remarkably efficient at quenching singlet oxygen, a highly reactive form of oxygen known for its mutagenic effects and potent stimulation of lipid peroxidation(52). It can arise through the transfer of energy from light to oxygen in a pigment-mediated process or it can be generated via lipid peroxidation. Sources of β-Carotene and related polyprenes include carrots and any diet containing chlorophyll. These molecules seem to serve as primary defense mechanisms against singlet oxygen, which forms as a byproduct from the interplay of light and chlorophyll in plants. Carotenoids' anticarcinogenic properties have been extensively demonstrated in rodents such as rats and mice(53). Carotenoids are also found in green and yellow vegetables, and they are believed to have potential anticarcinogenic effects in humans(54). Their protective roles in smokers against the high level of oxidants in both cigarette smoke and tar have also been observed(55). Carotenoids have been clinically useful in the management of many genetic diseases, including porphyrias, which is characterized by photosensitivity, presumably caused by singlet oxygen generation (Figure 13.5).

Furthermore, certain diets have been studied as chemopreventive agents, such as the following:

1. The Mediterranean diet is characterized by its emphasis on fruits, vegetables, whole grains, nuts, seeds, and healthy fats like olive oil and fatty fish. Research indicates that adhering to the Mediterranean diet could potentially lower the susceptibility to various cancer types, including breast and colorectal cancer.
2. The DASH (Dietary Approaches to Stop Hypertension) diet is a plant-focused eating plan characterized by its low saturated fat content and high inclusion of fruits, vegetables, whole grains, and lean protein sources. Research has indicated that following the DASH diet could potentially contribute to lowering the risk of various cancer types, including breast, colorectal, and prostate cancer.
3. Vegetarian and vegan diets, characterized by their emphasis on plant-based foods like fruits, vegetables, whole grains, and legumes while minimizing animal product consumption, have gained attention for their potential health benefits. Research indicates that adopting these diets may offer protective effects against specific cancer types, including colorectal and breast cancer.
4. Low-fat diets, which prioritize the consumption of fruits, vegetables, and whole grains while minimizing the intake of fats, have been investigated for their potential impact on cancer risk. Research findings indicate that such diets might contribute to a decreased risk of breast cancer in women.

13.3.2 ROLE OF DIETARY COMPONENTS IN INDUCTION OF CARCINOGENESIS

Plants synthesize harmful substances in large quantities, seemingly as a main defensive agent against the groups of fungal, bacterial, insect and other predators(56). The plants commonly incorporated into the human diet are not exempt from this consideration. Harmful chemicals generated by dietary plants have been extensively studied by organic chemists for more than a century, and ongoing research continues to unveil new compounds of concern(56). Nevertheless, only a very small percentage of them are being toxicologically studied. Quite a number of natural teratogens, mutagens, and carcinogens have been identified in human diets by current extensive use of short-term assessments for sensing mutagens. Some examples are highlighted in the following sections.

1) **Hydrazine:** Hydrazine has the chemical formula N2H4 and is an inorganic compound. It is a colorless, flammable liquid with an ammonia-like odor, and it is a simple pnictogen hydride(57). Edible mushrooms can contain a notable amount of carcinogenic hydrazines. A prime example is the widely consumed false morel (*Gyromitra esculenta*), which contains 11 hydrazines, with three of them identified as carcinogenic compounds(58). N-methyl-N-formylhydrazine (C2H6N2O, CID 12962) is one of them; it occurs at a concentration of 50 mg per 100 g; it is implicated in lung tumors in mice at a very negligible concentration of 20 ug per mouse per day. *Agaricus bisporus*, the most widely available mushroom in the market, contains around 300 mg of agaritine per 100 g of the mushroom. Agaritine is the 8-glutamyl derivative of 4-hydroxy methylphenyl hydrazine. Additionally, small quantities of the closely related carcinogen N-acetyl-4-hydroxymethylphenylhydrazine are also present in these mushrooms(59).

2) **Methyleugenol, estragole, safrole, and related compounds:** These compounds occur in many edible plants. They are reported to be carcinogenic in rodents and are mostly metabolized to mutagens(60). Oil of sassafras containing almost 75% safrole is applicable in "natural" sarsaparilla root beer. Black pepper also contains a negligible quantity of safrole and a high quantity (approximately 10% by weight) of piperine, which is an intimately related compound. Report showed that black pepper extracts resulted in tumors in mice at different parts of the body at a quantity equivalent 160 mg/kg per day in a 3-month experiment(61). The average human intake of black pepper is estimated to exceed 140 mg per day(61)

3) **Phenols and their quinones derivatives:** These compounds are commonly found in the human diet. Quinones can exhibit toxicity through their ability to act as electrophiles or by accepting a single electron to form semiquinone radicals, which can directly interact with DNA(62) or contribute in superoxide radical formation by shifting electron to O2. The superoxide radical and its metabolic product hydrogen peroxide (H2O2) participate in lipid oxidation within cell membranes and cellular organelles through a chain reaction called lipid peroxidation, consequently producing mutagenic and carcinogenic effects. Many dietary phenols and quinones have been reported to be mutagenic(63). Some of these are derivatives of mutagenic anthraquinone, which are present in mold toxins and in plants, including rhubarb. Several dietary phenols are capable of spontaneously autoxidizing to quinones, thereby producing hydrogen-peroxide simultaneously(64).

4) **Acrylamide:** Acrylamide is a compound present in plant-based foods such as potatoes and cereal grains. It is formed through a natural chemical reaction between sugars and asparagine, an amino acid. Acrylamide is generated when food is subjected to high temperatures during cooking processes like frying, roasting, or baking. Information about carcinogenic effect of acrylamide came to light over two decades ago by some Swedish scientists(65). Several experiments have confirmed the toxicity, carcinogenic, mutagenic, and teratogenic consequences of acrylamide in many experimental models(66–69).

5) **Benzo(a)pyrene:** Benzo-(a)-pyrene, a carcinogenic substance, is also present in food. This compound falls within the category of polycyclic aromatic hydrocarbons (PAHs) and is produced when organic materials like meat are cooked at elevated temperatures. The International Agency for Research on Cancer (IARC) has classified benzo-(a)-pyrene as a carcinogen. This classification is based on substantial evidence indicating its potential to induce cancer in humans. Various types of food, such as grilled or charred meat, smoked fish, and specific vegetable oils, may contain benzo-(a)-pyrene and other polycyclic aromatic hydrocarbons (PAHs). These compounds are present due to cooking methods

involving high temperatures, and their presence raises concerns about potential health risks. The levels of these compounds in food can vary depending on the cooking method and the type of food being cooked. For example, grilling or barbecuing meat can produce higher levels of PAHs compared to other cooking methods.

The consumption of foods rich in benzo(a)pyrene and other polycyclic aromatic hydrocarbons (PAHs) has been associated with an elevated risk of specific cancer types, including lung, bladder, and colon cancer. This underscores the importance of considering the cooking methods and food choices to minimize potential health risks. Nevertheless, it is crucial to acknowledge that the risk of cancer associated with the ingestion of these compounds through food is generally considerably lower compared to the risks posed by other sources, such as tobacco smoke or environmental contaminants. To reduce exposure to benzo(a)pyrene and other PAHs in food, it is recommended to avoid or limit consumption of charred or grilled meat, smoked fish, and other foods that are cooked at high temperatures. Cooking methods that involve lower temperatures, such as steaming, boiling, or baking, can help reduce the formation of these compounds. Additionally, using marinades that contain vinegar or lemon juice or adding herbs and spices to meat can help reduce the formation of PAHs during cooking.

13.4   CONCLUSION

Nutrition and diet have a noteworthy impact on both the emergence and management of cancer. Specific dietary elements, such as soy products and flaxseed, comprise substances that can imitate or obstruct hormonal influences within the body. Hormonal activity is implicated in the initiation of particular cancer types, like breast and prostate cancer. Moreover, persistent inflammation within the body can elevate the likelihood of cancer by fostering the proliferation of aberrant cells.

Some dietary factors, including trans fats and refined sugars, can promote inflammation, while certain dietary components can act as carcinogens, or cancer-causing agents. Certain essential nutrients, including folate, vitamin D, and calcium, exhibit a safeguarding influence against cancer. Insufficient levels of these nutrients can elevate the susceptibility to cancer and other prolonged ailments. The body's inherent mechanisms can generate detrimental molecules known as free radicals, which possess the potential to harm cells and heighten the likelihood of cancer.

However, antioxidants found in fruits, vegetables, and other foods can help neutralize these free radicals and protect cells from damage. In essence, nutrition assumes a pivotal role in the development of cancer, encompassing both its promotion and prevention. A chemopreventive agent refers to a substance capable of mitigating or diminishing the risk of cancer. Diets abundant in fruits, vegetables, whole grains, and lean proteins have demonstrated chemopreventive attributes.

Nonetheless, it's crucial to acknowledge that diet represents just a single facet among the myriad factors influencing cancer susceptibility. A comprehensive comprehension of the intricate interplay between diet and cancer prevention necessitates further investigative efforts.

REFERENCES

[1] International Agency for Research on Cancer (IARC), Acrylamide, IARC (1994). Monographs on the evaluation of carcinogenic risks to humans, some industrial chemicals. International Agency for Research on Cancer, Lyon, 60, 389–433.

[2] Willett, W. C. (2000). Diet and cancer. Oncologist, 5, 393–404.

[3] WCRF/AICR (1997). Food, nutrition and the prevention of cancer: A global perspective. USA: World Cancer Research Fund/American Institute for Cancer Research. New York, NY 10006-3111.

[4] Tannenbaum, A. (1940). Initiation and growth of tumors; introduction: Effects of underfeeding. American Journal of Cancer, 39, 335–350.

[5] WCRF/AICR (2018). Continuous update Project Expert Report 2018. Preservation and Processing of foods and the risk to cancer.

[6]   Duesberg, P., & Li, R. (2003). Multistep carcinogenesis: A chain reaction of aneuploidizations. Cell Cycle, 2(3), 201–209.

[7]   Siddiqui, I. A., Sanna, V., Ahmad, N., Sechi, M., & Mukhtar, H. (2015). Resveratrol nanoformulation for cancer prevention and therapy. Annals of the New York Academy of Sciences, 1348(1), 20–31.

[8]   Blagosklonny, M. V. 2005. Carcinogenesis, cancer therapy and chemoprevention. Cell Death & Differentiation, 12, 592–602.

[9]   Anand, P., Kunnumakkara, A. B., Sundaram, C., Harikumar, B., Tharakan, S. T., Lai, O. S., Sung, B., & Aggarwal, B. B. (September 2008). Cancer is a preventable disease that requires major lifestyle changes. Pharmaceutical Research, 25(9), 2097–2116.

[10] WHO (2017). Available at www.who.int/mediacentre/factsheets/fs297/en/, accessed on 04.02.2017

[11] Kiel, C., Yus, E., & Serrano, L. (2010). Engineering signal transduction pathways. Cell, 140(1), 33–47.

[12] Adjei, A. A. (2005). Intracellular signal transduction pathway proteins as targets for cancer therapy. Journal of Clinical Oncology, 23(23), 5386–5403.

[13] Lokker, N. A., Sullivan, C. M., Hollenbach, S. J., Israel, M. A., & Giese, N. A. (2002). Platelet-derived growth factor (PDGF) autocrine signaling regulates survival and mitogenic pathways in glioblastoma cells: Evidence that the novel PDGF-C and PDGF-D ligands may play a role in the development of brain tumors. Cancer Research, 62(13), 3729–3735.

[14] Derynck, R., Goeddel, D. V., Ullrich, A., Gutterman, J. U., Williams, R. D., Bringman, T. S., & Berger, W. H. (1987). Synthesis of messenger RNAs for transforming growth factors A and β and the epidermal growth factor receptor by human tumors. Cancer Research, 47(3), 707–712.

[15] Guo, G., Gong, K., Wohlfeld, B., Hatanpaa, K. J., Zhao, D., & Habib, A. A. (2015). Ligand-independent EGFR signaling. Cancer Research, 75(17), 3436–3441.

[16] Carnero, A. et al. (2008). The PTEN/PI3K/AKT signalling pathway in cancer, therapeutic implications. Current Cancer Drug Targets, 8, 187–198.

[17] Schwartzman, R. A., & Cidlowski, J. A. (1993). Apoptosis: The biochemistry and molecular biology of programmed cell death. Endocrine Reviews, 14(2), 133–151.

[18] Carneiro, B. A., & El-Deiry, W. S. (2020). Targeting apoptosis in cancer therapy. Nature Reviews Clinical Oncology, 17(7), 395–417.

[19] Blows, W. T. (2005). The biological basis of nursing: Cancer. London: Routledge.

[20] Van Gerpen, R. (2007). Pathophysiology. In Oncology nursing, M. E. Langhorne, J. S. Fulton, & S. E. Otto, Editors (pp. 3–16). Mosby: St. Louis.

[21] Bosman, F. T. (2006). Pathology. In nursing patients with cancer: Principles and practice, N. Kearney & A. Richardson, Editors. Elsevier: Edinburgh.

[22] Folkman, J. (2002). Role of angiogenesis in tumor growth and metastasis. Seminars in Oncology, 29(6), 15–18.

[23] Ferrara, N. (2002). VEGF and the quest for tumour angiogenesis factors. Nature Reviews Cancer, 2(10), 795–803.

[24] Wong, P. P., Bodrug, N., & Hodivala-Dilke, K. M. (2016). Exploring novel methods for modulating tumor blood vessels in cancer treatment. Current Biology, 26(21), R1161–R1166.

[25] Patel, A., Pathak, Y., Patel, J., & Sutariya, V. (2018). Role of nutritional factors in pathogenesis of cancer. Food Quality and Safety, 2(1), 27–36.

[26] Doll, R., & Peto, R. (1981). The causes of cancer: Quantitative estimates of avoidable risks of cancer in the United States today. JNCI: Journal of the National Cancer Institute, 66(6), 1192–1308.

[27] National Research Council (1982). Diet, nutrition and cancer. Washington, DC: National Academy Press.

[28] Donaldson, M. S. (2004). Nutrition and cancer: A review of the evidence for an anti-cancer diet. Nutrition Journal, 3(1), 1–21.

[29] Hartman, P. E. (1983). Putative mutagens and carcinogens in foods. I. Nitrate/nitrite ingestion and gastric cancer mortality. Environmental Mutagenesis, 5(1), 111–121.

[30] Totter, J. R. (1980). Spontaneous cancer and its possible relationship to oxygen metabolism. Proceedings of the National Academy of Sciences, 77(4), 1763–1767.

[31] Nagata, M. (2005). Inflammatory cells and oxygen radicals. Current Drug Targets-Inflammation & Allergy, 4(4), 503–504.

[32] Limón-Pacheco, J., & Gonsebatt, M. E. (2009). The role of antioxidants and antioxidant-related enzymes in protective responses to environmentally induced oxidative stress. Mutation Research/Genetic Toxicology and Environmental Mutagenesis, 674(1–2), 137–147.

[33] Wargovich, M. J. (2000). Anticancer properties of fruits and vegetables. HortScience, 35(4), 573–575.

[34] Kritchevsky, D. (1995). Epidemiology of fibre, resistant starch and colorectal cancer. European Journal of Cancer Prevention, 4(5), 345–352.

[35] Hunter, E. A., & Grimble, R. F. (1997). Dietary sulphur amino acid adequacy influences glutathione synthesis and glutathione-dependent enzymes during the inflammatory response to endotoxin and tumour necrosis factor-A in rats. Clinical Science, 92(3), 297–305.

[36] Wang, L. I., Giovannucci, E. L., Hunter, D., Neuberg, D., Su, L., & Christiani, D. C. (2004). Dietary intake of cruciferous vegetables, glutathione S-transferase (GST) polymorphisms and lung cancer risk in a Caucasian population. Cancer Causes & Control, 15(10), 977–985.

[37] Offord, E. A., Gautier, J. C., Avanti, O., Scaletta, C., Runge, F., Krämer, K., & Applegate, L. A. (2002). Photoprotective potential of lycopene, β-carotene, vitamin E, vitamin C and carnosic acid in UVA-irradiated human skin fibroblasts. Free Radical Biology and Medicine, 32(12), 1293–1303.

[38] Charalabopoulos, K., Karkabounas, S., Charalabopoulos, A. K., Papalimneou, V., Ioachim, E., & Giannakopoulos, X. (2003). Inhibition of benzo (a) pyrene-induced carcinogenesis by vitamin C alone and by vitamin C/vitamin E and selenium/glutathione. Biological Trace Element Research, 93(1), 201–211.

[39] Reddy, V. G., Khanna, N., & Singh, N. (2001). Vitamin C augments chemotherapeutic response of cervical carcinoma HeLa cells by stabilizing P53. Current Pharmaceutical Biotechnology, 282, 409–415. doi:10.1006/bbrc.2001.4593

[40] Martinotti, S., Ranzato, E., & Burlando, B. (2011). In vitro screening of synergistic ascorbate-drug combinations for the treatment of malignant mesothelioma. Toxicology in Vitro, 25, 1568–1574.

[41] Cieslak, J. A., Strother, R. K., Rawal, M., Du, J., Doskey, C. M., Schroeder, S. R., et al. (2015). Manganoporphyrins and ascorbate enhance gemcitabine cytotoxicity in pancreatic cancer. Free Radical Biology and Medicine, 83, 227–237.

[42] Xia, J., Xu, H., Zhang, X., Allamargot, C., Coleman, K. L., Nessler, R., et al. (2017). Multiple myeloma tumor cells are selectively killed by pharmacologically-dosed ascorbic acid. EBioMedicine, 18, 41–49.

[43] Hoffer, L. J., Robitaille, L., Zakarian, R., Melnychuk, D., Kavan, P., Agulnik, J., et al. (2015). High-dose intravenous vitamin C combined with cytotoxic chemotherapy in patients with advanced cancer: A phase I-II clinical trial. PLoS One, 10, e0120228.

[44] Monti, D. A., Mitchell, E., Bazzan, A. J., Littman, S., Zabrecky, G., Yeo, C. J., et al. (2012). Phase I evaluation of intravenous ascorbic acid in combination with gemcitabine and erlotinib in patients with metastatic pancreatic cancer. PLoS One, 7, e29794.

[45] Cieslak, J. A., & Cullen, J. J. (2015). Treatment of pancreatic cancer with pharmacological ascorbate. Current Pharmaceutical Biotechnology, 16, 759–770.

[46] Pryor, W. A. (1987). Cigarette smoke and the involvement of free radical reactions in chemical carcinogenesis. The British Journal of Cancer. Supplement, 8, 19.

[47] Bieri, J. G., Corash, L., & Hubbard, V. S. (1983). Medical uses of vitamin E. New England Journal of Medicine, 308(18), 1063–1071.

[48] Arnott, M. S., Van Eys, J., & Wang, Y. M. (1982). Molecular interrelations of nutrition and cancer. In Symposium on fundamental cancer research 1981: Anderson Hospital and Tumor Institute. New York: Raven Press.

[49] Wattenberg, L. W. (1983). Inhibition of neoplasia by minor dietary constituents. Cancer Research, 43(5 Suppl), 2448s–2453s.

[50] Ciolino, H. P., & Yeh, G. C. (1999). Inhibition of aryl hydrocarbon-induced cytochrome P-450 1A1 enzyme activity and CYP1A1 expression by resveratrol. Molecular Pharmacology, 56(4), 760–767.

[51] Riaz, M., Zia-Ul-Haq, M., & Dou, D. (2021). Chemistry of carotenoids. In Carotenoids: Structure and function in the human body (pp. 43–76). Cham: Springer.

[52] Telfer, A. (2014). Singlet oxygen production by PSII under light stress: Mechanism, detection and the protective role of β-carotene. Plant and Cell Physiology, 55(7), 1216–1223.

[53] Krinsky, N. I. (1994). The biological properties of carotenoids. Pure and Applied Chemistry, 66(5), 1003–1010.

[54] Khoo, H. E., Prasad, K. N., Kong, K. W., Jiang, Y., & Ismail, A. (2011). Carotenoids and their isomers: Color pigments in fruits and vegetables. Molecules, 16(2), 1710–1738.

[55] Gabriel, H. E., Liu, Z., Crott, J. W., Choi, S. W., Song, B. C., Mason, J. B., & Johnson, E. J. (2006). A comparison of carotenoids, retinoids, and tocopherols in the serum and buccal mucosa of chronic cigarette smokers versus nonsmokers. Cancer Epidemiology and Prevention Biomarkers, 15(5), 993–999.

[56] D'Mello, J. F., Duffus, C. M., & Duffus, J. H. (Eds.). (1991). Toxic substances in crop plants. Sawston, Cambridge: Woodhead Publishing.

[57] Chellappa, R., Dattelbaum, D., Daemen, L., & Liu, Z. (2014, May). High pressure spectroscopic studies of hydrazine (N2H4). Journal of Physics: Conference Series, 500(5), p. 052008.

[58] Sugimura, T., Miller, E. C., Miller, J. A., Hirono, I., & Takayama, S. (1979). Naturally occurring carcinogens – mutagens and modulators of carcinogenesis. In Naturally occurring genotoxic carcinogens (pp. 241–399). Baltimore: University Park Press.

[59] Lawson, T. (1987). Metabolism of arylhydrazines by cytochrome P-450 mixed function oxidases and prostaglandin (H) synthase from mouse lungs. Cancer Letters, 34(2), 193–200.

[60] Smith, R. L., Adams, T. B., Doull, J., Feron, V. J., Goodman, J. I., Marnett, L. J., . . . Sipes, I. G. (2002). Safety assessment of allylalkoxybenzene derivatives used as flavouring substances – methyl eugenol and estragole. Food and Chemical Toxicology, 40(7), 851–870.

[61] El-Mofty, M. M., Khudoley, V. V., & Shwaireb, M. H. (1991). Carcinogenic effect of force-feeding an extract of black pepper (Piper nigrum) in Egyptian toads (Bufo-regularis). Oncology, 48(4), 347–350.

[62] Yager, J. D. (2015). Mechanisms of estrogen carcinogenesis: The role of E2/E1–quinone metabolites suggests new approaches to preventive intervention–A review. Steroids, 99, 56–60.

[63] Kikugawa, K., & Kato, T. (1988). Formation of a mutagenic diazoquinone by interaction of phenol with nitrite. Food and Chemical Toxicology, 26(3), 209–214.

[64] Chand, R., Ince, N. H., Gogate, P. R., & Bremner, D. H. (2009). Phenol degradation using 20, 300 and 520 kHz ultrasonic reactors with hydrogen peroxide, ozone and zero valent metals. Separation and Purification Technology, 67(1), 103–109.

[65] Tareke, E., Rydberg, P., Karlsson, P., Eriksson, S., & Törnqvist, M. (2002). Analysis of acrylamide, a carcinogen formed in heated foodstuffs. Journal of Agricultural and Food Chemistry, 50(17), 4998–5006.

[66] Tyl, R. W. et al. (2003). Effects of acrylamide on rodent reproductive performance. Reproductive Toxicology, 17, 1–13.

[67] Rice, J. M. (2005). The carcinogenicity of acrylamide. Mutation Research, 580, 3–20.

[68] Ehling, U. H., & Neuhäuser-Klaus, A. (1992). Reevaluation of the induction of specific-locus mutations in spermatogonia of the mouse by acrylamide. Mutation Research Letters, 283(3), 185–191.

[69] Ghanayem, B. I., Witt, K. L., Kissling, G. E., Tice, R. R., & Recio, L. (2005). Absence of acrylamide-induced genotoxicity in CYP2E1-null mice: Evidence consistent with a glycidamide-mediated effect. Mutation Research/Fundamental and Molecular Mechanisms of Mutagenesis, 578(1–2), 284–297.

14 Lectins
(Glyco-)Proteins for Health and Longevity

Taiwo Scholes Adewole, Stanley Chukwuejim,
Titilayo Oluwaseun Agunbiade, and Adenike Kuku

14.1 INTRODUCTION

Lectins, also known as haemagglutinins or agglutinins, are common proteins or glycoproteins with no enzymatic activity that reversibly attach to carbohydrates (Enoma et al., 2023). In addition to this attribute, these molecules are also not of immune origin (Nilsson, 2007). They have long been thought to be involved in defence processes and are widely dispersed throughout prokaryotic and eukaryotic organisms, including higher plants, algae, fungi, marine corals, invertebrates, and vertebrates (Peumans and Van Damme, 1995; Adedoyin et al., 2021). Lectins interact with their saccharide ligands via specific pockets called the carbohydrates recognition domain (CRD) (López-Moreno et al., 2022). Each form of lectin has a distinctive structure and sugar selectivity, depending on its origin. For instance, animal lectins are more particular for multiplex sugar structures, while algal lectins are more specific for glycoconjugates such as glycoproteins. Bacteria and fungi lectins, on the other hand, are more specific for glycans and N-acetyl galactosamine, respectively, and lectins of plant origin mostly recognize simpler monosaccharides and oligosaccharides (Kilpatrick, 2002; López-Moreno et al., 2022).

Lectins play vital roles in the colonization processes of bacteria, archaea, protists, and fungi, serving as adhesion molecules (Gupta and Gupta, 2021; Lewis et al., 2022). They are also important in plant resistance systems and nodulation. Depending on their properties and distribution in tissues, lectins play key roles in a variety of animal processes, including hemolysis, cell motility and adhesion, opsonization, immunological responses, phagocytosis, and glycoprotein synthesis (Santos et al., 2014; Nubi et al., 2021; Nabi-Afjadi et al., 2022). The specific purpose of lectins in plants is still unresolved; however, they are considered to be involved in plant defence mechanisms (Berg et al., 2002). Aside from their beneficial roles, lectins are found in many of our meals, particularly seeds, tubers, cereals, and legumes, which are resistant to cooking and digestive enzymes, likely toxic, and potent inflammation agents (Sharon and Lis, 2004). Hence, this chapter discusses the different roles of lectins in their host organisms and their nutritional significance and further illuminates the biological and exploitable, health-promoting functions of these quintessential biomolecules.

14.2 CLASSIFICATION OF LECTINS

14.2.1 MICROBIAL LECTINS

Microbial lectins are heterogeneous glycoproteins found in microorganisms, including bacteria, fungi, and protozoa. Within their unique hosts, these lectins are mostly associated with microbe virulence, entry to host cell surfaces, and microbial association. These qualities make them an essential tool in a variety of disciplines, including biomedicine (Rubeena et al., 2021).

DOI: 10.1201/9781003361497-16

14.2.1.1 Bacteria Lectins

Bacteria lectins are also referred to as adhesins because they are used by microbes to begin their connection to host cells through specialized cell adhesion. The microbe eventually colonizes the host, begins to cause pathogenesis, and infects it as a result of its adhesion and adsorption. Consequently, altering the activity of lectins can be used to modify disease resistance, and it might serve as the foundation for new therapeutics to fight infectious diseases (Sharon and Ofek, 2000). The demonstration that bacterial cell surface lectins play a role in the attachment of the organisms to host cell surfaces during infection initiation took place in the 1970s. Additionally, it was shown that the inhibition of these lectins by the appropriate sugars can form the basis of an anti-adhesion therapy for bacterial infections (Sharon, 2008).

Bacterial lectins elicit diverse biological activities, including stimulation of murine lymphocytes (Nakae et al., 1994). As reviewed by Singh and Walia (2014), *Pseudomonas aeruginosa* is a bacterium species that has a high concentration of lectins with a sizable mitogenic potential. The PA-II lectin from *P. aeruginosa* stimulates the proliferation of T cells by interacting with mannose-bearing receptors. The activation of human peripheral lymphocytes and murine splenocytes by PA-II gets suppressed by L-fucose. Bacterial lectins from *P. aeruginosa*, PA-I, and PA-II have a preference for D-galactose and L-fucose, respectively, making them potential targets in the treatment of *P. aeruginosa* infections (Gilboa-Garber, 1982; Avichezer and Gilboa-Garber, 1987; Grishin et al., 2015). In a similar study, Lakhtin et al. (2006) reported the detection and isolation of lectin from different strains of *bifidobacteria* and *lactobacilli*. According to these authors, the lectins reacted with complex glycan structures such as mannan-alpha and GalNAc alpha-polysaccharide of mucin-like-type or galactan-beta and are implicated in signaling mechanisms regulating bacteria communication and association.

Many different bacterial strains produce surface lectins, frequently in the form of filamentous assemblies of protein components called fimbriae. The type 1 (mannose specific) fimbrial lectins of *Escherichia coli*, which are virtually entirely composed of one class of components with a molecular mass of 17 kDa, are among the best-studied of these. They have an extended combining site that is similar to a trisaccharide, and they prefer to bind oligomannose or hybrid carbohydrate units. Since aromatic A-mannosides greatly inhibit yeast agglutination by bacteria and their adhesion to pig ileal epithelial cells, type 1 fimbriae also have a hydrophobic area near the carbohydrate-binding site (Sharon, 1987). Pre-suspending the bacteria in a solution of A-methyl-D-mannoside, a sugar to which the bacteria do not attach, significantly reduced the amount of A-mannose-specific *E. coli* strain that infects mice bladders; however, glucose had no effect. Adhesion-inhibitory saccharides have been shown to have preventive effects in a variety of additional animal models, including *Helicobacter pylori* stomach infection in monkeys and *Pneumococcal pneumonia* in rats (Sharon, 2006).

14.2.1.2 Fungal Lectins

Recent years have seen a significant increase in interest in fungi, which includes yeasts, mushrooms, and microfungi (Adewole et al., 2022). They offer a promising source of new hemagglutinating proteins with distinct saccharide binding and the potential for use in biotechnological and medicinal purposes (Varrot et al., 2013). A plethora of fungal lectins has been documented, with more than 82%, 15%, and 3% from mushrooms, molds, and yeasts, respectively (Singh et al., 2011). Mushroom fruiting bodies and vegetative mycelia are both heavily populated with lectins. Mycelial lectins from *Basidiomycetes* have been isolated in various intracellular, extracellular, and surface forms (Nikitina et al., 2017; Adedoyin et al., 2021). Specific mushroom glycan-binding proteins have been documented to be specific to the inhibition of agglutination by one or more saccharide and/or their derivatives. These include lectins from *Agrocybe cylindracea* (lactose, sialic acid, and inulin), *Boletus edulis* (melibiose- and xylose-co-specific), *Ganoderma capense* (D+-galactose and D+-galactosamine), among others (Ng and Lam, 2002). Even though they frequently remain mysterious, several biological activities and physiological functions for fungal lectins in growth,

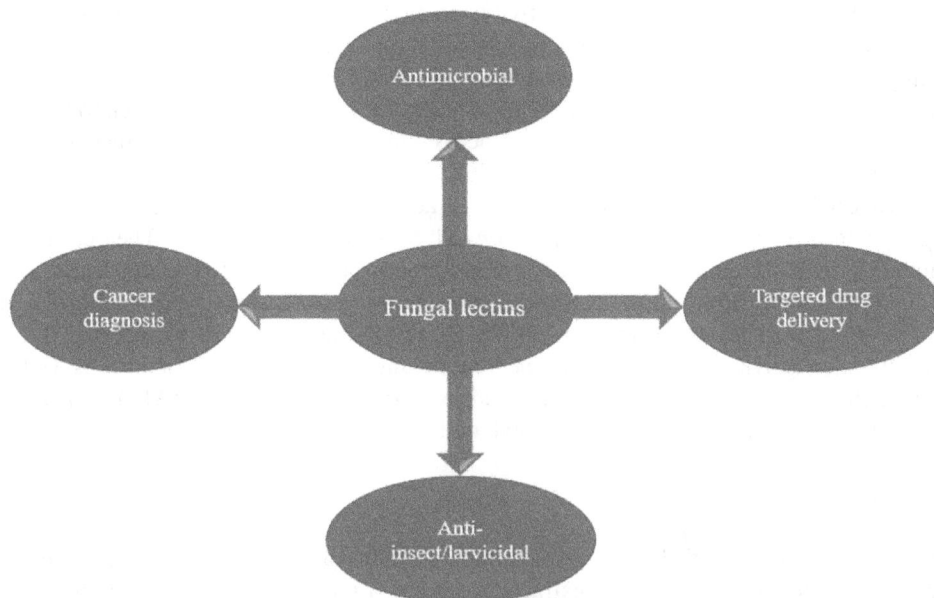

FIGURE 14.1 Fungal lectins and their exploitable applications.

development, morphogenesis, and defense have been hypothesized (Veelders et al., 2010; Díaz et al., 2011; Khan and Khan, 2011; Pujic et al., 2012), as shown in Figure 14.1.

Numerous lectins from yeasts and micro-fungi were demonstrated to take part in a direct function in the pathogenesis of human ailments. For instance, during all stages of infection, the N-acetylglucosamine-specific lectin paracoccin from *Paracoccidioides brasiliensis* binds to laminin, a component of the extracellular matrix, and induces macrophages to release TNF-A and nitric oxide, two substances that are important mediators in paracoccidioidomycosis (Coltri et al., 2006). *Aspergillus fumigatus* and *Candida glabrata* lectins, two fungi that cause serious nosocomial illnesses, have also recently shown specific binding to human oligosaccharides. The human blood type oligosaccharides that AFL1 from *A. fumigatus* binds to are located on the surface of conidia. When exogenous fucose is added, the lectin's potently pro-inflammatory impact on human bronchial cells may be reduced. On the other hand, there are several Epa epithelial adhesins/lectins, which are glycosylphosphatidylinositol-anchored cell wall proteins, in the pathogenic yeast *C. glabrata* (Maestre-Reyna et al., 2012).

14.2.1.3 Protozoa Lectins

Lectins are outstanding candidates to mediate contact between parasites and corresponding target-cell ligands, and as a result, they mediate a crucial function in cellular communications. Only 2.2% of all microbial lectins are protozoal lectins (Singh et al., 2016). Numerous protozoa, including *Trichomonas* (Roussel et al., 1991), *Entamoeba* (Petri et al., 1987), *Giardia* (Ward et al., 1990), *Cryptosporidium* (Joe et al., 1994), and *Plasmodium* (Jungery, 1985), among others, have hemagglutinating proteins. In these organisms, lectins facilitate parasitic attachment to host cellular components, and hence, facilitate a crucial function in a variety of cell-to-cell associations, erythrocyte attachment, and cytopathogenicity (Thea et al., 1992). Protozoan lectins preferentially interact with galactose/GalNAc moieties, which explains why they can bind to human erythrocytes that have these groups. *Entamoeba histolytica* and *C. parvum* have both been found to produce lectins that are specific for Gal/GalNAc (Ravdin and Guerrant, 1981; Joe et al., 1994).

Parasitic lectins typically have their activity increased when treated with enzymes. *Giardia lamblia* trophozoites' surface membrane-associated lectin eagerly adheres to rabbit erythrocytes, especially following trypsin treatment (Farthing et al., 1986). By eliminating the glycol layer from the surface of the erythrocyte, protease treatment causes the underlying cryptantigen to become *de novo* exposed. According to the available evidence, *G. lamblia* lectin has the distinctive ability to activate with minimal proteolysis (Lev et al., 1986).

Selective erythrocyte agglutination was displayed at the intrusive sporozoite phase, while oocyst and sporozoite hemagglutinins from *C. parvum* exhibit non-precise activity (Thea et al., 1992). The glutaraldehyde-fixed rabbit erythrocytes showed the strongest reactivity to this lectin. Human ABO and erythrocytes from rabbit, pig, sheep, and rat are agglutinated by the trophozoite lectin of *E. histolytica* (Kobiler and Mirelman, 1980). However, Kato et al. (2015) reported the weak hemagglutination activity of the lectin intermediate subunit toward horse red blood cells. Unlike *E. histolytica*, *Acanthamoeba* hemagglutinin elicited a strong specificity for Man(A1–3)Man units and methyl-A-mannopyranoside (Garate et al., 2004; da Rocha-Azevedo et al., 2010).

14.2.2 PLANT LECTINS

Lectins were initially identified in plants more than a century ago when Stillmark discovered that castor bean (*Ricinus communis*) seed extracts contained a protein that could agglutinate animal red blood cells (Stillmark, 1888). Plant lectins can be categorized into four types based on their molecular makeup: merolectins, hololectins, chimerolectins, and superlectins. Merolectins are composed of just one lectin domain. Hololectins and superlectins, on the other hand, have several lectin domains. A superlectin consists of many lectin domains with distinct capacities for binding carbohydrates. Chimerolectins are lectins that combine a lectin domain with one or more protein domains that have different functions (Peumans and Van Damme, 1995). Research on plant lectins in the 1980s focused on storage tissues as a rich source of proteins that bind to carbohydrates (particularly bark, rhizomes, bulbs, and corms) (Van Damme et al., 1998). Since their isolation and purification, new lectins displaying a wide range of molecular arrangements and sugar-binding characteristics were discovered, allowing lectin research to advance from seeds to other plant tissues (Johnny et al., 2016; Oladokun et al., 2019; Nubi et al., 2021).

The first group of copious lectins is sometimes called "classical lectins". These proteins/glycoproteins are present in many commonly consumed plant foods, including vegetables, cereals, fruits, pulses, and legumes, among others (Vasconcelos and Oliveira, 2004). In recent times, it has been conclusively demonstrated that, in addition to these groups of lectins, plants usually produce trace quantities of hemagglutinating proteins that bind to carbohydrates when they are subjected to stressful conditions like drought, high salt content, hormone treatment, pathogen attack, or insect herbivory (Lannoo and Van Damme, 2010). These lectins are known as "inducible" lectins because they exhibit no detectable lectin activity under normal growth conditions but exhibit a definite upregulation in response to stress. These inducible hemagglutinins can be found at different subcellular structures of plant cells, as opposed to the vacuole or cell wall, as in the case of the classical lectins. Based on research findings, it was hypothesized that the cytoplasm and nucleus's lectin-mediated protein-carbohydrate interactions are crucial to the plant cell's stress physiology (Smith et al., 2010).

14.2.3 ANIMAL LECTINS

Animal lectins were found before plant lectins; however, most have remained unrecognized as proteins that bind to carbohydrates for many years after their first discovery (Kilpatrick, 2002). Although the main architectures of animal and plant lectins are not identical, they both prefer to bind to the myriads of glycans (Ghazarian et al., 2011). In variance to immunoglobulins or catalytic proteins, animal lectins are neither immunological initiators nor catalysts, and they can recognize

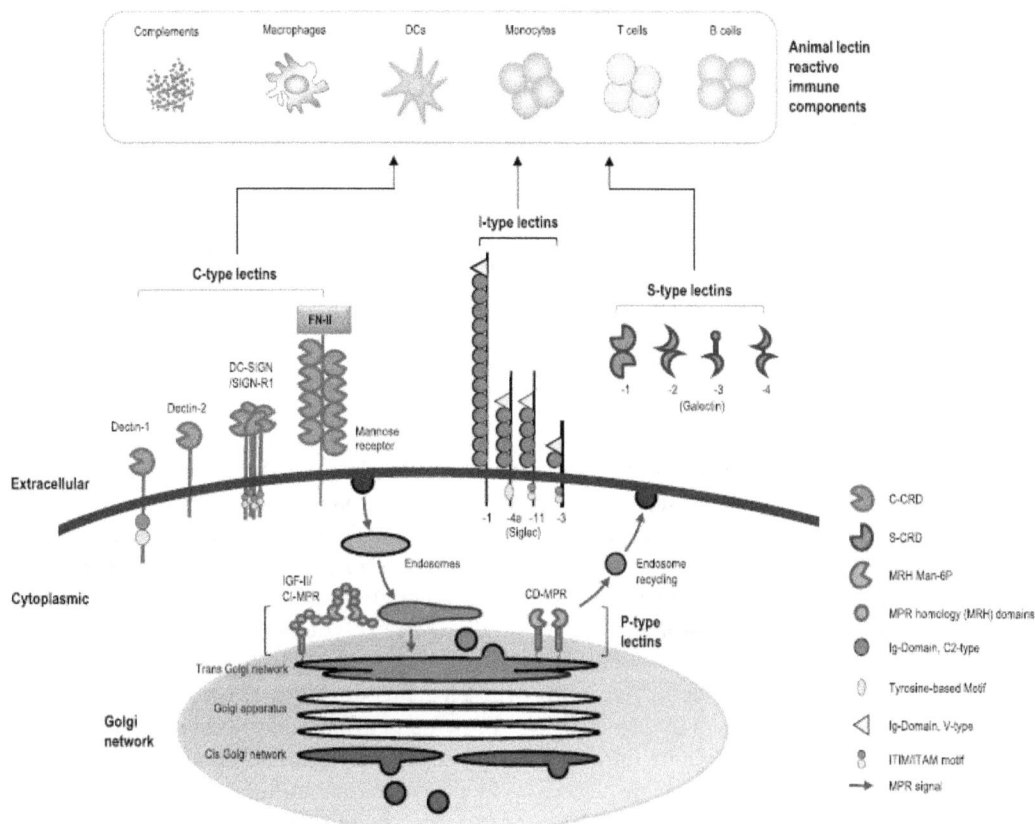

FIGURE 14.2 The composition, cellular distribution, and immune-reactive elements of animal lectins (Loh et al., 2017).

or bind sophisticated glycan structures, particularly via the CRD (Anderson et al., 2008). Animal lectin activity has been linked to an amazing variety of basic structures (Kilpatrick, 2002).

There are at least 12 structural families that bind substances other than carbohydrates through interactions between proteins, lipids, or nucleic acids. Cell adhesion, cell migration, cell signaling, morphogenesis, complement activation, and cell recognition are some of their functions in glycol-recognition systems (Figure 14.2).

Animal lectins can also support defense systems, particularly by recognizing the carbohydrate of a pathogen. Additionally, they can attach to different cells or microbial pathogens by binding to the target cells' superficial glycan types (Matsumoto et al., 2001; Anderson et al., 2008).

Over the past few decades, marine creatures have been thoroughly investigated as possible sources of novel physiologically active chemicals, and substantial study has been done on lectins. Lectins originating from marine creatures have a variety of structural characteristics and biological activities and are distinct from those found in terrestrial organisms (Cheung et al., 2015). One of the first hemagglutinins used in blood typing was from the European eel, *Anguilla anguilla* (Honda et al., 2000). But it was not until very recently that the main structure's entirety was established, resulting in the identification of a new family of animal lectins (Kilpatrick, 2002).

Lectins from marine species can interact specifically with the saccharide residues on the pathogen exterior necessary for binding to the integumental cells. Ottinger et al. (1999) isolated a mannose-specific lectin from *Salmo sala* serum that demonstrated opsonizing action for a highly pathogenic *Aeromonas salmonicida*. Programmed cell death initiation in human tumor cells by an aquatic sponge hemagglutinin was the subject of research by Rabelo et al. (2012). These authors extracted the lectin (CaL) from *Cinachyrella apion*, a sea sponge, and investigated its antiproliferative effects on three different human carcinoma cell lines. Their findings demonstrated that CaL had the strongest growth-inhibitory action against HeLa cells in a concentration-related order. Additionally, Rabelo and colleagues showed that CaL most likely caused programmed cell death in target cells by boosting the production of the apoptotic-inducing protein Bax, improving mitochondrial membrane porosity, activating specific cysteine proteases, and causing cell cycle incapacitation at the "synthesis stage". Ashraf et al. (2015) also documented a β-galactoside-specific galectin isolated from the goat heart muscle elicited potent hemolytic activity and was moderately inhibited by lactose and sucrose.

14.3   DIETARY LECTINS: BENEFICIAL AND HAZARDOUS IMPLICATIONS

Foods contain several lectin kinds, and individuals respond to them in a variety of ways. It is conceivable that someone with a preexisting digestive sensitivity, such as irritable bowel syndrome, may be more susceptible to unpleasant side effects from lectin ingestion. Legume lectins have been the subject of lectin study for a while now because they are so prevalent in legume seeds (Sharon and Lis, 1990). Several hazardous lectins were identified shortly after ricin was discovered. However, it became clear that not all lectins are harmful as more and more lectins were isolated. Proof for nonlethal lectins from the *Leguminosae* family was provided by Landsteiner and Raubitschek (1907) from beans, vetch, pea, and lentil.

Heterotrophs including humans are frequently exposed to functionally active lectins (Vasconcelos and Oliveira, 2004). Numerous of these lectins have been found to particularly bind to the sialic acid and N-acetylglucosamine-containing O- and N-linked sugar moieties that are ubiquitously found on the exterior of the epithelial cells displayed on the digestive tract of higher and lower animals, respectively (Peumans et al., 2000). These glycans are accessible to food proteins/lectins, making them possible binding sites for lectins from ingested plants. However, lectin might have negative or hazardous consequences ranging from mild discomfort to fatal poisoning if binding to these receptors has an unfavorable outcome, which sometimes includes alteration of the gut microbiota, epithelial membrane damage, and triggering of systemic inflammation (Van Damme, 2008; Zarate et al., 2009; Vandenborre et al., 2011).

Following their capacity to bind immunoglobulin E (IgE), degranulate mast cells and basophils, and initiate interleukin responses in a variety of allergic patients, many plant lectins, particularly those derived from wheat, chestnut, avocado, pawpaw, tomatoes, etc., have been identified as possible food allergens (Haas et al., 1999; Moreno et al., 2003; Barre et al., 2020). Some outbreaks of food poisoning have been attributed to the availability of nutritionally notable quantities of active hemagglutinating proteins/glycoproteins as well as the unavailability of widespread awareness regarding the negative significance of these lectins on the stomach and human well-being. For instance, toxins found in raw or only partially cooked kidney beans (*Phaseolus vulgaris*) were blamed for seven instances involving 43 people (Noah et al., 1980). The oral severe lethality of lectins in exposed people is typically characterized by nausea, bloating, vomiting, and diarrhea. Evident signs include appetite loss, weight reduction, and in due course, mortality, as evidenced in laboratory animals placed on plant lectin diets (Duranti and Gius, 1997; Lajolo and Genovese, 2002).

Studies on animals and cells have shown that active lectins can also obstruct the uptake of minerals, including calcium, iron, phosphorus, and zinc. These minerals are frequently found in cereals and legumes; hence, the presence of lectins may inhibit the body from absorbing and using these minerals. Additionally, the binding of lectins to the cells in the digestive tract can induce dysbiosis (Banwell et al., 1988). Similarly, dietary lectins reportedly diminish the activities of jejunal digestive enzymes, reduce gastric acid secretions, and alter the structural integrity of the microvilli (Kordás et al., 2001; Nciri et al., 2015; Nciri and Cho, 2018). Inflammatory disorders, including rheumatoid arthritis and type 1 diabetes, are thought to be influenced by the long-lasting cell-binding properties of lectins to immunoglobulin molecules, which have the potential to trigger an autoimmune reaction (Freed, 1999; Barre et al., 2020). Supporting the autoimmune theory of dietary lectins, Lambert and Vojdani (2017) discovered that individuals with IgG antibodies to wheat germ agglutinin were more likely to have higher autoantibodies to several tissue components than individuals without these antibodies.

Despite all of these scenarios, there is very little human research on the number of active lectins taken in the diet and their long-term consequences on health. The diets of underdeveloped nations, where malnutrition is common or where food diversity is relatively restricted and whole grains and legumes are significant daily mainstays, are those where anti-nutrients, particularly lectins, are most frequently investigated (Gibson et al., 2010; Roos et al., 2013). In addition, it is crucial to keep in mind that consuming meals with a high concentration of active lectins is uncommon. This is because lectins are most effective when they are fresh, but most people do not eat their lectin-containing foods uncooked. Most food lectins can be rendered inactive by cooking, particularly when moist high-heat techniques like boiling or stewing are used, as well as by soaking in water for several hours. Lectins are normally present on the outer surface of food crops and are water-soluble, so they are removed when the food is exposed to water (Petroski and Minich, 2020).

Lectins can function as antioxidants, shielding cells from the harm that free radicals can do. Additionally, they slow down digestion and glucose absorption, which may lessen the likelihood of significant blood sugar and insulin spikes. Early studies are also examining the use of non-toxic, low doses of specific lectins to aid in stimulating gut cell growth in patients who are unable to eat for a period as well as in anticancer therapies due to their capacity to trigger cancer cell death (Liu et al., 2013). Legumes, whole grains, and nuts are lectin-rich foods that have been linked to lower incidences of type 2 diabetes, heart disease, and weight loss in numerous large population studies. These foods are abundant in healthy fibres, protein, minerals, and B vitamins. Because of this, eating these foods is believed to have much greater health benefits than any potential risks from their lectin content (Liu et al., 1999; De Munter et al., 2007; Aune et al., 2013). The effects of dietary lectins on autoimmune, inflammation, or gastrointestinal disease have not yet been thoroughly studied, and there isn't enough evidence to say that they cause any particular disorders. Even though it is wise to avoid consuming lectins in their raw, uncooked forms, properly cooked lectin-containing foods are believed to not necessarily pose a health risk to everyone (Lucius, 2020).

14.4 BIOLOGICAL ACTIVITIES OF LECTINS

Lectins stand out in remedial functions due to their many characteristic properties, driving their potential applications. The principal of this is their ability to bind glycoconjugates, making them vital tools in biological science research. They are quite prevalent in plants (Table 14.1) and affect cells in several different ways, including cell aggregation, mitogenic stimulation, redistribution of cell surface components, modification of the activity of membrane catalytic proteins, and defence against microbial growth, among others (Li et al 2008, Araújo et al., 2013, Silva et al., 2016a).

Due to their saccharide specificity, lectins can identify tissues and support illness detection. These fundamental biomolecules have been demonstrated to trigger a variety of biological processes, such as cell identification and labeling, antibacterial, fungal, insecticidal, viral, inflammatory, and nociceptive effects, among others (Mishra et al., 2019).

14.4.1 ANTI-INSECT AND LARVICIDAL ACTIVITY

Lectins function as a vital larvicidal and/or insecticidal biomolecule for a vast array of insects. They are being proposed as a bio-inspired substitute for classical insect control (Santos et al., 2014; Hamid et al., 2013; Adedoyin et al., 2021). By interfering with their regular physiological activities, lectins have been shown to have negative impacts on specific life stages of insects, including nymph, adult, and oviposition (Sadeghi et al., 2006; Lagarda-Diaz et al., 2017). In our previous studies,

TABLE 14.1

Tissue-Specific Localization of Plant Lectins with Corresponding Biological Functions

Tissues	Biological activities	References
Seeds	Anticoagulant, antiplatelet aggregation properties; coagulant, mitogenic, antibacterial, antifungal, antitumor activities	(Wong et al., 2006; Singha et al., 2007; Sitohy et al., 2007; Santos et al., 2009; Brustein et al., 2012, Silva et al., 2014)
Bark	Antifungal and insecticidal activities	(Vaz et al., 2010, de Araújo et al., 2012)
Hartwood	Termiticidal activity	(Vaz et al., 2010, de Araújo et al., 2012)
Stem	Antiviral and apoptosis-inducing activities	(Sa et al., 2008)
Leaves	Antiviral, antibacterial, and antifungal activities	(Peng et al., 2009)
Fruits	Mitogenic and antiviral activities	(Costa et al., 2010)
Roots	Antifungal and termiticidal activities	(Souza et al., 2011)
Tubers	Insecticidal and antitumor activities	(Kaur et al., 2005)
Bulbs	Proteolytic activities	(Parisi et al., 2008)
Rhizomes	Antiproliferative, immunostimulatory, antiviral, antifungal, antitumor, and apoptosis-inducing activities	(Yao et al., 2010)

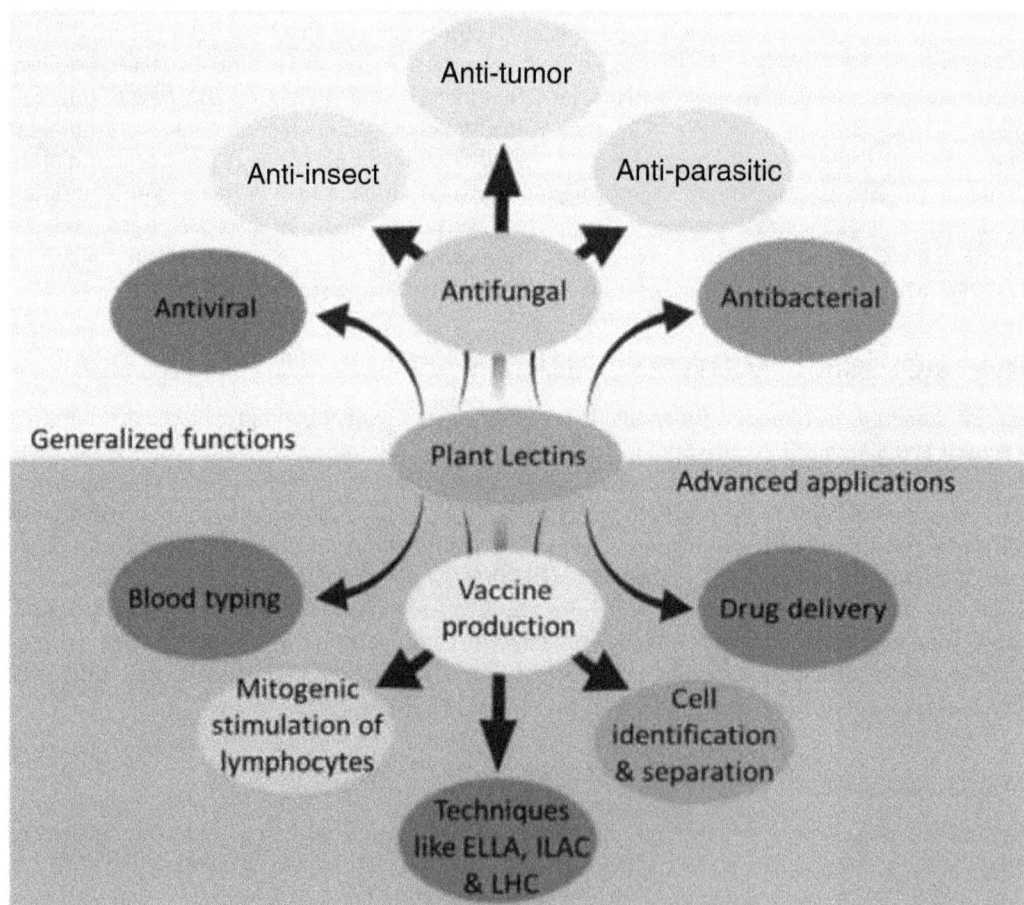

FIGURE 14.3 Overview of the application of plant lectins (Mishra et al., 2019).

we reported the homodimeric glucose/N-acetyl-D-glucosamine-specific lectin from *Dioscorea mangenotiana* tuber (DML 1) was toxic to the second instar larva stage of *Eldana saccharina*, a major pest of sugarcane. This lectin dramatically alters the levels of the enzymes acetylcholine esterase, alkaline phosphatase, and acid phosphatase in the insects placed on a diet containing DML 1. This tuber lectin also elongated the duration of development as well as significantly slowed the pupation and emergence of *E. saccharina* in a concentration-dependent order (Akinyoola et al., 2016). Similarly, we showed, in our recent study, that a 16.6 kDa lectin isolated from the woodland mushroom, *Agaricus semotus*, was lethal to the larva of *Culex quinquefasciatus* – a medically significant insect (Adedoyin et al., 2021).

According to earlier research on entomotoxic lectins, the death brought on by these proteins typically involves a number of intricate mechanisms, such as the induction of programmed cell death and association with particular saccharide residues of essential catalytic proteins, particularly those involved in metabolic reactions and toxin clearance. They can cross-link glycoconjugates arranged on the cellular surface or promote specific macromolecular arrangements of glycan-associated signal-mediating receptors as a result of their multivalent assembly, which may slow down their rate of biosynthesis and degradation (Hamshou et al. 2012). Their insecticidal/larvicidal effect has also been linked to morphological damage to the gut brought on by excessive protein degradation in target insects (Coelho et al. 2009).

Other studies have shown that the subcellular marks of lectins reduce food assimilation by tethering to the peritrophic matrix or the mid-gut epithelium. Given the abundance of glycoproteins on their surfaces, epithelial cells provide excellent lectin-binding targets. Regardless of the mechanism involving the connection between lectin and insect cells, lectins mostly avoid being proteolytically degraded by food-metabolizing enzymes and exhibit defiance to insect assimilatory proteins to exhibit their harmful impact. The capacity of lectins to bind to insect gut glycoconjugates determines the degree of resistance to digestive enzymes (Lagarda-Diaz et al., 2017).

14.4.2 ANTI-FUNGAL ACTIVITY

Lectins exert anti-fungal activity by adhering to chitins and other polysaccharide moieties on fungal surfaces, which has an impact on the existence of the fungus and other associated processes. Similarly, these quintessential proteins/glycoproteins tether to hyphae and interfere with spore development and nutrient uptake (Hamid et al., 2013). Lectin tethering impairs cell-wall chitin formation and/or arrangements, preventing fungal development. In addition to these processes, they also cause many structural modifications that increase the susceptibility of the fungi to various stressors. Some low molecular weight hemagglutinins can permeate the fungal extracellular matrices; they bind to the active sites of the crucial enzymes to inhibit their catalysis. A typical example of lectin associated with these mechanisms is wheat germ agglutinin (WGA), which is lethal to *Trichoderma viride* (Kumar et al., 2012).

Several studies have established this bioactivity; for example, *Ophiopogon japonicus*'lectin demonstrated antifungal efficacy against *Gibberella saubinetii* and *Rhizoctonia solani*. Similarly, *Exserohilum turicicum*, *Fusarium oxysporum*, and *Colectrotrichum cassiicola* are reportedly inhibited by *Curcuma longa* lectin (Petnual et al., 2010). *Fusarium moniliforme* and *Saccharomyces cerevisiae* showed growth suppression in response to two new chitin-specific lectins of *Artocarpus integrifolia* (Karnchanatat, 2012). Plants like Mongolian milkvetch, runner bean, jeering, orchid tree, soybean, Himalayan indigo, and groundnut contain lectins that have been shown to have promising fungicidal activity (Chen et al., 2009).

In addition to having a direct impact on the development of fungi, genes encoding lectins also provide immunity against fungal infection in genetically engineered plants. Typically, the introduction of the stinging nettle isolectin I precursor gene into the *Nicotiana tabacum* plant reduced the spore development of *Trichoderma viride*, *Colletotrichum lindemuthianum*, and *Botrytis cinerea* (Qadir et al., 2013).

14.4.3 Anti-Viral Activity

Lectins can bind the glycans found on the viral envelope glycoproteins, inhibiting the spread of the virus and its host entry (Barton et al., 2014; Akkouh et al., 2015). Additionally, they conjoin viral surface carbohydrate residues to stop co-receptor associations. Plant lectins' antiviral action is dependent on their glycan specificity and differs among lectins. In cases of severe acute respiratory syndrome, coronavirus was shown to be susceptible to mannose-binding lectins. These lectins inhibit the development of viruses by attaching and interfering with viral binding in the early stages of the replication process (Keyaerts et al., 2007). Wang et al. (2021) revealed that lentil lectin from *Lens culinaris*, which preferentially binds to oligomannose-type glycans and GlcNAc at the non-reducing end terminal, exhibited the strongest and most widespread antiviral efficacy against a panel of mutant viral strains and variations, including the Sars-Cov-2. Griffithsin (GRFT), cyanovirin (CV-N), and banana lectin (BanLec) are non-legume lectins that have been shown to have antiviral action (Swanson et al., 2010). According to Lusvarghi and Bewley (2016), these lectins are frequently used in gels, lotions, and suppositories to stop the spread of HIV. The lectins incapacitate viruses and prevent infection by obstructing viral entry and attachment into host cells. In addition, specific hemagglutinins from the autumn bean and the macrofungi *Russula delica* carry out an antiviral mechanism by inhibiting HIV-1 reverse transcriptase, which prevents the virus from converting its RNA to DNA and entering the host's nucleus (Zhao et al., 2009).

14.4.4 Anti-Parasitic Activity

Specific lectins of plant origin have been documented to be quite lethal to infection-causing parasites such as those belonging to the Genus *Trypanosoma* spp., *Leishmania* spp., *Tetrahymena* spp., and *Giardia* spp. Their toxicity to these parasites has been attributed to their adjuvant-forming nature and their glycan/glycoconjugate-binding specificities, especially those present on the parasite's surface, hence, triggering various biochemical/biological effects (Iordache et al., 2015). It is worth mentioning that a very minute proportion of plant hemagglutinins elicit this bioactivity. For example, jacalin, a lectin from jackfruit with the ability to modulate immune response, has been reported to induce massive immunoglobulin production against *Trypanosoma cruzi* or its antigens (Jandú et al., 2017).

In their research, Wang et al. (2017) showed that the *Helicoverpa armigera* C-type lectin HaCTL3 plays a role in parasite defense, and specifically, in nematodes' adherence. According to these authors, research conducted in vitro and in vivo shows that the lectin promotes hemocytic encapsulation and melanization, whereas *H. armigera* β-integrin, which is found on the surface of hemocytes, takes a role in encapsulation. HaCTL3 interacts with Haβ-integrin, as shown by co-immunoprecipitation studies, and Haβ-integrin knockdown results in reduced encapsulation of HaCTL3-coated beads. These findings suggest that, during the encapsulation event, HaCTL3 binds to the hemocytic receptor Haβ-integrin.

14.4.5 Anti-Bacterial Activity

The capacity of lectins to bind with a range of complex carbohydrates, including lipopolysaccharides (LPS), peptidoglycans, and teichoic acids found on the surface of bacteria, is thought to be the basis for their anti-bacterial activity. This interaction changes the morphology of bacteria, causing severe structural damage to the outer membrane components of these organisms (Hamid et al., 2013; Lagarda-Diaz et al., 2017). Additionally, lectins bind with N-acetylglucosamine (NAG), N-acetylmuramic acid (NAM), and tetrapeptides connected to N-acetylmuramic acid or lipopolysaccharides located on bacteria surfaces to exert their microbicidal activity. Further research revealed that lectins can prevent bacterial adherence and invasion. For example, lectins from the soft, fleshy part of *Punica granatum* testa reduced the attachment and invasion of various pathogenic bacteria, including *Staphylococcus aureus* (Silva et al., 2016b).

According to Hasan et al. (2014), *Shigella boydii, Salmonella enteritidis, Escherichia coli*, and *Listeria monocytogenes* were all successfully eradicated by lectins obtained from a potato cultivar from Bangladesh that particularly binds to chitin. A different lectin, found in the seeds of *Apuleia leiocarpa*, reportedly inhibited the development of *Bacillus cereus, Bacillus subtilis, Micrococcus luteus, Enterococcus faecalis, Streptococcus pyogenes, Staphylococcus aureus, Salmonella enteritidis, Pseudomonas aeruginosa*, and *Escherichia coli* (de Souza Carvalho et al., 2015).

Some lectins also reduce the permeability of bacterial cell walls. For instance, a study by Moura et al. (2017) showed that internal proteins leaked as a result of the loss of wall/membrane integrity produced by the application of *Moringa oleifera* lectin against pathogenic bacterial strains. Specific lectins also prevent the development of bacterial biofilms in addition to their bactericidal and bacteriostatic effects. It is necessary to conclude that using hemagglutinins in this situation would be beneficial to successfully decrease or manage issues of biofilm. This is because these extracellular structures significantly contribute to microbial resistance to antimicrobial agents, hence increasing the infectivity and virulence of these pathogens. *Streptococcus mutans* has been shown to be inhibited from forming biofilms by several of the key lectins from the *Fabaceae* family (Islam and Khan, 2012).

14.4.6 Inflammatory and Anti-Nociceptive Activities

Depending on the assay's delivery method, many lectins have shown anti- or pro-inflammatory effects in mouse models. These lectins caused neutrophil migration and paw edema when administered locally. On the other hand, they displayed an anti-inflammatory effect and improved cellular permeability when given systemically, encouraging neutrophil migration. In a study by Assreuy et al. (1997), all lectins tested except for ConBr, a lectin from *Canavalia brasiliensis*, had an anti-inflammatory effect. Research by Pinto et al. (2013) has confirmed this finding, which has been linked to slight structural variations between these lectins that may include interactions with glycans. In our previous research, we also reported that *Tetracarpidium conoforum* lectin elicited promising anti-nociceptive activity (Oladokun et al., 2019).

14.5 CONCLUSION AND PROSPECTS

The ubiquity of lectins in nature cannot be over-emphasized. While some of these proteins are beneficial, others can be quite lethal, eliciting potent hazards. Understanding their biological activities and structural biology is highly fundamental to their potential applications. Efforts must be improved in the field of lectin biochemistry regarding the use of modern equipment in lectin isolation, purification, and characterization. This will contribute to the potential application of these proteins in drug discovery processes, especially in designing structural mimetics/analogs of morbific microbial/viral lectins to mitigate the infectivity and pathogenicity of disease-causing organisms and vectors. Furthermore, caution must be exercised when consuming raw or active dietary lectins, as conventional processes, including cooking at elevated temperatures, fermentation, microwaving, sprouting, and enzymatic digestion, among others, have been implicated in lowering lectin content in food sources.

REFERENCES

Adedoyin, I. O., Adewole, T. S., Agunbiade, T. O., Adewoyin, F. B., & Kuku, A. (2021). A purified lectin with larvicidal activity from a woodland mushroom, *Agaricus semotus* Fr. *Acta Biologica Szegediensis, 65*(1), 65–73. https://doi.org/10.14232/abs.2021.1.65-73

Adewole, T. S., Ogidi, C. O., & Kuku, A. (2022). Bioactivities of *Calocybe indica* Protein combined with cell-free supernatant of lactobacilli from a fermented cereal against free radicals and microorganisms. *Journal of Food Bioactives, 18*. https://doi.org/10.31665/jfb.2022.18314

Akinyoola, K. A., Odekanyin, O. O., Adenike, K. U. K. U., & Sosan, M. B. (2016). Anti-insect potential of a lectin from the tuber, Dioscorea mangenotiana towards Eldana saccharina (Lepidoptera: Pyralidae).

Journal of Agricultural Biotechnology and Sustainable Development, 8(3), 16. https://doi.org/10.5897/jabsd2015.0249

Akkouh, O., Ng, T. B., Singh, S. S., Yin, C., Dan, X., Chan, Y. S., Pan, W., & Cheung, R. C. F. (2015). Lectins with anti-HIV activity: A review. *Molecules*, 20(1), 648–668. https://doi.org/10.3390/molecules20010648

Anderson, K., Evers, D., & Rice, K. G. (2008). Structure and function of mammalian carbohydrate-lectin interactions. *Glycoscience*, 2445. https://doi.org/10.1007/978-3-540-30429-6_63

Araújo, L. C. C., Aguiar, J. S., Napoleão, T. H., Mota, F. V. B., Barros, A. L. S., Moura, M. C., Coriolano, M. C., Coelho, L. C. B. B., Silva, T. G., & Paiva, P. M. G., 2013. Evaluation of cytotoxic and anti-inflammatory activities of extracts and lectins from *Moringa oleifera* seeds. *PloS One*, 8(12), p.e81973. https://doi.org/10.1371/journal.pone.0081973

Ashraf, G. M., Perveen, A., Zaidi, S. K., Tabrez, S., Kamal, M. A., & Banu, N. (2015). Studies on the role of goat heart galectin-1 as an erythrocyte membrane perturbing agent. *Saudi Journal of Biological Sciences*, 22(1), 112–116. https://doi.org/10.1016/j.sjbs.2014.09.018

Assreuy, A. M. S., Shibuya, M. D. D., Martins, G. J., De Souza, M. L. P., Cavada, B. S., Moreira, R. A., Oliveira, J. T. A., Ribeiro, R. D. A., & Flores, C. A. (1997). Anti-inflammatory effect of glucose – mannose binding lectins isolated from Brazilian beans. *Mediators of Inflammation*, 6(3), 201–210. https://doi.org/10.1080/09629359791695

Aune, D., Norat, T., Romundstad, P., & Vatten, L. J. (2013). Whole grain and refined grain consumption and the risk of type 2 diabetes: A systematic review and dose–response meta-analysis of cohort studies. *European journal of epidemiology*, 28(11), 845–858.

Avichezer, D., & Gilboa-Garber, N. (1987). PA-II, the L-fucose and D-mannose binding lectin of Pseudomonas aeruginosa stimulates human peripheral lymphocytes and murine splenocytes. *FEBS Letters*, 216(1), 62–66. https://doi.org/10.1016/0014-5793(87)80757-3

Banwell, J. G., Howard, R., Kabir, I., & Costerton, J. W. (1988). Bacterial overgrowth by indigenous microflora in the phytohemagglutinin-fed rat. *Canadian Journal of Microbiology*, 34(8), 1009–1013. https://doi.org/10.1139/m88-177

Barre, A., Damme, E. J. V., Simplicien, M., Benoist, H., & Rougé, P. (2020). Are dietary lectins relevant allergens in plant food allergy? *Foods*, 9(12), 1724. https://doi.org/10.3390/foods9121724

Barton, C., Kouokam, J. C., Lasnik, A. B., Foreman, O., Cambon, A., Brock, G., Montefiori, D. C., Vojdani, F., McCormick, A. A., O'Keefe, B. R., & Palmer, K. E. (2014). Activity of and effect of subcutaneous treatment with the broad-spectrum antiviral lectin griffithsin in two laboratory rodent models. *Antimicrobial Agents and Chemotherapy*, 58(1), 120–127. https://doi.org/10.1128/AAC.01407-13

Berg, J. M., Tymoczko, J. L., & Stryer, L. (2002). *Biochemistry*. New York: W. H. Freeman and Company.

Brustein, V. P., Souza-Araújo, F. V., Vaz, A. F. M., Araújo, R. V. S., Paiva, P. M. G., Coelho, L. C. B. B., Carneiro-Leão, A. M. A., Teixeira, J. A., Carneiro-da-Cunha, M. G., & Correia, M. T. S. (2012). A novel antimicrobial lectin from *Eugenia malaccensis* that stimulates cutaneous healing in mice model. *Inflammopharmacology*, 20(6), 315–322.

Chen, J., Liu, B., Ji, N., Zhou, J., Bian, H. J., Li, C. Y., Chen, F., & Bao, J. K. (2009). A novel sialic acid-specific lectin from *Phaseolus coccineus* seeds with potent antineoplastic and antifungal activities. *Phytomedicine*, 16(4), 352–360. https://doi.org/10.1016/j.phymed.2008.07.003

Cheung, R. C. F., Wong, J. H., Pan, W., Chan, Y. S., Yin, C., Dan, X., & Ng, T. B. (2015). Marine lectins and their medicinal applications. *Applied Microbiology and Biotechnology*, 99(9), 3755–3773. https://doi.org/10.1007/s00253-015-6518-0

Coelho, J. S., Santos, N. D., Napoleão, T. H., Gomes, F. S., Ferreira, R. S., Zingali, R. B., Coelho, L. C., Leite, S. P., Navarro, D. M., & Paiva, P. M. (2009). Effect of *Moringa oleifera* lectin on development and mortality of *Aedes aegypti* larvae. *Chemosphere*, 77(7), 934–938. https://doi.org/10.1016/j.chemosphere.2009.08.022

Coltri, K. C., Casabona-Fortunato, A. S., Gennari-Cardoso, M. L., Pinzan, C. F., Ruas, L. P., Mariano, V. S., Martinez, R., Rosa, J. C., Panunto-Castelo, A. and Roque-Barreira, M. C. (2006). Paracoccin, a GlcNAc-binding lectin from *Paracoccidioides brasiliensis*, binds to laminin and induces TNF-A production by macrophages. *Microbes and Infection*, 8(3), 704–713. https://doi.org/10.1016/j.micinf.2005.09.008

Costa, R. M., Vaz, A. F., Oliva, M. L., Coelho, L. C., Correia, M. T., & Carneiro-da-Cunha, M. G. (2010). A new mistletoe *Phthirusa pyrifolia* leaf lectin with antimicrobial properties. *Process Biochemistry*, 45(4), 526–533. https://doi.org/10.1016/j.procbio.2009.11.013

da Rocha-Azevedo, B., Jamerson, M., Cabral, G. A., & Marciano-Cabral, F. (2010). *Acanthamoeba culbertsoni*: Analysis of amoebic adhesion and invasion on extracellular matrix components collagen I and laminin-1. *Experimental Parasitology*, 126(1), 79–84. https://doi.org/10.1016/j.exppara.2009.08.004

de Araújo, R. M. S., da Silva Ferreira, R., Napoleão, T. H., das Graças Carneiro-da-Cunha, M., Coelho, L. C. B. B., dos Santos Correia, M. T., Oliva, M. L. V., & Paiva, P. M. G. (2012). *Crataeva tapia* bark lectin is an affinity adsorbent and insecticidal agent. *Plant Science, 183*, 20–26. https://doi.org/10.1016/j.plantsci.2011.10.018

De Munter, J. S. L., Hu, F. B., Spiegelman, D., Franz, M., & van Dam, R. M. (2007). Whole grain, bran, and germ intake and risk of type 2 diabetes: A prospective cohort study and systematic review. *PLoS Medicine, 4*(8), e261. https://doi.org/10.1371/journal.pmed.0040261

de Souza Carvalho, A., da Silva, M. V., Gomes, F. S., Paiva, P. M. G., Malafaia, C. B., da Silva, T. D., de Melo Vaz, A. F., da Silva, A. G., de Souza Arruda, I. R., Napoleão, T. H., & dos Santos Correia, M. T. (2015). Purification, characterization and antibacterial potential of a lectin isolated from *Apuleia leiocarpa* seeds. *International Journal of Biological Macromolecules, 75*, 402–408. https://doi.org/10.1016/j.ijbiomac.2015.02.001

Díaz, E. M., Vicente-Manzanares, M., Sacristan, M., Vicente, C., & Legaz, M. E. (2011). Fungal lectin of *Peltigera canina* induces chemotropism of compatible Nostoc cells by constriction-relaxation pulses of cyanobiont cytoskeleton. *Plant Signaling & Behavior, 6*(10), 1525–1536. https://doi.org/10.4161/psb.6.10.16687

Duranti, M., & Gius, C. (1997). Legume seeds: Protein content and nutritional value. *Field Crops Research, 53*(1–3), 31–45. https://doi.org/10.1016/s0378-4290(97)00021-x

Enoma, S., Adewole, T. S., Agunbiade, T. O., & Kuku, A. (2023). Antimicrobial activities and phylogenetic study of Erythrina senegalensis DC (Fabaceae) seed lectin. *BioTechnologia. Journal of Biotechnology Computational Biology and Bionanotechnology, 104*(1).

Farthing, M. J., Pereira, M. E., & Keusch, G. T. (1986). Description and characterization of a surface lectin from *Giardia lamblia. Infection and Immunity, 51*(2), 661–667. https://doi.org/10.1128/iai.51.2.661-667.1986

Freed, D. L. (1999). Do dietary lectins cause disease?: The evidence is suggestive – and raises interesting possibilities for treatment. *BMJ, 318*(7190), 1023–1024. https://doi.org/10.1136/bmj.318.7190.1023

Garate, M., Cao, Z., Bateman, E., & Panjwani, N. (2004). Cloning and characterization of a novel mannose-binding protein of Acanthamoeba. *Journal of Biological Chemistry, 279*(28), 29849–29856. https://doi.org/10.1074/jbc.m402334200

Ghazarian, H., Idoni, B., & Oppenheimer, S. B. (2011). A glycobiology review: Carbohydrates, lectins and implications in cancer therapeutics. *Acta histochemica, 113*(3), 236–247.

Gibson, R. S., Bailey, K. B., Gibbs, M., & Ferguson, E. L. (2010). A review of phytate, iron, zinc, and calcium concentrations in plant-based complementary foods used in low-income countries and implications for bioavailability. *Food and Nutrition Bulletin, 31*(2_suppl2), S134-S146. https://doi.org/10.1177/15648265100312s206

Gilboa-Garber, N. (1982). [32] *Pseudomonas aeruginosa* lectins. In *Methods in enzymology* (Vol. 83, pp. 378–385). Ramat Gan, Israel: Bar-Ilan University, Academic Press. https://doi.org/10.1016/0076-6879(82)83034-6

Grishin, A. V., Krivozubov, M. S., Karyagina, A. S., & Gintsburg, A. L. (2015*). Pseudomonas aeruginosa* lectins as targets for novel antibacterials. *Acta Naturae (англоязычная версия), 7*(2 (25)), 29–41. https://doi.org/10.32607/20758251-2015-7-2-29-41

Gupta, A., & Gupta, G. S. (2021). Status of mannose-binding lectin (MBL) and complement system in COVID-19 patients and therapeutic applications of antiviral plant MBLs. *Molecular and Cellular Biochemistry, 476*(8), 2917–2942. https://doi.org/10.1007/s11010-021-04107-3

Haas, H., Falcone, F. H., Schramm, G., Haisch, K., Gibbs, B. F., Klaucke, J., Pöppelmann, M., Becker, W. M., Gabius, H.J., & Schlaak, M. (1999). Dietary lectins can induce in vitro release of IL-4 and IL-13 from human basophils. *European Journal of Immunology, 29*(3), 918–927. https://doi.org/10.1002/(sici)1521-4141(199903)29:03<918::aid-immu918>3.0.co;2-t

Hamid, R., Masood, A., Wani, I. H., & Rafiq, S. (2013). Lectins: Proteins with diverse applications. *Journal of Applied Pharmaceutical Science, 3*(4), S93–S103. http://doi.org/10.7324/JAPS.2013.34.S18

Hamshou, M., Van Damme, E. J., Vandenborre, G., Ghesquiere, B., Trooskens, G., Gevaert, K., & Smagghe, G. (2012). GalNAc/Gal-binding *Rhizoctonia solani* agglutinin has antiproliferative activity in *Drosophila melanogaster* S2 cells via MAPK and JAK/STAT signaling. *PLoS One, 7*(4), e33680. https://doi.org/10.1371/journal.pone.0033680

Hasan, I., Ozeki, Y., & Kabir, S. R. (2014). Purification of a novel chitin-binding lectin with antimicrobial and antibiofilm activities from a Bangladeshi cultivar of potato (*Solanum tuberosum*). *Indian Journal of Biochemistry & Biophysics, 51*, 142–148.

Honda, S., Kashiwagi, M., Miyamoto, K., Takei, Y., & Hirose, S. (2000). Multiplicity, structures, and endocrine and exocrine natures of eel fucose-binding lectins. *Journal of Biological Chemistry, 275*(42), 33151–33157. https://doi.org/10.1074/jbc.m002337200

Iordache, F., Ionita, M., Mitrea, L. I., Fafaneata, C., & Pop, A. (2015). Antimicrobial and antiparasitic activity of lectins. *Current Pharmaceutical Biotechnology*, *16*(2), 152–161. https://doi.org/10.2174/138920101 602150112151907

Islam, B., & Khan, A. U. (2012). Lectins: To combat infections. *Protein Purification*, *1*, 167–188.

Jandú, J. J., Moraes Neto, R. N., Zagmignan, A., de Sousa, E. M., Brelaz-de-Castro, M. C., dos Santos Correia, M. T., & da Silva, L. C. (2017). Targeting the immune system with plant lectins to combat microbial infections. *Frontiers in Pharmacology*, *8*, 671. https://doi.org/10.3389/fphar.2017.00671

Joe, A., Hamer, D. H., Kelley, M. A., Pereira, M. E., Keusch, G. T., Tzipori, S., & Ward, H. D. (1994). Role of a Gal/GalNAc-specific sporozoite surface lectin in Cryptosporidium parvum-host cell interaction. *The Journal of Eukaryotic Microbiology*, *41*(5), 44S-44S. https://doi.org/10.1128/iai.62.6.2208-2213.1994

Johnny, I. I., Kuku, A., Odekanyin, O. O., & Adesina, S. K. (2016). A lectin with larvicidal potential from the fresh leaves of *Agelanthus brunneus* (Engl.) Van Tiegh *Loranthaceae*. *British Journal of Pharmaceutical Research*, *13*(3), 1–9. https://doi.org/10.9734/bjpr/2016/28577

Jungery, M. (1985). Studies on the biochemical basis of the interaction of the merozoites of *Plasmodium falciparum* and the human red cell. *Transactions of the Royal Society of Tropical Medicine and Hygiene*, *79*(5), 591–597. https://doi.org/10.1016/0035-9203(85)90164-6

Karnchanatat, A. (2012). Antimicrobial activity of lectins from plants. *Antimicrobial Agents. InTech*, 145–178.

Kato, K., Yahata, K., Gopal Dhoubhadel, B., Fujii, Y., & Tachibana, H. (2015). Novel hemagglutinating, hemolytic and cytotoxic activities of the intermediate subunit of Entamoeba histolytica lectin. *Scientific Reports*, *5*(1), 1–13. https://doi.org/10.1038/srep13901

Kaur, A., Singh, J., Kamboj, S. S., Sexana, A. K., Pandita, R. M., & Shamnugavel, M. (2005). Isolation of an N-acetyl-D-glucosamine specific lectin from the rhizomes of Arundo donax with antiproliferative activity. *Phytochemistry*, *66*(16), 1933–1940. https://doi.org/10.1016/j.phytochem.2005.06.026

Keyaerts, E., Vijgen, L., Pannecouque, C., Van Damme, E., Peumans, W., Egberink, H., Balzarini, J. & Van Ranst, M. (2007). Plant lectins are potent inhibitors of coronaviruses by interfering with two targets in the viral replication cycle. *Antiviral Research*, *75*(3), 179–187. https://doi.org/10.1016/j.antiviral.2007.03.003

Khan, F., & Khan, M. I. (2011). Fungal lectins: Current molecular and biochemical perspectives. *International Journal of Biological Chemistry*, *5*(1), 1–20. https://doi.org/10.3923/ijbc.2011.1.20

Kilpatrick, D. C. (2002). Animal lectins: A historical introduction and overview. *Biochimica et Biophysica Acta (BBA)-General Subjects*, *1572*(2–3), 187–197. https://doi.org/10.1016/s0304-4165(02)00308-2

Kobiler, D., & Mirelman, D. (1980). Lectin activity in Entamoeba histolytica trophozoites. *Infection and Immunity*, *29*(1), 221–225. https://doi.org/10.1128/iai.29.1.221-225.1980

Kordás, K., Szalmay, G., Bardocz, S., Pusztai, Á., & Varga, G. (2001). Phytohaemagglutinin inhibits gastric acid but not pepsin secretion in conscious rats. *Journal of Physiology-Paris*, *95*(1–6), 309–314. https://doi.org/10.1016/s0928-4257(01)00043-2

Kumar, K. K., Chandra, K. L. P., Sumanthi, J., Reddy, G. S., Shekar, P. C., & Reddy, B. V. R. (2012). Biological role of lectins: A review. *Journal of orofacial sciences*, *4*(1), 20. https://doi.org/10.4103/0975-8844.99883

Lagarda-Diaz, I., Guzman-Partida, A. M., & Vazquez-Moreno, L. (2017). Legume lectins: Proteins with diverse applications. *International Journal of Molecular Sciences*, *18*(6), 1242. https://doi.org/10.3390/ijms18061242

Lajolo, F. M., & Genovese, M. I. (2002). Nutritional significance of lectins and enzyme inhibitors from legumes. *Journal of Agricultural and Food Chemistry*, *50*(22), 6592–6598. https://doi.org/10.1021/jf020191k

Lakhtin, V. M., Lakhtin, M. V., Pospelova, V. V., & Shenderov, B. A. (2006). *Lactobacilli* and *bifidobacteria* lectins as possible signal molecules regulating intra-and inter-population bacteria–bacteria and host–bacteria relationships. Part I. Methods of bacterial lectin isolation, physico-chemical characterization and some biological activity investigation. *Microbial Ecology in Health and Disease*, *18*(1), 55–60. https://doi.org/10.1080/08910600600799646

Lambert, J., & Vojdani, A. (2017). Correlation of tissue antibodies and food immune reactivity in randomly selected patient specimens. *Journal of Clinical and Cellular Immunology*, *8*(521), 2. https://doi.org/10.4172/2155-9899.1000521

Landsteiner, K., & Raubitschek, H. (1907). Beobachtungen über hämolyse und hämagglutination. *Zbl Bakt I Abt Orig*, *45*, 600–607.

Lannoo, N., & Van Damme, E. J. (2010). Nucleocytoplasmic plant lectins. *Biochimica et Biophysica Acta (BBA)-General Subjects*, *1800*(2), 190–201. https://doi.org/10.1016/j.bbagen.2009.07.021

Lev, B., Ward, H., Keusch, G. T., & Pereira, M. E. (1986). Lectin activation in *Giardia lamblia* by host protease: A novel host-parasite interaction. *Science*, *232*(4746), 71–73. https://doi.org/10.1126/science.3513312

Lewis, A. L., Kohler, J. J., & Aebi, M. (2022). Microbial lectins: Hemagglutinins, adhesins, and toxins. In *Essentials of Glycobiology [Internet]*. 4th edition.

Li, Y. R., Liu, Q. H., Wang, H. X., & Ng, T. B. (2008). A novel lectin with potent antitumor, mitogenic and HIV-1 reverse transcriptase inhibitory activities from the edible mushroom *Pleurotus citrinopileatus*. *Biochimica et Biophysica Acta (BBA)-General Subjects*, *1780*(1), 51–57. https://doi.org/10.1016/j.bbagen.2007.09.004

Liu, S., Stampfer, M. J., Hu, F. B., Giovannucci, E., Rimm, E., Manson, J. E., Hennekens, C. H., & Willett, W. C. (1999). Whole-grain consumption and risk of coronary heart disease: Results from the Nurses' Health Study. *The American Journal of Clinical Nutrition*, *70*(3), 412–419. https://doi.org/10.1093/ajcn/70.3.412

Liu, Z. 1., Luo, Y., Zhou, T. T., & Zhang, W. Z. (2013). Could plant lectins become promising anti-tumour drugs for causing autophagic cell death? *Cell Proliferation*, *46*(5), 509–515. https://doi.org/10.1111/cpr.12054

Loh, S. H., Park, J. Y., Cho, E. H., Nah, S. Y., & Kang, Y. S. (2017). Animal lectins: Potential receptors for ginseng polysaccharides. *Journal of Ginseng Research*, *41*(1), 1–9. https://doi.org/10.1016/j.jgr.2015.12.006

López-Moreno, M., Garcés-Rimón, M., & Miguel, M. (2022). Antinutrients: Lectins, goitrogens, phytates and oxalates, friends or foe? *Journal of Functional Foods*, *89*, 104938.

Lucius, K. (2020). Dietary lectins: Gastrointestinal and immune effects. *Alternative and Complementary Therapies*, *26*(4), 168–174. https://doi.org/10.1089/act.2020.29286.klu

Lusvarghi, S., & Bewley, C. A. (2016). Griffithsin: An antiviral lectin with outstanding therapeutic potential. *Viruses*, *8*(10), 296. https://doi.org/10.3390/v8100296

Maestre-Reyna, M., Diderrich, R., Veelders, M. S., Eulenburg, G., Kalugin, V., Brückner, S., Keller, P., Rupp, S., Mösch, H. U., & Essen, L. O. (2012). Structural basis for promiscuity and specificity during *Candida glabrata* invasion of host epithelia. *Proceedings of the National Academy of Sciences*, *109*(42), 16864–16869.

Matsumoto, J., Nakamoto, C., Fujiwara, S., Yubisui, T., & Kawamura, K. (2001). A novel C-type lectin regulating cell growth, cell adhesion and cell differentiation of the multipotent epithelium in budding tunicates. *Development*, *128*(17), 3339–3347. https://doi.org/10.1242/dev.128.17.3339

Mishra, A., Behura, A., Mawatwal, S., Kumar, A., Naik, L., Mohanty, S. S., Manna, D, Dokania, D., Mishra, A., Patra, S. K., & Dhiman, R. (2019). Structure-function and application of plant lectins in disease biology and immunity. *Food and Chemical Toxicology*, *134*, 110827.

Moreno, A. N., Jamur, M. C., Oliver, C., & Roque-Barreira, M. C. (2003). Mast cell degranulation induced by lectins: Effect on neutrophil recruitment. *International Archives of Allergy and Immunology*, *132*(3), 221–230. https://doi.org/10.1159/000074303

Moura, M. C., Trentin, D. S., Napoleão, T. H., Primon-Barros, M., Xavier, A. S., Carneiro, N. P., Paiva, P. M. G., Macedo, A.J. & Coelho, L. C. B. B. (2017). Multi-effect of the water-soluble *Moringa oleifera* lectin against *Serratia marcescens* and *Bacillus* sp.: Antibacterial, antibiofilm and anti-adhesive properties. *Journal of Applied Microbiology*, *123*(4), 861–874. https://doi.org/10.1111/jam.13556

Nabi-Afjadi, M., Heydari, M., Zalpoor, H., Arman, I., Sadoughi, A., Sahami, P., & Aghazadeh, S. (2022). Lectins and lectibodies: Potential promising antiviral agents. *Cellular & Molecular Biology Letters*, *27*(1), 1–25.

Nakae, H., Yumoto, H., Matsuo, T., & Ebisu, S. (1994). Mitogenic stimulation of murine B lymphocytes by the N-acetyl-D-galactosamine specific bacterial lectin-like substance from *Eikenella corrodens*. *FEMS Microbiology Letters*, *116*(3), 349–353. https://doi.org/10.1111/j.1574-6968.1994.tb06726.x

Nciri, N., & Cho, N. (2018). New research highlights: Impact of chronic ingestion of white kidney beans (Phaseolus vulgaris L. var. Beldia) on small-intestinal disaccharidase activity in Wistar rats. *Toxicology Reports*, *5*, 46–55. https://doi.org/10.1016/j.toxrep.2017.12.016

Nciri, N., Cho, N., Bergaoui, N., Mhamdi, F. E., Ammar, A. B., Trabelsi, N., Zekri, S., Guémira, F., Mansour, A. B., Sassi, F. H., & Aissa-Fennira, F. B. (2015). Effect of white kidney beans (Phaseolus vulgaris L. var. Beldia) on small intestine morphology and function in Wistar rats. *Journal of Medicinal Food*, *18*(12), 1387–1399. https://doi.org/10.1089/jmf.2014.0193

Ng, T. B., & Lam, Y. W. (2002). Isolation of a novel agglutinin with complex carbohydrate binding specificity from fresh fruiting bodies of the edible mushroom *Lyophyllum shimeiji*. *Biochemical and Biophysical Research Communications*, *290*(1), 563–568. https://doi.org/10.1006/bbrc.2001.6235

Nikitina, V. E., Loshchinina, E. A., & Vetchinkina, E. P. (2017). Lectins from mycelia of basidiomycetes. *International Journal of Molecular Sciences*, *18*(7), 1334. https://doi.org/10.3390/ijms18071334

Nilsson, C. L. (2007). Lectins: Analytical tools from nature. In *Lectins* (pp. 1–13). Amsterdam, Netherlands: Elsevier Science BV.

Noah, N. D., Bender, A. E., Reaidi, G. B., & Gilbert, R. J. (1980). Food poisoning from raw red kidney beans. *British Medical Journal*, *281*(6234), 236–237.

Nubi, T., Adewole, T. S., Agunbiade, T. O., Osukoya, O. A., & Kuku, A. (2021). Purification and erythrocyte-membrane perturbing activity of a ketose-specific lectin from *Moringa oleifera* seeds. *Biotechnology Reports*, *31*, e00650. https://doi.org/10.1016/j.btre.2021.e00650

Oladokun, B. O., Omisore, O. N., Osukoya, O. A., & Kuku, A. (2019). Anti-nociceptive and anti-inflammatory activities of *Tetracarpidium conophorum* seed lectin. *Scientific African*, *3*, e00073. https://doi. org/10.1016/j.sciaf.2019.e00073

Ottinger, C. A., Johnson, S. C., Ewart, K. V., Brown, L. L., & Ross, N. W. (1999). Enhancement of anti-*Aeromonas salmonicida* activity in Atlantic salmon (*Salmo salar*) macrophages by a mannose-binding lectin. *Comparative Biochemistry and Physiology Part C: Pharmacology, Toxicology and Endocrinology*, *123*(1), 53–59. https://doi.org/10.1016/s0742-8413(99)00009-2

Parisi, M. G., Moreno, S., & Fernández, G. (2008). Isolation and characterization of a dual function protein from *Allium sativum* bulbs which exhibits proteolytic and hemagglutinating activities. *Plant Physiology and Biochemistry*, *46*(4), 403–413. https://doi.org/10.1016/j.plaphy.2007.11.003

Peng, H., Lv, H., Wang, Y., Liu, Y. H., Li, C. Y., Meng, L., Chen, F., & Bao, J. K. (2009). *Clematis montana* lectin, a novel mannose-binding lectin from traditional Chinese medicine with antiviral and apoptosis-inducing activities. *Peptides*, *30*(10), 1805–1815. https://doi.org/10.1016/j.peptides.2009.06.027

Petnual, P., Sangvanich, P., & Karnchanatat, A. (2010). A lectin from the rhizomes of turmeric (*Curcuma longa* L.) and its antifungal, antibacterial, and A-glucosidase inhibitory activities. *Food Science and Biotechnology*, *19*(4), 907–916. https://doi.org/10.1007/s10068-010-0128-5

Petri, W. A., Smith, R. D., Schlesinger, P. H., Murphy, C. F., & Ravdin, J. I. (1987). Isolation of the galactose-binding lectin that mediates the in vitro adherence of *Entamoeba histolytica*. *The Journal of Clinical Investigation*, *80*(5), 1238–1244. https://doi.org/10.1172/jci113198

Petroski, W., & Minich, D. M. (2020). Is there such a thing as "anti-nutrients"? A narrative review of perceived problematic plant compounds. *Nutrients*, *12*(10), 2929. https://doi.org/10.3390/nu12102929

Peumans, W. J., & Van Damme, E. J. (1995). Lectins as plant defense proteins. *Plant Physiology*, *109*(2), 347. https://doi.org/10.1104/pp.109.2.347

Peumans, W. J., Barre, A., Hao, Q., Rougé, P., & Van Damme, E. J. (2000). Higher plants developed structurally different motifs to recognize foreign glycans. *Trends in Glycoscience and Glycotechnology*, *12*(64), 83–101.

Pinto, N. V., Santos, C. F., Cavada, B. S., Nascimento, K. S. D., Junior, F. N. P., de Freitas Pires, A., & Assreuy, A. M. S. (2013). Homologous *Canavalia* lectins elicit different patterns of antinociceptive responses. *Natural product communications*, *8*(11), 1934578X1300801130. https://doi.org/10.1177/1934578x1300801130

Pujic, P., Fournier, P., Alloisio, N., Hay, A. E., Maréchal, J., Anchisi, S., & Normand, P. (2012). Lectin genes in the *Frankia alni* genome. *Archives of Microbiology*, *194*(1), 47–56. https://doi.org/10.1007/s00203-011-0770-1

Qadir, S., Wani, I. H., Rafiq, S., Ganie, S. A., Masood, A., & Hamid, R. (2013). Evaluation of the antimicrobial activity of a lectin isolated and purified from *Indigofera heterantha*. *Advances in Bioscience and Biotechnology*, *4*(11), 999. http://dx.doi.org/10.4236/abb.2013.411133

Rabelo, L., Monteiro, N., Serquiz, R., Santos, P., Oliveira, R., Oliveira, A., Rocha, H., Morais, A. H., Uchoa, A., & Santos, E. (2012). A lactose-binding lectin from the marine sponge *Cinachyrella apion* (Cal) induces cell death in human cervical adenocarcinoma cells. *Marine Drugs*, *10*(4), 727–743. https://doi.org/10.3390/md10040727

Ravdin, J. I., & Guerrant, R. L. (1981). Role of Adherence in Cytopathogenic Mechanisms of *Entamoeba Histolytica*. *Journal of Clinical Investigation*, *68*(5), 1305–1313. https://doi.org/10.1172/jci110377 https://doi.org/10.1172/jci110377

Roos, N., Sørensen, J. C., Sørensen, H., Rasmussen, S. K., Briend, A., Yang, Z., & Huffman, S. L. (2013). Screening for anti-nutritional compounds in complementary foods and food aid products for infants and young children. *Maternal & Child Nutrition*, *9*, 47–71. https://doi.org/10.1111/j.1740-8709.2012.00449.x

Roussel, F., De Carli, G., & Brasseur, P. H. (1991). A cytopathic effect of Trichomonas vaginalis probably mediated by a mannose/N-acetyl-glucosamine binding lectin. *International journal for parasitology*, *21*(8), 941–944. https://doi.org/10.1016/0020-7519(91)90170-c

Rubeena, A. S., Abraham, A., & Aarif, K. M. (2021). Microbial Lectins. In *Lectins* (pp. 131–146). Springer, Singapore. https://doi.org/10.1007/978-981-16-7462-4_7

Sa, R. A., Napoleao, T. H., Santos, N. D., Gomes, F. S., Albuquerque, A. C., Xavier, H. S., Coelho, L. C., Bieber, L. W., & Paiva, P. M. (2008). Induction of mortality on *Nasutitermes corniger* (Isoptera, *Termitidae*) by *Myracrodruon urundeuva* heartwood lectin. *International Biodeterioration & Biodegradation*, *62*(4), 460–464. https://doi.org/10.1016/j.ibiod.2008.04.003

Sadeghi, A., Van Damme, E. J., Peumans, W. J., & Smagghe, G. (2006). The deterrent activity of plant lectins on cowpea weevil *Callosobruchus maculatus* (F.) oviposition. *Phytochemistry*, *67*(18), 2078–2084. https://doi.org/10.1016/j.phytochem.2006.06.032

Santos, A. F., Da Silva, M. D. C., Napoleão, T. H., Paiva, P. M. G., Correia, M. D. S., & Coelho, L. C. B. B. (2014). Lectins: Function, structure, biological properties and potential applications. *Current Topics in Peptide and Protein Research*, *15*, 41–62. https://hdl.handle.net/1822/43440

Santos, A. F., Luz, L. A., Argolo, A. C., Teixeira, J. A., Paiva, P. M., & Coelho, L. C. (2009). Isolation of a seed coagulant *Moringa oleifera* lectin. *Process Biochemistry*, *44*(4), 504–508. https://doi.org/10.1016/j.procbio.2009.01.002

Sharon, N. (1987). Bacterial lectins, cell-cell recognition and infectious disease. *FEBS Letters*, *217*(2), 145–157. https://doi.org/10.1016/0014-5793(87)80654-3

Sharon, N. (2006). Carbohydrates as future anti-adhesion drugs for infectious diseases. *Biochimica et Biophysica Acta (BBA)-General Subjects*, *1760*(4), 527–537. https://doi.org/10.1016/j.bbagen.2005.12.008

Sharon, N. (2008). Lectins: Past, present and future 1. *Biochemical Society Transactions*, *36*(6), 1457–1460. https://doi.org/10.1042/bst0361457

Sharon, N., & Lis, H. (1990). Legume lectins – a large family of homologous proteins. *The FASEB journal*, *4*(14), 3198–3208. https://doi.org/10.1096/fasebj.4.14.2227211

Sharon, N., & Lis, H. (2004). History of lectins: From hemagglutinins to biological recognition molecules. *Glycobiology*, *14*(11), 53R–62R. https://doi.org/10.1093/glycob/cwh122

Sharon, N., & Ofek, I. (2000). Safe as mother's milk: Carbohydrates as future anti-adhesion drugs for bacterial diseases. *Glycoconjugate Journal*, *17*(7), 659–664.

Silva, M. C., de Paula, C. A., Ferreira, J. G., Paredes-Gamero, E. J., Vaz, A. M., Sampaio, M. U., Correia, M. T. S., & Oliva, M. L. V. (2014). *Bauhinia forficata* lectin (BfL) induces cell death and inhibits integrin-mediated adhesion on MCF7 human breast cancer cells. *Biochimica et Biophysica Acta (BBA)-General Subjects*, *1840*(7), 2262–2271. https://doi.org/10.1016/j.bbagen.2014.03.009

Silva, P. M., Lima, A. L., Silva, B. V., Coelho, L. C., Dutra, R. F., & Correia, M. T. (2016a). *Cratylia mollis* lectin nanoelectrode for differential diagnostic of prostate cancer and benign prostatic hype rplasia based on label-free detection. *Biosensors and Bioelectronics*, *85*, 171–177. https://doi.org/10.1016/j.bios.2016.05.004

Silva, P. M., Napoleão, T. H., Silva, L. C., Fortes, D. T., Lima, T. A., Zingali, R. B., Pontual, E. V., Araújo, J. M., Medeiros, P. L., Rodrigues, C. G. & Gomes, F. S. (2016b). The juicy sarcotesta of *Punica granatum* contains a lectin that affects growth, survival as well as adherence and invasive capacities of human pathogenic bacteria. *Journal of Functional Foods*, *27*, 695–702. https://doi.org/10.1016/j.jff.2016.10.015

Singh, R. S., & Walia, A. K. (2014). Microbial lectins and their prospective mitogenic potential. *Critical Reviews in Microbiology*, *40*(4), 329–347. https://doi.org/10.3109/1040841x.2012.733680

Singh, R. S., Bhari, R., & Kaur, H. P. (2011). Characteristics of yeast lectins and their role in cell–cell interactions. *Biotechnology Advances*, *29*(6), 726–731. https://doi.org/10.1016/j.biotechadv.2011.06.002

Singh, R. S., Walia, A. K., & Kanwar, J. R. (2016). Protozoa lectins and their role in host–pathogen interactions. *Biotechnology Advances*, *34*(5), 1018–1029. https://doi.org/10.1016/j.biotechadv.2016.06.002

Singha, B., Adhya, M., & Chatterjee, B. P. (2007). Multivalent II [β-d-Galp-(1→ 4)-β-d-GlcpNAc] and TA [β-d-Galp-(1→ 3)-A-d-GalpNAc] specific *Moraceae* family plant lectin from the seeds of *Ficus bengalensis* fruits. *Carbohydrate Research*, *342*(8), 1034–1043. https://doi.org/10.1016/j.carres.2007.02.012

Sitohy, M., Doheim, M., & Badr, H. (2007). Isolation and characterization of a lectin with antifungal activity from Egyptian *Pisum sativum* seeds. *Food Chemistry*, *104*(3), 971–979. https://doi.org/10.1016/j.foodchem.2007.01.026

Smith, D. F., Song, X., & Cummings, R. D. (2010). Use of glycan microarrays to explore specificity of glycan-binding proteins. *Methods in Enzymology*, *480*, 417–444. https://doi.org/10.1016/s0076-6879(10)80033-3

Souza, J. D., Silva, M. B., Argolo, A. C., Napoleão, T. H., Sá, R. A., Correia, M. T., Paiva, P. M., Silva, M. D., & Coelho, L. C. (2011). A new *Bauhinia monandra* galactose-specific lectin purified in milligram quantities from secondary roots with antifungal and termiticidal activities. *International Biodeterioration & Biodegradation*, *65*(5), 696–702. https://doi.org/10.1016/j.ibiod.2011.02.009

Stillmark, H. (1888). Über Ricin ein giftiges Ferment aus den Samen von *Ricinus communis* L. und einige anderen Euphorbiaceen. Inaugural dissertation Dorpat, Tartu.

Swanson, M. D., Winter, H. C., Goldstein, I. J., & Markovitz, D. M. (2010). A lectin isolated from bananas is a potent inhibitor of HIV replication. *Journal of Biological Chemistry*, *285*(12), 8646–8655. https://doi.org/10.1074/jbc.M109.034926

Thea, D. M., Pereira, M. E., Kotler, D., Sterling, C. R., & Keusch, G. T. (1992). Identification and partial purification of a lectin on the surface of the sporozoite of Cryptosporidium parvum. *The Journal of Parasitology*, 886–893. https://doi.org/10.2307/3283323

VanDamme,E.J.(2008).Plant lectins as part of the plant defense system against insects. In *Induced Plant Resistance to Herbivory* (pp. 285–307). Dordrecht: Springer. https://doi.org/10.1007/978-1-4020-8182-8_14

Van Damme, E. J. V., Peumans, W. J., Barre, A., & Rougé, P. (1998). Plant lectins: A composite of several distinct families of structurally and evolutionary related proteins with diverse biological roles. *Critical Reviews in Plant Sciences, 17*(6), 575–692. https://doi.org/10.1080/07352689891304276

Vandenborre, G., Smagghe, G., & Van Damme, E. J. (2011). Plant lectins as defense proteins against phytophagous insects. *Phytochemistry, 72*(13), 1538–1550. https://doi.org/10.1016/j.phytochem.2011.02.024

Varrot, A., Basheer, S. M., & Imberty, A. (2013). Fungal lectins: Structure, function and potential applications. *Current Opinion in Structural Biology, 23*(5), 678–685. https://doi.org/10.1016/j.sbi.2013.07.007

Vasconcelos, I. M., & Oliveira, J. T. A. (2004). Antinutritional properties of plant lectins. *Toxicon, 44*(4), 385–403. https://doi.org/10.1016/j.toxicon.2004.05.005

Vaz, A. F., Costa, R. M., Melo, A. M., Oliva, M. L., Santana, L. A., Silva-Lucca, R. A., Coelho, L. C., & Correia, M. T. (2010). Biocontrol of *Fusarium* species by a novel lectin with low ecotoxicity isolated from *Sebastiania jacobinensis*. *Food Chemistry, 119*(4), 1507–1513. https://doi.org/10.1016/j.foodchem.2009.09.035

Veelders, M., Brückner, S., Ott, D., Unverzagt, C., Mösch, H. U., & Essen, L. O. (2010). Structural basis of flocculin-mediated social behavior in yeast. *Proceedings of the National Academy of Sciences, 107*(52), 22511–22516. https://doi.org/10.1073/pnas.1013210108

Wang, P., Zhuo, X. R., Tang, L., Liu, X. S., Wang, Y. F., Wang, G. X., Yu, X. Q., & Wang, J. L. (2017). C-type lectin interacting with β-integrin enhances hemocytic encapsulation in the cotton bollworm, *Helicoverpa armigera*. *Insect Biochemistry and Molecular Biology, 86*, 29–40. https://doi.org/10.1016/j.ibmb.2017.05.005

Wang, W., Li, Q., Wu, J., Hu, Y., Wu, G., Yu, C., Xu, K., Liu, X., Wang, Q., Huang, W., & Wang, L. (2021). Lentil lectin derived from *Lens culinaris* exhibit broad antiviral activities against SARS-CoV-2 variants. *Emerging Microbes & Infections, 10*(1), pp. 1519–1529. https://doi.org/10.1080/22221751.2021.1957720

Ward, H. D., Keusch, G. T., & Pereira, M. E. (1990). Induction of a phosphomannosyl binding lectin activity in *Giardia*. *BioEssays, 12*(5), 211–215. https://doi.org/10.1002/bies.950120504

Wong, J. H., Wong, C. C., & Ng, T. B. (2006). Purification and characterization of a galactose-specific lectin with mitogenic activity from pinto beans. *Biochimica et Biophysica Acta (BBA)-General Subjects, 1760*(5), 808–813. https://doi.org/10.1016/j.bbagen.2006.02.015

Yao, Q., Wu, C. F., Luo, P., Xiang, X. C., Liu, J. J., Mou, L., & Bao, J. K. (2010). A new chitin-binding lectin from rhizome of Setcreasea purpurea with antifungal, antiviral and apoptosis-inducing activities. *Process Biochemistry, 45*(9), 1477–1485. https://doi.org/10.1016/j.procbio.2010.05.026

Zarate, G., & Perez Chaia, A. (2009). Dairy bacteria remove in vitro dietary lectins with toxic effects on colonic cells. *Journal of Applied Microbiology, 106*(3), 1050–1057. https://doi.org/10.1111/j.1365-2672.2008.04077.x

Zhao, J. K., Wang, H. X., & Ng, T. B. (2009). Purification and characterization of a novel lectin from the toxic wild mushroom *Inocybe umbrinella*. *Toxicon, 53*(3), 360–366.

15 Biomedical Prospects of Lectins in Cancer, Infectious Diseases, and Neurodegenerative Diseases

Taiwo Scholes Adewole, Stanley Chukwuejim,
Titilayo Oluwaseun Agunbiade, Gbenga
Emmanuel Ogundepo, and Adenike Kuku

15.1 INTRODUCTION

Cancer and infectious diseases caused by pathogenic microbes are one of the leading causes of morbidity and mortality globally. The World Health Organization estimated the annual global deaths due to cancer in 2020 to be approximately 10 million (www.who.int/news-room/fact-sheets/detail/cancer), with a significant quota of burden fatality being felt in developing countries with low income (Kocarnik et al., 2022). Corroboratively, the COVID-19 pandemic, which has had a devastating effect on lives and livelihoods around the world, is only one of a wave of severe infectious disease epidemics that have occurred in the twenty-first century (Baker et al., 2022). While death and morbidity linked to communicable diseases and malaria remain high, the burden of infectious diseases is still significant in developing nations, especially those with high poverty rates (Baker et al., 2022). To complicate issues, several pathogenic microbes (viruses, parasites, bacteria, and fungi) and cancer cells frequently alter and modify their structures and biochemistry to ensure their survival, hence, encouraging infectivity and drug resistance (Konozy et al., 2022; Rezayatmand et al., 2022). The downstream consequences of drug resistance have been linked to the progressing fatalities characterized by these pathologies, and if left unchecked, antimicrobial resistance alone might impose strict economic hardship on developing countries and cause the global death of 10 million people by 2050 (WHO, 2014; Pulingam et al., 2022).

Similarly, millions in the world's population are afflicted by neurodegenerative illnesses, which are characterized by the progressive onset of cognitive dysfunction and movement disability brought on by neuronal damage and death. These groups of diseases are often considered incurable due to the inadequate understanding of their pathogenesis, therefore limiting treatment options; hence, the search for novel prognostic and diagnostic tools (Ramos-Martínez et al., 2022).

In order to proffer novel solutions to these health menaces, natural products such as lectins are being explored as a veritable sustainable alternative to combat these pathologies, especially in the area of diagnosis and drug design (Araújo et al., 2020; Konozy et al., 2022; Enoma et al., 2023). In this chapter, we discuss the prospective and potential biomedical applications of lectins in the diagnosis and treatment of infectious diseases, cancer, and neurodegenerative diseases.

15.2 OVERVIEW OF LECTINS

Lectins are non-immune carbohydrate-binding proteins or glycoproteins that are widely distributed in nature (Konozy et al., 2022). Their name was coined from the Latin word *Legere*, literally meaning

DOI: 10.1201/9781003361497-17

"to select". They are also called hemagglutinins and originate from the glycoprotein superfamily and elicit closely related characteristics, especially in their sugar-binding specificities, without altering the covalent arrangements of their bound ligands (Manning et al., 2017). Coupled with their selective and reversible saccharide-binding features, lectins are also capable of cell agglutination, a property distinguishing them from other carbohydrate-binding proteins (Chettri et al., 2021). The three-dimensional organization of lectins determines their specificity structurally, indicating the presence of an evolutionarily preserved amino acid sequence. They are made up of a carbohydrate-binding domain (CBD) or carbohydrate-recognition domain (CRD) that is non-enzymatic (Hamid et al., 2013).

CBDs/CRDs are domains that can be found in larger multi-domain proteins or as standalone proteins (Figure 15.1). They usually identify the end groups of saccharides, which fit inside the narrow but distinct recognition domains (Taylor et al., 2022). When a hemagglutinin is only made up of its sugar-binding pocket, many of its roles rely on multivalency ability, allowing them to cross-link glycan-containing structures (Varki et al., 2009). These domains have hydrophobic and metal ion binding sites, which aid to improve binding affinity and specificity by arranging amino acid residues in their proper positions within the CBD and preserving subunit integrity (Lakhtin et al., 2011).

Lectins have also been shown to be a valuable biological tool for the purification and subsequent characterization of glycoproteins due to their carbohydrate-binding recognition capabilities (Nabi-Afjadi et al., 2022). These ubiquitous biomolecules are structurally diverse from each other and might be generally classified based on their origins – plant, animal, and microbial lectin (Jagdale and Devkatte, 2006; Adedoyin et al., 2021). Similarly, lectins can also be classified based on their structure, carbohydrate recognition domain, sugar specificity, and phylogenetic relationship (Radhakrishnan et al., 2021). Depending on their structure, binding preferences, and calcium dependence, lectins are further divided into different families, such as C-type lectins, I-type lectins, F-type lectins, intelectins, rhamnose-binding lectins, galectins, and Lily-type lectins (Vibhute et al., 2022), as shown in Figure 15.2.

Lectins play vital roles in the colonization processes of bacteria, archaea, protists, and fungi, serving as adhesion molecules (Gupta and Gupta, 2021; Lewis et al., 2022). They are also important in plant resistance systems and nodulation. Depending on their properties and distribution in tissues, lectins function in diverse animal processes, such as hemolysis, cell motility and adhesion, opsonization, immunological responses and phagocytosis, and glycoprotein synthesis (Santos et al., 2014; Nubi et al., 2021; Nabi-Afjadi et al., 2022). The specific purpose of lectins in plants is still unresolved; however, they are considered to be involved in plant defense mechanisms (Berg et al., 2002). Lectin research has attracted a lot of interest, especially in the field of biotechnology, medicine, and drug discovery, especially toward pathogenic microbes and cancer cells (Huo et al., 2022;

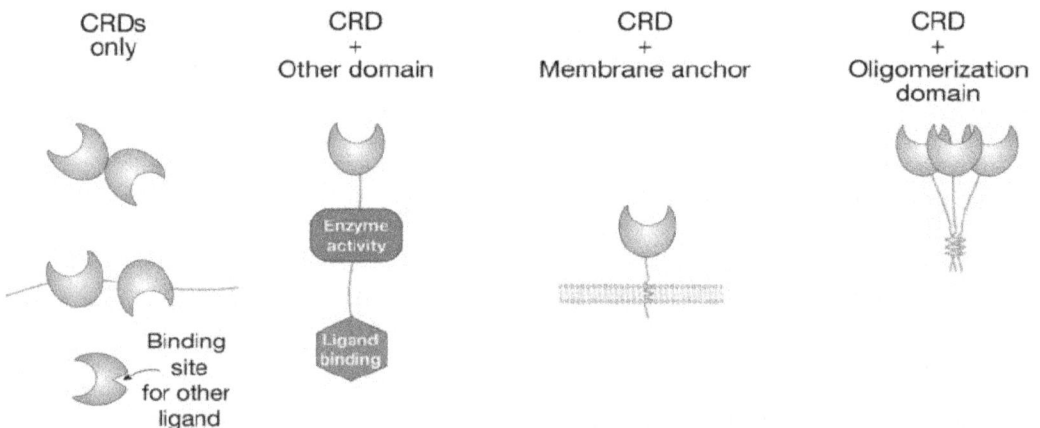

FIGURE 15.1 Carbohydrate-recognition domain (CRD) arrangements in lectins (Varki et al., 2009).

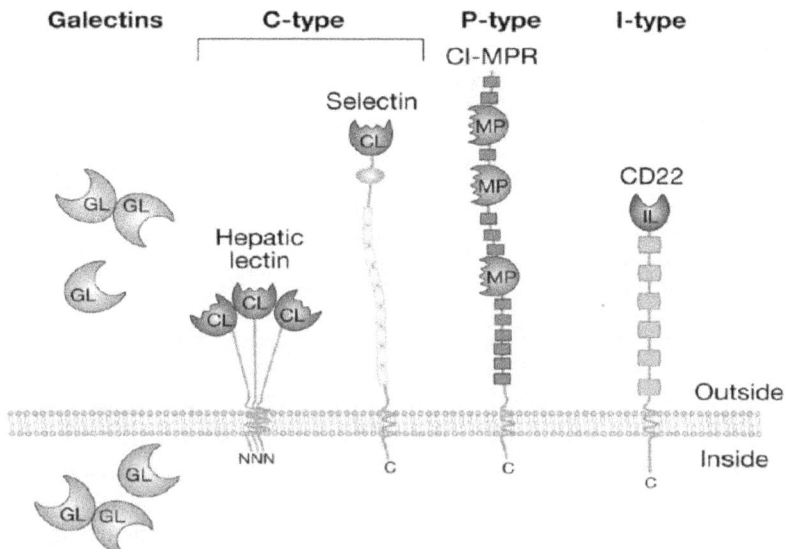

FIGURE 15.2 Typical members of four main animal lectin families. The identified carbohydrate-binding domains (CRDs) are displayed as follows: galectin, (MP) P-type lectin, (IL) I-type lectin, (CL) C-type lectin, and (GL) galectin (Varki et al., 2009).

Naseri et al., 2022). These emerging prospects have been linked with key interactions between diverse arrays of carbohydrates on cancer cells and pathogenic microbes, fostering specific, exploitable lectin-sugar interactions in the diagnosis and therapy of these pathologies (da Silva et al., 2023; Kusuma and Kottapalli, 2023). Also, due to their capacity to alter molecular targets in the central nervous system that may be connected to neuroplasticity, neurobehavioral effects, and neuroprotection, this distinct category of sugar-binding proteins has potential in the treatment/management of neurodegenerative illnesses (Araújo et al., 2020).

15.3 LECTINS AND CANCER THERAPY

Lectins are valuable in glycobiology research due to their high degree of specificity. The role they play in health and cancer research is because of the numerous interactions between lectins and sugar moieties located at the cell surface. The major forces driving these interactions are hydrogen bonding, Vander Waals interaction, and hydrophobic forces (Hamid et al., 2013). Various lectins have been employed in the past with success as anti-tumor agents or anti-neoplastic drugs against different cancer types, such as leukemia, prostate, sarcoma, lung, hepatoma, and breast cancer (Yau et al., 2015).

In addition to their therapeutic applications, the expression profiles of carbohydrates, the patterns of metastatic distribution, and the prognosis of lymphatic invasion of cancer cells may all be studied using lectins (Wang et al., 2000). It is also possible that the enhancement of the immune system of the host is another mechanism that underlies lectin antitumor action. *Vicia faba* agglutinin, often known as VFA, is a lectin that may be found in broad beans. These lectins caused colon cancer cells to clump together, accelerated their morphological differentiation, and decreased their aggressive character. According to Jordinson et al. (1999), a monoclonal antibody directed against epithelial cell adhesion molecule (epCAM) has the potential to prevent cancer cells from aggregating in response to VFA. These authors hypothesized that the mechanism by which VFA exerts its effect is either by binding directly to the N-glycosylated form of epCAM or via a route that involves epCAM.

A new class of bioactive glycan-binding proteins, known as galectins, has evolved, with the potential to influence a variety of immune system functions, from inflammation and cell-matrix associations to transport, cell survival, growth control, cytokine mobilization, and metastasis. Glycoconjugates on the cell surface may be crosslinked by galectins because of their multiple valences. The strong affinity with which these lectins bind polylactosamine-containing glycoproteins makes them an excellent choice for cancer-drug screening. Contrasting effects of galectins on cell growth and proliferation are crucial to understanding how they work. More than a dozen galectins have been found in the tissues of at least 13 mammalian species. It has been shown that galectin-carbohydrate interactions influence cell death and cellular communications (Rabinovich et al., 2002).

Characterization of the phenotype and function of membrane-associated glycoproteins that are produced on cancer cells is made possible by the carbohydrate-binding specificity of lectins. For instance, wheat germ agglutinin (WGA) has been demonstrated to have a repressive impact on the rat pancreatic tumor cell line AR42J, which was followed by a slight reduction in the amount of beta-amylase that was secreted (Mikkat et al., 2001). Aside from general cytotoxicity toward cancer cells, the specialized anticancer mechanism of lectins encompasses its capacity to limit tumor growth by triggering apoptosis and autophagy, downregulating telomerase activity as well as preventing angiogenesis.

15.3.1 Anticancer/Anti-Tumor Mechanisms of Lectins

15.3.1.1 Triggering Apoptosis

Nearly all of the major classes of plant lectins have been investigated for their role in cancer apoptosis to better understand how plant lectins work against cancer (Bhutia et al., 2019). Plant lectins are cytotoxic to a variety of cancer cells by focusing on apoptotic, necrotic, and autophagic cell death, which is implicated in numerous important signaling pathways, thanks to their unique structural makeup and capacity to bind sugar receptors. Understanding the biochemical and molecular complexity of the apoptotic and autophagic pathways will lead to the development of novel therapeutic approaches building on the numerous laboratory results already obtained. The health-promotional properties and hazardous side effects of these proteins are the focus of biomedical researchers to drive innovation on realistic diagnostic and anti-tumor agents (Lei and Chang, 2009). Surface-death receptors or the release of cytochrome c from the mitochondria trigger the energy-dependent, regulated kind of cell death known as apoptosis. Diverse cell surface receptors, including TNF-R, bind to particular molecules to initiate the extrinsic apoptotic pathway. Next, apoptotic signals like TNF-R type 1-associated death domain protein (TRADD) and Fas-associated protein with death domain are activated and transmitted, which dimerizes and switches on the death-inducing signaling complex (DISC); by dimerizing the pro-apoptotic proteins Bax and Bak before cytochrome c is released, intracellular stimuli that encourage mitochondrial outer membrane permeabilization (MOMP) cause intrinsic apoptosis. Caspase-9 and caspase-3 are activated by cytochrome c by binding to apoptotic protein activating factor-1 (Mukhopadhyay et al., 2014, Gamie et al., 2017).

Different lectins alter several signaling pathways that are connected to apoptosis in various malignancies. Typically, lectins of plant origin have undergone in-depth research, including Concanavalin A (Con A), the lectins of mistletoe (*V. album*), and *Polygonatum cyrtonema* lectin (PCL). In both human melanoma A375 cells and human hepatocellular carcinoma HepG2 cells, ConA, the first described legume lectin, reportedly triggers a mitochondrial transmembrane collapse, facilitating cytochrome c release and caspase activation, ultimately resulting in mitochondria-umpired cell death (Jiang et al., 2015). The mannose/sialic acid lectin *Polygonatum cyrtonema* (PCL), a member of the *Galanthus nivalis* agglutinin (GNA) family initially isolated from *P. cyrtonema*, also elicited a similar mechanism. This lectin triggers cell death in melanoma A375 cells and involves control of the Bax, B cell lymphoma-extra-large (Bcl-xL) and B cell lymphoma-2 (Bcl-2) proteins as well as the collapse of mitochondrial membrane permeabilization, which results in the release of cytochrome c and activation of caspases. PCL inhibits the proliferation of cervical cancer HeLa cells and promotes apoptosis, and it activates caspase to cause apoptosis in human breast cancer MCF-7 cells. Through a caspase-dependent apoptotic mechanism, PCL also causes apoptosis in fibrosarcoma L929 cells, together with activation of caspases-3/-8/-9 (Jiang et al., 2015).

15.3.1.2 Targeting Autophagic Signaling Pathway

In certain circumstances, autophagy results from a stress-induced response to avoiding cell death; an alternate sort of cell death, known as autophagic cell death, can also occur, leading to cellular demise (Lei and Chang, 2009). Autophagy and apoptosis have a complicated interaction. Common triggers can initiate both autophagy and apoptosis, which can occasionally happen together. At other times, the development of autophagy and apoptosis is mutually exclusive (Jiang et al., 2015).

Depending on concentration and time, Con A reportedly interacts with mannose moiety found on the cellular surface. This binding generally inhibits growth and induces cell mortality. A high concentration of Con A is toxic to cancer cells, while a low dose practically inhibits the growth of tumor cell lines (Lei and Chang, 2009). Varied cell lines have different Con A sensitivity-levels. However, Con A is a T-cell mitogen for lymphocytes at concentrations of 1–10 μg/ml, while a larger concentration is still cytotoxic. Because they have a higher concentration of mannosylated or glucosylated components on their cell surface, immune cells demonstrated heightened response relative to the cancerous cells.

Con A may initially cause a non-specific immune response in tumor cells, but when tumor cells are eliminated, a tumor-specific immune induction takes place, which leads to a tumor-cell-specific response later on. Necrotic autophagic mortality of cancer cells induced by Concanavalin A can also trigger a tumor cell-specific immunological response. This lectin is, thus, a potential innovative form of endogenous cancer vaccine immunotherapy. The interplay of initial autophagic activation on cancer cells and subsequent immunomodulating effect on lymphocytes via the mannose/glucose tumor cells association will result in an original inflammatory response and secondary anti-tumor response (Lei and Chang, 2009).

According to Chang et al. (2007), Con A promotes autophagy in hepatoma cells through the BNIP3-mitochondrial pathway. BNIP3 mediates mitochondrial pore formation. BNIP3 promotes mitochondrial depolarization and Con A permeabilization, beginning autophagy. Additionally, pro-inflammatory cytokine MIF has a function in Con A-induced autophagy in hepatoma cells. MIF inhibitors limit autophagic Concanavalin A-induced cell mortality, and short hairpin RNAs validate MIF's role in both. MIF contributes to Con A's antitumor effect by regulating STAT3-MIF-BNIP3-dependent autophagy (Lai et al., 2015). IFN-gamma induces IRGM1 translocation to lysosomes and prolongs Con A-treated hepatoma cell activity (Chang et al., 2011). When treated with Con A, U87 glioblastoma cells upregulated BNIP3, ATG12, and ATG3, but this was reversed when the MT1-MMP gene was silenced (Pratt et al., 2012). Con A-induced autophagy in U87 cells involves the interaction between STAT3 and MT1-MMP (Pratt and Annabi, 2014). Con A activates autophagy in HeLa cells by reducing PI3K/AKT/mTOR levels and activating MEK/ERK (Roy et al., 2014).

Lectins from *Dioclea reflexa* and *Canavalia bonariensis* have also been reported to cause autophagy-associated cell death in glioma cells (Cavada et al., 2018; Wolin et al., 2023). In their research findings, Mukhopadhyay et al. (2014) and Panda et al. (2014) reported the lectins PNA (peanut agglutinin) and SBL (soybean lectin) reduced tumor cell growth in DL mice by inducing autophagy and programmed cell death. In vitro tests showed that these two lectins exploit these biochemical mechanisms to induce fatality in HeLa cells by producing ROS, whereas N-acetylcysteine (NAC) inhibited these processes (Mukhopadhyay et al., 2014, Panda et al., 2014).

15.3.1.3 Inhibition of Angiogenesis and Immunomodulation

Checkmating angiogenic gene expressions is a potent mechanism of lectin-induced anti-tumor activity. *Dolichos lablab* lectin exhibits cytotoxic activity against cancer cells by regressing the proliferation of solid tumor cells and slowing the pre-angiogenic signals, particularly vascular endothelial growth factor, hypoxia-inducible factor, nuclear factor kappa B, and matrix metalloproteinase. This contributes to tumor regression and points toward the valuable role *Dolichos lablab* lectin will play in cancer therapeutics. Cancer cell lines overexpressing mannose can become targeted by mannose-binding lectins, functioning both as an anticancer and diagnostic agent. Algal lectin, particularly mannose-specific seaweed lectin, has both cytotoxic and anti-viral properties (Barre et al., 2019). Due to their ability to exclusively engage with the viral envelope glycoprotein gp120 and stop HIV-1 virion infectivity toward the host CD4+ T-lymphocyte cells in vitro, mannose-specific seaweed lectins have been employed extensively as potent human-immunodeficiency-virus-(HIV-1)-inactivating proteins.

It has been proven that Abrus lectins-derived peptide fractions (AGG) exert their cytotoxic bioactivity via the apoptotic induction and stimulation of Th1 immunomodulation. This cytotoxic efficacy of AGG has been studied in many cancer cells (Ghosh and Maiti, 2007; Bhutia et al., 2009, Ghosh et al., 2009). Interestingly, due to their association with the glycosylated structures, domiciled on the surface of immune cells, a number of plant lectins are capable of inducing immunomodulatory activity. This, in turn, causes the production of cytokines, which are responsible for exerting tumoricidal activity in cancer cells (Souza et al., 2013).

15.3.1.4 Lectin-Based Drug Delivery System

One of the major challenges encountered in drug delivery is the effectiveness of the active agent, and it is usually correlated to the mode of administration (oral, gastrointestinal, ocular). Typically, when proteins and peptides are ingested orally, there are no major clear-cut interactions between the macromolecule and the membrane topology (Višnjar et al., 2019). The ability of proteins and drugs to be absorbed usually depends on passive diffusion, availability, and solubility. The transit time of the active agent in the lumen of the small intestine is also important because the active agent is usually cleared from the small intestine to the large intestine. The surface lining of the mucosa membrane as well as gastrointestinal enzymes also play a huge part in drug delivery by making the active agent available for specific receptors and monitoring the release rate as well. The availability of the active ingredients can be increased by using small-scale cargo delivery systems, which include nanoparticles and dendrimers, among others. The accessibility of the active ingredients to the mucosal surface and the length of time the medication stays in the digestive tract may be reduced with some nanocarriers (Mishra et al., 2019).

Lectins can be utilized in the drug-delivery system to overcome some of the challenges that are encountered in conventional drug delivery (Nubi et al., 2021). The major targets of lectins are the carbohydrate residues in glycolipids and glycoproteins, and the interactions of lectin with these residues channel a downstream effect that brings about physiological changes. A drug delivery system, including haptens that are recognized and implicated by cell-surface internally-generated lectins, constitutes the first scenario (glycotargeting) (Yau et al., 2015). In this scenario, the drug is prepared and coated with suitable haptens that will interact favorably with endogenous lectins, and this interaction will trigger downstream effects that translate to physiological changes. Another scenario involves targeting cell-surface glycolipids, glycoproteins, or cell surfaces expressing complex carbohydrates. The goal of the second scenario (reverse lectin-targeting technique) is to direct the drug delivery system to glycolipids, glycoproteins, or other carbohydrates that are resident on the cellular exterior by using exogenous lectins as targeting moieties (Višnjar et al., 2019). These tactics can therefore lengthen the period that a drug stays in the target region, allowing for intimate interactions between the therapeutic agent and the membrane exterior and speeding up the transepithelial cargo trafficking (the movement of a drug or nanocarrier across a cell membrane). Because of their great selectivity for membrane-bound receptors on epithelial cells, lectins have been utilized in bioadhesive systems. They can identify cell-surface carbohydrates (also known as mucins), have demonstrated resistance to enzymatic degradation, and can bind to specific cell surfaces. The relevance of these ligands for gene therapy has increased over the years, as evidenced by their use as mediators of therapeutics trafficking through the intestinal epithelium by glycan-mediated endocytosis or lectin-conjugated drug-delivery system (e.g., liposome) targeting for gene vector transfer to airway epithelial cells in which the transfected cell can express (Mishra et al., 2019).

Della Giovampaola et al. (2017) constructed doxorubicin-loaded liposomes conjugated with *Lotus tetragonolobus* lectin on two cancer cell lines, and the delivery was monitored in vivo and in vitro by confocal and electron microscopy. The uptake and delivery of the functionalized lectin loaded with doxorubicin to the cancer cell line significantly increased when compared to unmodified doxorubicin-loaded liposomes. The functionalized lectin, loaded with doxorubicin, decreases non-specific toxicity by specifically delivering doxorubicin to the cytoplasm of the cancer cells. The distinct structure of the urothelium makes it a difficult barrier to cross. The major challenge faced by the pharmaceutical industry in designing a drug to target bladder cancer cells is the low concentration of active ingredients in the malignant cells due to the barrier created by the urothelium (Apfelthaler et al., 2017). Coupling WGA with poly-L-glutamic acid (PGA) as the backbone for active pharmaceutical ingredients improves the specificity of the interaction between the conjugate and cell surface (Apfelthaler et al., 2017). Optimizing WGA-PGA-Doxorubicin conjugates and introducing these conjugates to urothelial cell monolayers increases the cell binding affinity and residence time, inhibiting cell viability up to 99% (Apfelthaler et al., 2018). This is a promising strategy in intravesical chemotherapy because this combination has a higher binding affinity to cancer cells, with proven cytotoxicity.

15.4 LECTINS AND NEURODEGENERATIVE DISEASES

There are a number of neurodegenerative disorders that affect the nervous system as a whole, including Alzheimer's disease, Parkinson's disease, Huntington's disease, multiple sclerosis, and amyotrophic lateral sclerosis (ALS) (Chen et al., 2016; Dorothée, 2018). These abnormalities in human brains may, over time, cause a patient to experience a decrease in their cognitive or functional abilities. Inflammation is thought to be a common feature in neurodegenerative illnesses, in which neurodegeneration and the course of these diseases are both contributed to by prolonged responses to inflammation (Amor et al., 2010).

To regulate the inflammatory feedback, galectins have been suggested as a promising drug candidate (Liu et al., 2012; Rabinovich and Croci, 2012). These galectins would respond to the molecular alteration in the sugar phenotype and induce signaling cascades that are at the root of the cellular response to externally generated impulses. It has been discovered that galectins participate in the control of several disorders characterized by chronic inflammation (Di Lella et al., 2011; Vasta et al., 2012). There has been a significant amount of research conducted on galectin-1 and galectin-3 in the CNS; it has been demonstrated that galectin-1 inhibits the inflammatory feedback, while galectin-3 promotes inflammation (Sasaki, 2004; Starossom et al., 2012; Shin, 2013). In addition to this, these galectins take part in the internal regulation of the various intracellular signaling pathways, which influences the modulation of the cellular response (Dhirapong et al., 2009; Rabinovich and Croci, 2012).

Neuroinflammation is a factor that is present in all forms of neurodegenerative illness. In the treatment of neurodegenerative illnesses, galectin-1 and galectin-3 serve as therapeutic targets, since they are two of the most important regulators of the inflammatory response. As a result, galectin-1 overexpression or therapy in instances of inflammation-mediated neuronal injury may assist in the neuromodulation and repair of injured neuronal tissues and/or postpone the neurodegenerative processes generated by neuroinflammation. Consequently, inhibiting galectin-3 may assist in lowering the inflammatory response and, as a consequence, reducing the amount of neurodegeneration that takes place (Ramírez Hernández et al., 2020).

The expression of galectin-1 in the central nervous system boosts neural stem/progenitor cell growth. Recombinant galectin-1 improves neural regeneration by inhibiting astrocyte growth and producing BDNF, which prevents neuronal loss (Huang, 2007). Galectin-1 engages in acute inflammation and has anti-inflammatory effects on microglia and astrocytes. When the expression level of this galectin is increased, there is regeneration of axons in the nerves of the periphery following axotomy and neural stem cell proliferation in the subventricular zone (Horie et al., 2004). Given its immunoregulatory functions, galectin-1 has been recommended as a possibility for innovative anti-inflammatory medications as a target for neurodegenerative illnesses (Ramírez Hernández et al., 2020).

Galectin-3 is proinflammatory, unlike galectin-1. Galectin-3 has multiple activities based on cell type and location and is elevated during inflammation, cell proliferation, and cell differentiation (Inohara et al., 1998). In neurodegenerative disorders, galectin-3 seems to regulate inflammation in the CNS. In response to proinflammatory stimuli, galectin-3 activates microglia and astrocytes by activating the JAK-STAT-signaling cascade, and it works as an endogenous paracrine TLR4 ligand (Zhou et al., 2018). Thus, galectin-3 expression leads to proinflammatory activity, which improves microglial survival under neuroinflammatory stimuli and neurodegeneration (Ramírez Hernández et al., 2020).

15.5   LECTINS AND INFECTIOUS DISEASES

Lectins play vital roles, especially as key mediators of immune response, by recognizing glycan structural components of pathogenic viruses, bacteria, fungi, and parasites. Intracellularly, these molecules function as pattern-recognition receptors, and their antimicrobial activities toward pathogenic bacteria and fungi depend on their interactions with cell wall components of the target organisms via their CRD. These interactions usually result in secondary downstream effects, such as membrane puncture or inhibition of vital cell wall components (Mayer et al., 2017; Breitenbach et al., 2018). Lectins are potential biologics that can be used to treat a variety of pathogenic microorganisms, such as viruses that are causing epidemics and pose a threat from treatment resistance. Since glycans with mannose residues are frequently used in viral entry mechanisms, mannose-binding lectins, for example, are now being exploited and proposed as new antiviral agents against a number of viruses, including SARS-COV-2 and HIV (Koharudin and Gronenborn, 2014; Watanabe et al., 2020). In their anti-HIV mechanism, lectins bind to highly mannosylated gp120 on the viral surface, inducing a conformational change of the virus. On the other hand, lectins also have a high affinity for the mannosylated spike protein receptor, therefore preventing SARS-COV-2 from binding to its major receptor, angiotensin-converting enzyme 2. By aggregating and eliminating oral-resistant microbes, salivary agglutinin, another lectin, contributes significantly to the human innate immune system. By attaching to the component of the HIV gp120 envelope glycoprotein, fragments of this lectin decreased the ability of HIV to infect people (Kallenbach et al., 2007). Other lectins that have shown potent antiviral activities include lectins from banana (BanLec) (Markovitz et al., 2019), balsam apple (MOMO30) (Powell and Gbodossou, 2020), *Nostoc ellipsosporum* (cyanovirin-N) (Mayo et al., 2009), mistletoe (Lentzen and Witthohn, 2016), *Sambucus nigra* (Hotchen, 2002), among others.

To capture viral particles and prevent their reproduction and dissemination, specific lectins can also be fixed onto immobile surfaces (Carneiro et al., 2022). By activating carboxyl groups on the surface of specialized raw material, the lectin concanavalin A (Con A) was, for example, immobilized on the microspheres. The HIV membrane glycoprotein gp120 was captured with around 90% efficiency in the resulting embodiment, and the HIV infectious value was decreased by 70%. Mitsuru et al. (1998) advised using it in aerosol spray, lotions, solid preparations, and materials with molded surfaces. Similar to this, the biodegradable, electrospun polymer was coupled to the lectin griffithsin via an amide bond via a chemical cross-linker. This allowed for the capture and inactivation of viral particles (Steinbach-Rankins et al., 2016).

Some infections brought on by pathogenic bacteria and fungi may be treated or prevented with the help of mannan-binding lectin (MBL). MBL generally includes three CRDs, and by identifying mannose glycans from microbial pathogens and activating the complement proteins, these CRDs play a significant role in human first-line defense. More vulnerability to infectious illnesses is linked to mutations in MBL that result in its deficit (Fischer, 2004). The recombinant 20 kDa human mannose-binding lectin ZG16 reportedly elicited potent antifungal activities against pathogenic fungi (Atsushi and Hiroaki, 2010). According to these authors, ZG16 bioactivity was mediated by the ability of this lectin to bind specific cell surface glycans. Lectins can also function as opsonin when they are linked to antibodies, hence recruiting phagocytic immune cells for the clearance of microbial pathogens (Mayer et al., 2018). We also recently reported the antimicrobial activity of a lactose-binding lectin from *Erythrina senegalensis* seeds (Enoma et al., 2023). This lectin inhibited the growth of *Erwinia carotovora, Pseudomonas aeruginosa, Klebsiella pneumonia, Staphyloccocus aureus, Aspergillus niger, Penicillium camemberti*, and *Scopulariopsis brevicaulis*. Typically, after cell-surface glycan-binding, the downstream antifungal effect of lectins includes hyphae binding and inhibition of spore germination (Coelho et al., 2017),

Lectins incorporated into drug delivery systems, such as liposomes, have been demonstrated to increase the specificity of cargo delivery and the antibacterial activity of antibiotics (Weiming et al., 2016). This technique has been tested against *Listeria monocytogenes*, which was found to be susceptible to antimicrobial peptide delivered by liposome coated with wheat germ agglutinin and concanavalin A (Chuanfen and Wenting, 2017).

15.6 CONCLUSION AND FUTURE PROSPECTS

Lectins are a subclass of proteins/glycoproteins that can reversibly attach to certain carbohydrates without changing their covalent structure. They function in biological recognition processes involving proteins and cells, defending the biosystem from particular threats. These biomolecules are so-named hemagglutinins because they can bind to and agglutinate erythrocytes, which is a useful property for blood typing. Lectins are employed in research to gain an understanding of important biological processes, including microbial infection, leukocyte homing and trafficking, leukocyte arrest, apoptosis, neoplasm cell metastasis, and cell proliferation. Lectins are also frequently utilized for cell characterization and separation as well as for research on glycoconjugates. Additionally, lectins are used in novel data-storing methods where carbohydrates are used as the hardware for information coding as well as in microarrays for a high-throughput examination of glycans and glycoproteins. The biomedical significance cannot be overemphasized, as these biomolecules are now finding a place as emerging biologics, therapeutic drug analogs, or molecular drug targets; hence, intensified efforts should be directed toward their isolation and characterization from non-conventional sources to foster their full exploitation. However, utmost attention must be given to addressing issues regarding their toxicity.

REFERENCES

Adedoyin, I. O., Adewole, T. S., Agunbiade, T. O., Adewoyin, F. B., & Kuku, A. (2021). A purified lectin with larvicidal activity from a woodland mushroom, *Agaricus semotus* Fr. *Acta Biologica Szegediensis, 65*(1), 65–73. https://doi.org/10.14232/abs.2021.1.65-73

Amor, S., Puentes, F., Baker, D., & van der Valk, P. (2010). Inflammation in neurodegenerative diseases. *Immunology, 129*(2), 154–169. https://doi.org/10.1111/j.1365-2567.2009.03225.x

Apfelthaler, C., Anzengruber, M., Gabor, F., & Wirth, M. (2017). Poly–(1)–glutamic acid drug delivery system for the intravesical therapy of bladder cancer using WGA as targeting moiety. *European Journal of Pharmaceutics and Biopharmaceutics, 115*, 131–139. https://doi.org/10.1016/j.bbagen.2017.01.015

Apfelthaler, C., Skoll, K., Ciola, R., Gabor, F., & Wirth, M. (2018). A doxorubicin loaded colloidal delivery system for the intravesical therapy of non-muscle invasive bladder cancer using wheat germ agglutinin as targeter. *European Journal of Pharmaceutics and Biopharmaceutics, 130*, 177–184. https://doi.org/10.1016/j.ejpb.2018.06.028

Araújo, J. R. C., Coelho, C. B., Campos, A. R., de Azevedo Moreira, R., & de Oliveira Monteiro-Moreira, A. C. (2020). Animal galectins and plant lectins as tools for studies in neurosciences. *Current Neuropharmacology, 18*(3), 202–215.

Atsushi, H., & Hiroaki, T. (2010). Antifungal agent (Japan). JP2010150187thA

Baker, R. E., Mahmud, A. S., Miller, I. F., Rajeev, M., Rasambainarivo, F., Rice, B. L., . . . Metcalf, C. J. E. (2022). Infectious disease in an era of global change. *Nature Reviews Microbiology*, *20*(4), 193–205. https://doi.org/10.1038/s41579-021-00639-z

Barre, A., Simplicien, M., Benoist, H., Van Damme, E. J., & Rougé, P. (2019). Mannose-specific lectins from marine algae: Diverse structural scaffolds associated to common virucidal and anti-cancer properties. *Marine Drugs*, *17*(8), 440. https://doi.org/10.3390/md17080440

Berg, J. M., Tymoczko, J. L., & Stryer, L. (2002). *Biochemistry*. New York: W. H. Freeman and Company.

Bhutia, S. K., Mallick, S. K., & Maiti, T. K. (2009). In vitro immunostimulatory properties of Abrus lectins derived peptides in tumor bearing mice. *Phytomedicine*, *16*(8), 776–782. https://doi.org/10.1016/j.phymed.2009.01.006

Bhutia, S. K., Panda, P. K., Sinha, N., Praharaj, P. P., Bhol, C. S., Panigrahi, D. P., Mahapatra, K. K., Saha, S., Patra, S., Mishra, S. R., Behera, B. P., Patil, S., & Maiti, T. K. (2019). Plant lectins in cancer therapeutics: Targeting apoptosis and autophagy-dependent cell death. *Pharmacological Research*, *144*(1), 8–18. https://doi.org/10.1016/j.phrs.2019.04.001

Breitenbach Barroso Coelho, L. C., Marcelino dos Santos Silva, P., Felix de Oliveira, W., De Moura, M. C., Viana Pontual, E., Soares Gomes, F., . . . dos Santos Correia, M. T. (2018). Lectins as antimicrobial agents. *Journal of Applied Microbiology*, *125*(5), 1238–1252. https://doi.org/10.1111/jam.14055

Carneiro, D. C., Fernandez, L. G., Monteiro-Cunha, J. P., Benevides, R. G., & Cunha Lima, S. T. (2022). A patent review of the antimicrobial applications of lectins: Perspectives on therapy of infectious diseases. *Journal of Applied Microbiology*, *132*(2), 841–854. https://doi.org/10.1111/jam.15263

Cavada, B. S., Mayara, S., Silva, J., Pinto-Junior, Vanir Reis, Paula, A., Alessandra, I., Heinrich, I. A., Nobre, Moreira, C. G., & Lossio, C. F. (2018). *Canavalia bonariensis* lectin: Molecular bases of glycoconjugates interaction and antiglioma potential. *International Journal of Biological Macromolecules*, *106*(1), 369–378.

Chang, C. P., Yang, M. C., & Lei, H. Y. (2011). Concanavalin A/IFN-gamma triggers autophagy-related necrotic hepatocyte death through IRGM1-mediated lysosomal membrane disruption. *PLoS ONE*, *6*(12), e28323. https://doi.org/10.1371/journal.pone.0028323

Chang, C. P., Yang, M. C., Liu, H. S., Lin, Y. S., & Lei, H. Y. (2007). Concanavalin A induces autophagy in hepatoma cells and has a therapeutic effect in a murine in situ hepatoma model. *Hepatology (Baltimore, Md.)*, *45*(2), 286–296. https://doi.org/10.1002/hep.21509

Chen, W. W., Zhang, X., & Huang, W. J. (2016). Role of neuroinflammation in neurodegenerative diseases (Review). *Molecular Medicine Reports*, *13*(4), 3391–3396. https://doi.org/10.3892/mmr.2016.4948

Chettri, D., Boro, M., Sarkar, L., & Verma, A. K. (2021). Lectins: Biological significance to biotechnological application. *Carbohydrate Research*, *506*, 108367. https://doi.org/10.1016/j.carres.2021.108367

Chuanfen, P., & Wenting, T. (2017). Applications of lectin-modified anchovy antibacterial peptide liposome in inhibition of *Listeria monocytogenes* and biofilm thereof (China). CN106360250A

Coelho, L. C. B. B., Silva, P. M. D. S., Lima, V. L. D. M., Pontual, E. V., Paiva, P. M. G., Napoleao, T. H., & Correia, M. T. D. S. (2017). Lectins, interconnecting proteins with biotechnological/pharmacological and therapeutic applications. *Evidence-Based Complementary and Alternative Medicine*, *2017*. https://doi.org/10.1155/2017/1594074

da Silva, S. P., da Silva, J. D. F., da Costa, C. B. L., da Silva, P. M., de Freitas, A. F. S., da Silva, C. E. S., . . . Napoleão, T. H. (2023). Purification, characterization, and assessment of antimicrobial activity and toxicity of Portulaca elatior leaf lectin (PeLL). *Probiotics and Antimicrobial Proteins*, *15*(2), 287–299. https://doi.org/10.1007/s12602-021-09837-w

Della Giovampaola, C., Capone, A., Ermini, L., Lupetti, P., Vannuccini, E., Finetti, F., . . . Bonechi, C. (2017). Formulation of liposomes functionalized with Lotus lectin and effective in targeting highly proliferative cells. *Biochimica et Biophysica Acta (BBA)-General Subjects*, *1861*(4), 860–870. https://doi.org/10.1016/j.bbagen.2017.01.015

Dhirapong, A., Lleo, A., Leung, P., Gershwin, M. E., & Liu, F. T. (2009). The immunological potential of galectin-1 and -3. *Autoimmunity Reviews*, *8*(5), 360–363. https://doi.org/10.1016/j.autrev.2008.11.009

Di Lella, S., Sundblad, V., Cerliani, J. P., Guardia, C. M., Estrin, D. A., Vasta, G. R., & Rabinovich, G. A. (2011). When galectins recognize glycans: From biochemistry to physiology and back again. *Biochemistry*, *50*(37), 7842–7857. https://doi.org/10.1021/bi201121m

Dorothée, G. (2018). Neuroinflammation in neurodegeneration: Role in pathophysiology, therapeutic opportunities and clinical perspectives. *Journal of Neural Transmission*, *125*(5), 749–750. https://doi.org/10.1007/s00702-018-1880-6

Enoma, S., Adewole, T. S., Agunbiade, T. O., & Kuku, A. (2023). Antimicrobial activities and phylogenetic study of Erythrina senegalensis DC (Fabaceae) seed lectin. *BioTechnologia. Journal of Biotechnology Computational Biology and Bionanotechnology*, *104*(1): 21–32. https://doi.org/10.5114/bta.2023.125083

Fischer, P. (2004). Mannan-binding lectin (MBL) treatment of infections in individuals treated with TNF-alpha inhibitors (United States). US20040029785A1

Gamie, Z., Kapriniotis, K., Papanikolaou, D., Haagensen, E., Da Conceicao Ribeiro, R., Dalgarno, K., Krippner-Heidenreich, A., Gerrand, C., Tsiridis, E., & Rankin, K. S. (2017). TNF-related apoptosis-inducing ligand (TRAIL) for bone sarcoma treatment: Pre-clinical and clinical data. *Cancer Letters*, *409*(1), 66–80. https://doi.org/10.1016/j.canlet.2017.08.036

Ghosh, D., & Maiti, T. K. (2007). Immunomodulatory and anti-tumor activities of native and heat denatured Abrus agglutinin. *Immunobiology*, *212*(7), 589–599. https://doi.org/10.1016/j.imbio.2007.03.005

Ghosh, D., Bhutia, S. K., Mallick, S. K., Banerjee, I., & Maiti, T. K. (2009). Stimulation of murine B and T lymphocytes by native and heat-denatured Abrus agglutinin. *Immunobiology*, *214*(3), 227–234. https://doi.org/10.1016/j.imbio.2008.08.002

Gupta, A., & Gupta, G. S. (2021). Status of mannose-binding lectin (MBL) and complement system in COVID-19 patients and therapeutic applications of antiviral plant MBLs. *Molecular and Cellular Biochemistry*, *476*(8), 2917–2942. https://doi.org/10.1007/s11010-021-04107-3

Hamid, R., Masood, A., Wani, I. H., & Rafiq, S. (2013). Lectins: Proteins with diverse applications. *Journal of Applied Pharmaceutical Science*, *3*(4), S93–S103. http://doi.org/10.7324/JAPS.2013.34.S18

Horie, H., Kadoya, T., Hikawa, N., Sango, K., Inoue, H., Takeshita, K., Asawa, R., Hiroi, T., Sato, M., Yoshioka, T., & Ishikawa, Y. (2004). Oxidized galectin-1 stimulates macrophages to promote axonal regeneration in peripheral nerves after axotomy. *The Journal of Neuroscience*, *24*(8), 1873–1880. https://doi.org/10.1523/JNEUROSCI.4483-03.2004

Hotchen, M. (2002). Antiviral composition incorporating lectins (France). WO2002100424A1.

Huang, Q. (2007). Volatile of alkyd varnish inhibits the expression of neuronal growth associated protein-43 in mice. *Neural Regeneration Research*, *2*(6), 331–334. https://doi.org/10.1016/s1673-5374(07)60060-7

Huo, F., Zhang, Y., Li, Y., Bu, H., Zhang, Y., Li, W., Guo, Y., Wang, L., Jia, R., Huang, T., & Zhang, W. (2022), Mannose-targeting concanavalin A-epirubicin conjugate for targeted intravesical chemotherapy of bladder cancer. *Chemistry–An Asian Journal, 17*(16), p.e202200342. https://doi.org/10.1002/asia.202200342

Inohara, H., Akahani, S., & Raz, A. (1998). Galectin-3 Stimulates Cell Proliferation. *Experimental Cell Research*, *245*(2), 294–302. https://doi.org/10.1006/excr.1998.4253

Jagdale, Y. D., & Devkatte, A. (2006). Lectin–An astonishing protein that is both a boon and a bane for humanity. *Integration*, *15*, 10.

Jiang, Q. L., Zhang, S., Tian, M., Zhang, S. Y., Xie, T., Chen, D. Y., . . . Jiang, X. (2015). Plant lectins, from ancient sugar-binding proteins to emerging anti-cancer drugs in apoptosis and autophagy. *Cell Proliferation*, *48*(1), 17–28. https://doi.org/10.1111/cpr.12155

Jordinson, M., El-Hariry, I., Calnan, D. A., Calam, J., & Pignatelli, M. (1999). *Vicia faba* agglutinin, the lectin present in broad beans, stimulates differentiation of undifferentiated colon cancer cells. *Gut*, *44*(5), 709–714. https://doi.org/10.1136/gut.44.5.709

Kallenbach, N., Malamud, D., Liu, Z., Abrams, W., & Arora, P. (2007). Polyvalent multimeric composition containing active polypeptides, pharmaceutical compositions and methods of using the same. US20070053934A1

Kocarnik, J. M., Compton, K., Dean, F. E., Fu, W., Gaw, B. L., Harvey, J. D., . . . Dhimal, M. (2022). Cancer incidence, mortality, years of life lost, years lived with disability, and disability-adjusted life years for 29 cancer groups from 2010 to 2019: A systematic analysis for the global burden of disease study 2019. *JAMA Oncology*, *8*(3), 420–444.

Koharudin, L. M., & Gronenborn, A. M. (2014) Antiviral lectins as potential HIV microbicides. *Current Opinion in Virology*, 7, 95–100. https://doi.org/10.1016/j.coviro.2014.05.006

Konozy, E. H. E., Osman, M. E. F. M., & Dirar, A. I. (2022). Plant lectins as potent Anti-coronaviruses, Anti-inflammatory, antinociceptive and antiulcer agents. *Saudi Journal of Biological Sciences*, 103301. https://doi.org/10.1016/j.sjbs.2022.103301

Konozy, E. H. E., Osman, M. E. F. M., Dirar, A. I., & Ghartey-Kwansah, G. (2022). Plant lectins: A new antimicrobial frontier. *Biomedicine & Pharmacotherapy*, *155*, 113735. https://doi.org/10.1016/j.biopha.2022.113735

Kusuma, V., & Kottapalli, S. (2023). Purification and characterization of a novel anti-tumour galactose binding lectin from Euphorbia caducifolia latex. *bioRxiv*, 2023–03. https://doi.org/10.1101/2023.03.10.532027

Lai, Y. C., Chuang, Y. C., Chang, C. P., & Yeh, T. M. (2015). Macrophage migration inhibitory factor has a permissive role in concanavalin A-induced cell death of human hepatoma cells through autophagy. *Cell Death & Disease*, *6*(12), e2008–e2008. https://doi.org/10.1038/cddis.2015.349

Lakhtin, V., Lakhtin, M., & Alyoshkin, V. (2011). Lectins of living organisms. The overview. *Anaerobe*, *17*(6), 452–455. https://doi.org/10.1016/j.anaerobe.2011.06.004

Lei, H. Y., & Chang, C. P. (2009). Lectin of Concanavalin A as an anti-hepatoma therapeutic agent. *Journal of Biomedical Science*, *16*(1), 1–12. https://doi.org/10.1186/1423-0127-16-10

Lentzen, H., & Witthohn, K. (2016). Antiviral agent comprising recombinant mistletoe lectins. US20160175390A1.

Lewis, A. L., Kohler, J. J., & Aebi, M. (2022). Microbial lectins: Hemagglutinins, adhesins, and toxins. In Varki A, Cummings RD, Esko JD, et al., (eds): *Essentials of Glycobiology [Internet]*. 4th edition. Cold Spring Harbor, NY: Cold Spring Harbor Laboratory Press.

Liu, F. T., Yang, R. Y., & Hsu, D. K. (2012). Galectins in acute and chronic inflammation. *Annals of the New York Academy of Sciences*, *1253*(1), 80–91. https://doi.org/10.1111/j.1749-6632.2011.06386.x

Manning, J. C., Romero, A., Habermann, F. A., García Caballero, G., Kaltner, H., & Gabius, H. J. (2017). Lectins: A primer for histochemists and cell biologists. *Histochemistry and Cell Biology*, *147*(2), 199–222. https://doi.org/10.1007/s00418-016-1524-6

Markovitz, D. M., Stuckey, J. A., Boudreaux, D. M., Meagher, J., Al-Hashimi, H., & Salmon, L. (2019). Lectins and uses thereof (United States). US10450355.

Mayer, S., Moeller, R., Monteiro, J. T., Ellrott, K., Josenhans, C., & Lepenies, B. (2018). C-type lectin receptor (CLR)–Fc fusion proteins as tools to screen for novel CLR/bacteria interactions: An exemplary study on preselected Campylobacter jejuni isolates. *Frontiers in Immunology*, *9*, 213. https://doi.org/10.3389/fimmu.2018.00213

Mayer, S., Raulf, M. K., & Lepenies, B. (2017). C-type lectins: Their network and roles in pathogen recognition and immunity. *Histochemistry and Cell Biology*, *147*, 223–237. https://doi.org/10.1007/s00418-016-1523-7

Mayo, S. L., Keeffe, J., & Perryman, A. L. (2009). Engineered lectins for viral inactivation (United States). US20090297516A1

Mikkat, U., Damm, I., Kirchhoff, F., Albrecht, E., Nebe, B., & Jonas, L. (2001). Effects of lectins on CCK-8–stimulated enzyme secretion and differentiation of the rat pancreatic cell line AR42J. *Pancreas*, *23*(4), 368–374. https://doi.org/10.1097/00006676-200111000-00006

Mishra, A., Behura, A., Mawatwal, S., Kumar, A., Naik, L., Mohanty, S. S., Manna, D, Dokania, D., Mishra, A., Patra, S. K., & Dhiman, R. (2019). Structure-function and application of plant lectins in disease biology and immunity. *Food and Chemical Toxicology*, *134*, 110827.

Mitsuru, A., Masanori, B., & Makoto, O. (1998). Antiviral materials (Japan). EP0883993A1

Mukhopadhyay, S., Panda, P. K., Behera, B., Das, C. K., Hassan, M. K., Das, D. N., Sinha, N., Bissoyi, A., Pramanik, K., Maiti, T. K., & Bhutia, S. K. (2014). *In vitro* and *in vivo* antitumor effects of Peanut agglutinin through induction of apoptotic and autophagic cell death. *Food and Chemical Toxicology*, *64*(1), 369–377. https://doi.org/10.1016/j.fct.2013.11.046

Nabi-Afjadi, M., Heydari, M., Zalpoor, H., Arman, I., Sadoughi, A., Sahami, P., & Aghazadeh, S. (2022). Lectins and lectibodies: Potential promising antiviral agents. *Cellular & Molecular Biology Letters*, *27*(1), 1–25.

Naseri, M., Maliha, M., Dehghani, M., Simon, G. P., & Batchelor, W. (2022). Rapid detection of gram-positive and-negative bacteria in water samples using mannan-binding lectin-based visual biosensor. *ACS Sensors*, *7*(4), 951–959.

Nubi, T., Adewole, T. S., Agunbiade, T. O., Osukoya, O. A., & Kuku, A. (2021). Purification and erythrocyte-membrane perturbing activity of a ketose-specific lectin from *Moringa oleifera* seeds. *Biotechnology Reports*, *31*, e00650. https://doi.org/10.1016/j.btre.2021.e00650

Panda, P. K., Mukhopadhyay, S., Behera, B., Bhol, C. S., Dey, S., Das, D. N., Sinha, N., Bissoyi, A., Pramanik, K., Maiti, T. K., & Bhutia, S. K. (2014). Antitumor effect of soybean lectin mediated through reactive oxygen species-dependent pathway. *Life Sciences*, *111*(1–2), 27–35. https://doi.org/10.1016/j.lfs.2014.07.004

Powell, M. D., & Gbodossou, E. V. A. (2020). Antiviral compositions and methods (United States). WO2020132062A1

Pratt, J., & Annabi, B. (2014). Induction of autophagy biomarker BNIP3 requires a JAK2/STAT3 and MT1-MMP signaling interplay in Concanavalin-A-activated U87 glioblastoma cells. *Cellular Signalling*, *26*(5), 917–924. https://doi.org/10.1016/j.cellsig.2014.01.012

Pratt, J., Roy, R., & Annabi, B. (2012). Concanavalin-A-induced autophagy biomarkers requires membrane type-1 matrix metalloproteinase intracellular signaling in glioblastoma cells. *Glycobiology*, *22*(9), 1245–1255. https://doi.org/10.1093/glycob/cws093

Pulingam, T., Parumasivam, T., Gazzali, A. M., Sulaiman, A. M., Chee, J. Y., Lakshmanan, M., Chin, C. F., & Sudesh, K. (2022). Antimicrobial resistance: Prevalence, economic burden, mechanisms of resistance and strategies to overcome. *European Journal of Pharmaceutical Sciences*, *170*, 106103. ttps://doi. org/10.1016/j.ejps.2021.106103

Rabinovich, G. A., & Croci, D. O. (2012). Regulatory circuits mediated by lectin-glycan interactions in autoimmunity and cancer. *Immunity*, *36*(3), 322–335. https://doi.org/10.1016/j.immuni.2012.03.004

Rabinovich, G. A., Ramhorst, R. E., Rubinstein, N., Corigliano, A., Daroqui, M. C., Kier-Joffe, E. B., & Fainboim, L. (2002). Induction of allogenic T-cell hyporesponsiveness by galectin-1-mediated apoptotic and non-apoptotic mechanisms. *Cell Death & Differentiation*, *9*(6), 661–670. https://doi.org/10.1038/sj.cdd.4401009

Radhakrishnan, A., Park, K., Kwak, I. S., Jaabir, M., & Sivakamavalli, J. (2021). Classification of lectins. In *Lectins* (pp. 51–72). Singapore: Springer. https://doi.org/10.1007/978-981-16-7462-4_3

Ramírez Hernández, E., Sánchez-Maldonado, C., Mayoral Chávez, M. A., Hernández-Zimbrón, L. F., Patricio Martínez, A., Zenteno, E., & Limón Pérez de León, I. D. (2020). The therapeutic potential of galectin-1 and galectin-3 in the treatment of neurodegenerative diseases. *Expert Review of Neurotherapeutics*, *20*(5), 439–448. https://doi.org/10.1080/14737175.2020.1750955

Ramos-Martínez, E., Ramos-Martínez, I., Sánchez-Betancourt, I., Ramos-Martínez, J. C., Peña-Corona, S. I., Valencia, J., . . . Cerbón, M. (2022). Association between galectin levels and neurodegenerative diseases: Systematic review and meta-analysis. *Biomolecules*, *12*(8), 1062. https://doi.org/10.3390/biom12081062

Rezayatmand, H., Razmkhah, M., & Razeghian-Jahromi, I. (2022). Drug resistance in cancer therapy: The Pandora's Box of cancer stem cells. *Stem Cell Research & Therapy*, *13*(1), 181. https://doi.org/10.1186/s13287-022-02856-6

Roy, B., Pattanaik, A. K., Das, J., Bhutia, S. K., Behera, B., Singh, P., & Maiti, T. K. (2014). Role of PI3K/Akt/mTOR and MEK/ERK pathway in Concanavalin A induced autophagy in HeLa cells. *Chemico-Biological Interactions*, *210*(1), 96–102. https://doi.org/10.1016/j.cbi.2014.01.003

Santos, A. F., Da Silva, M. D. C., Napoleão, T. H., Paiva, P. M. G., Correia, M. D. S., & Coelho, L. C. B. B. (2014). Lectins: Function, structure, biological properties and potential applications. *Current Topics in Peptide and Protein Research*, *15*, 41–62. https://hdl.handle.net/1822/43440

Sasaki, T. (2004). Galectin-1 induces astrocyte differentiation, which leads to production of brain-derived neurotrophic factor. *Glycobiology*, *14*(4), 357–363. https://doi.org/10.1093/glycob/cwh043

Shin, T. (2013). The pleiotropic effects of galectin-3 in neuroinflammation: A review. *Acta Histochemica*, *115*(5), 407–411. https://doi.org/10.1016/j.acthis.2012.11.010

Souza, M. A., Carvalho, F. C., Ruas, L. P., Ricci-Azevedo, R., & Roque-Barreira, M. C. (2013). The immunomodulatory effect of plant lectins: A review with emphasis on ArtinM properties. *Glycoconjugate Journal*, *30*(7), 641–657. https://doi.org/10.1007/s10719-012-9464-4

Starossom, Sarah C., Mascanfroni, Ivan D., Imitola, J., Cao, L., Raddassi, K., Hernandez, Silvia F., Bassil, R., Croci, Diego O., Cerliani, Juan P., Delacour, D., Wang, Y., Elyaman, W., Khoury, Samia J., & Rabinovich, Gabriel A. (2012). Galectin-1 Deactivates Classically Activated Microglia and Protects from Inflammation-Induced Neurodegeneration. *Immunity*, *37*(2), 249–263. https://doi.org/10.1016/j.immuni.2012.05.023

Steinbach-Rankins, J., & Palmer, K. (2016). Microbicidal compositions and methods for treatment of viral infections (United States). US2016361382A1.

Taylor, M., Drickamer, K., Imberty, A., van Kooyk, Y., Schnaar, R., Etzler, M., & Varki, A. (2022). Discovery and classification of glycan-binding proteins. *Essentials of Glycobiology*. 4th edition. Cold Spring Harbor, NY: Cold Spring Harbor Laboratory Press. doi: 10.1101/glycobiology.4e.28

Varki, A., Etzler, M. E., Cummings, R. D., & Esko, J. D. (2009). Discovery and classification of glycan-binding proteins. *Essentials of Glycobiology*, *2*. https://doi.org/10.1134/s0006297909090156

Vasta, G. R., Ahmed, H., Nita-Lazar, M., Banerjee, A., Pasek, M., Shridhar, S., Guha, P., & Fernández-Robledo, J. A. (2012). Galectins as self/non-self-recognition receptors in innate and adaptive immunity: An unresolved paradox. *Frontiers in Immunology*, *3*(1). https://doi.org/10.3389/fimmu.2012.00199

Vibhute, P., Radhakrishnan, A., Sivakamavalli, J., Chellapandian, H., & Selvin, J. (2022). Antimicrobial and immunomodulatory role of fish lectins. *Aquatic Lectins*, 257–286. https://doi.org/10.1007/978-981-19-0432-5_12

Višnjar, T., Romih, R., & Zupančič, D. (2019). Lectins as possible tools for improved urinary bladder cancer management. *Glycobiology*, *29*(5), 355–365. https://doi.org/10.1093/glycob/cwz001

Wang, H., Ng, T. B., Ooi, V. E., & Liu, W. K. (2000). Effects of lectins with different carbohydrate-binding specificities on hepatoma, choriocarcinoma, melanoma and osteosarcoma cell lines. *The International Journal of Biochemistry & Cell Biology*, *32*(3), 365–372. https://doi.org/10.1016/s1357-2725(99)00130-2

Watanabe, Y., Allen, J. D., Wrapp, D., McLellan, J. S., & Crispin, M. (2020) Site-specific glycan analysis of the SARS-CoV-2 spike. *Science*, 369(6501), 330–333. https://doi.org/10.1126/scien ce.abb9983

Weiming, D., Xucheng, H., Guiling, L., Xinru, L., & Yansha, M. (2016). Multi-function lipid composition with drug-resisting bacteria resisting activity and preparation method of multi-function lipid composition (China). CN105879039A

Wolin, I. A., Nascimento, A. P. M., Seeger, R., Poluceno, G. G., Zanotto-Filho, A., Nedel, C. B., . . . Leal, R. B. (2023). The lectin DrfL inhibits cell migration, adhesion and triggers autophagy-dependent cell death in glioma cells. *Glycoconjugate Journal*, 40(1), 47–67. https://doi.org/10.1007/s10719-022-10095-3

World Health Organization. (2014). *Antimicrobial Resistance: Global Report on Surveillance*. Geneva, Switzerland: World Health Organization. ISBN 978 92 4 156474 8.

Yau, T., Dan, X., Ng, C. C. W., & Ng, T. B. (2015). Lectins with potential for anti-cancer therapy. *Molecules*, 20(3), 3791–3810. https://doi.org/10.3390/molecules20033791

Zhou, W., Chen, X., Hu, Q., Chen, X., Chen, Y., & Huang, L. (2018). Galectin-3 activates TLR4/NF-κB signaling to promote lung adenocarcinoma cell proliferation through activating lncRNA-NEAT1 expression. *BMC Cancer*, 18(1). https://doi.org/10.1186/s12885-018-4461-z

16 Molecular Mechanism Underlying Nutritional Influence on the Onset of Infectious Diseases

*Taoheed Olawale Bello, Fatima Alaba Ibrahim,
Johnson Olaleye Oladele, and Adenike Temidayo Oladiji*

16.1 INTRODUCTION

Nutrition is a fundamental feature of life that is linked to varieties of components, systems, and activities, including those that manifest during diseases such as infection (Rodriguez-Morales *et al.*, 2016). Nutrition, being a vital aspect of life, will be examined in relation to infection in this context. According to Rodriguez-Morales *et al.* (2016), malnutrition raises the vulnerability of the host to viral diseases, which, in turn, have unfavorable feedback effects on the metabolism of the host, exacerbating the nutritional situation.

In other words, malnutrition causes an enhanced response of the host to infectious diseases, while infections cause malnutrition to rise. Farhadi and Ovchinnikov (2018) reported that this malnutrition-infection complex/cycle can be linked to significant morbidity and death worldwide, especially in poor or less developed countries, where children are disproportionately affected by cases of food insecurity and malnutrition. As a result, Farhadi and Ovchinnikov (2018) also claimed that children below five years of age are among the most vulnerable groups, with infectious diseases accounting for more than half of their mortality.

According to Rodriguez-Morales *et al.* (2016), a bidirectional relation between infection and malnutrition can be established, with infectious disorders such as giardiasis compromising intestinal absorption for digested food substances. In the case of parasitoses, several epidemiological studies have found strong links between helminthic diseases (such as hookworm, ascariasis, strongyloidiasis, trichuriasis, and so on) and protozoan infections (such as amoebiasis, giardiasis, and so on) (Farhadi & Ovchinnikov, 2018).

Micronutrient deficits and infections are linked in a complex way, with consequences manifested as stunted growth, poor intellectual performance, and susceptibility to infection (mostly bacterial, viral, and parasitic). In reality, poor nutrition may be to blame for a massive global impact of parasitic infections. Consumption of polluted food and water has a significant impact on public health, political development, and economic development in many countries (Chatterjee & Abraham, 2017).

16.2 NUTRITION AND INFECTION

The potential of nutrition to resist or trigger the occurrence of infectious diseases is central to the link between nutrition and infection. For the first time, it was stated in a WHO monograph titled "Interaction of Nutrition and Infection" (Scrimshaw *et al.*, 1968) that the interaction between nutrition (malnutrition) and infection is synergistic in nature (Figure 16.1). Evidence was presented in

DOI: 10.1201/9781003361497-18

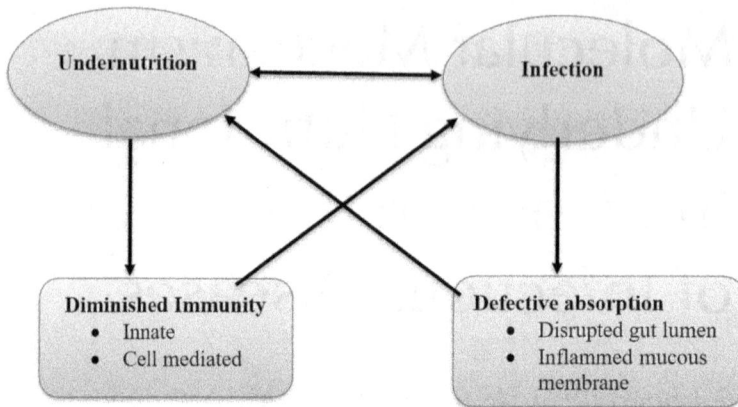

FIGURE 16.1   Interaction between malnutrition and infection.

detail about both the negative impacts of infections on nutritional status and the vulnerability to infection by malnourished people, which are both intensified by the other.

The link between malnutrition and infectious disease (famine-pestilence) has been known from the dawn of time, but it was not until the late 1950s that this relationship was scientifically proven (Warren & Mahmoud, 1984). While early accounts of kwashiorkor noted the presence of infection, the function of infection in the development of malnutrition was often neglected. Nutrition-infection interactions were studied using both synergistic and antagonistic models (Scrimshaw *et al.*, 1968; Warren & Mahmoud, 1984).

Malnutrition intensifies the outcome of infection, and infection, in turn, intensifies nutritional insufficiency, thereby resulting in a consequence that is reportedly higher than the total of both variables. Synergism is more common in developing countries, where infectious diseases are common and nutrition typically demonstrates deficiencies in quality or quantity. Conversely, a deficit of one or more nutrients required by an infectious pathogen may obstruct its proliferation process, resulting in an antagonistic relationship (Murray & Murray, 1977).

16.3   EFFECTS OF NUTRITION ON RESISTANCE TO INFECTIOUS DISEASES

Reduced lymphoid cells, poor T and B lymphocyte activity, and reduced complement and secretory IgA production have all been reported to be experienced in severely malnourished children (Chandra & Newbeme, 1977; Suskind, 1977). Infections affect undernourished children with higher severity, chronicity, and mortality. In comparison to well-nourished persons, the duration of infectious disease and the carrier state of particular agents is often longer within undernourished individuals (Good & Fernandes, 1980). According to Arroyave and Calcano (1979), it was submitted that the depletion of the immune system during extreme food deprivation (malnutrition) may suppress infection rather than prevent it, and starving people can suffer acute infectious disease after nutritional recovery. On the other hand, Targett (1980) reported that infection might boost immunity or cause secondary immunodeficiency or immunological paralysis. Increased clinical symptoms, a longer course, and increased death from infectious disease are the public health implications (Scrimshaw *et al.*, 1968; Mata, 1978; Chen *et al.*, 1980).

16.4   EFFECTS OF MALNUTRITION ON INFECTIONS

Malnutrition has been found to manifest a close relationship with the emergence of infection, labeled as a synergistic pattern of diseases by WHO in 1968 (Scrimshaw *et al.*, 1968; Katona

& Katona-Apte, 2008). The established association between malnutrition and the cell-mediated immune system was described as a metabolic consequence of infection in a report by Keusch (2003). The role of protein-energy malnutrition in the spread of infectious diseases is one example of destructive consequences of malnutrition. When there is protein malnutrition, microbial contamination poses a health risk to the entire child population. Vitamin A, which is one of the most significant immune-system boosters, should be supplemented to the diet in such poor societies where vitamin A insufficiency is common (Katona & Katona-Apte, 2008). Protein and vitamin A deficiencies have resulted in widespread infections in the poorest places in the world (Sanson et al., 2018).

16.5 IMPACT OF NUTRITION ON THE ONSET OF INFECTIOUS DISEASES

Food poisoning and digestive diseases are two diseases that can be caused by contaminated food. People are susceptible to a variety of food poisonings, including microbial contamination, which can occur at any time of year. Cholera is one of the most common and severe intestinal infections in hot weather (Davis et al., 2017). Consumption of contaminated foods can result in a wide range of disorders caused by numerous pathogens (viruses, bacteria, fungi, and parasites) (Rodriguez-Morales et al., 2016). It's never a good idea to eat rotten canned foods. Typhoid fever is another potentially fatal disease spread by contaminated food and water (Farhadi & Hashemian, 2017). Salmonella species produce it, and because the causative agent is antibiotic resistance, it poses a lot of complications for patients (Farhadi & Hashemian, 2017).

Along with severe diarrhea and viral diseases in children, microbial contamination of food and water can also induce these conditions (Chatterjee et al., 2017). Being exposed to contaminated water or food can transmit brucellosis, an infectious disease that affects both humans and animals. Brucella bacteria can make sheep, cows, goats, pigs, and dogs sick (Singh et al., 2018). Brucella infection occurs when humans consume unpasteurized milk or any undercooked products from infected animals (Singh et al., 2018). Close contact with infected animal secretions can potentially spread the virus to humans (Singh et al., 2018). Amoebiasis is a serious disease associated with drinking polluted water or eating infected food. Toxoplasmosis is also spread through the consumption of undercooked or raw meat. The parasitic cyst is released by gastric acid as it enters the human stomach, absorbed into the liver through the intestinal mucosa, and then, into the lymph nodes (Greenwood, 2012). Another parasitic condition that spreads through food is pinworm infection. The infection is widespread in almost all countries, presenting children with a higher frequency than adults. Inappropriate diet can also lead to parasitic worm diseases like hookworm and taeniasis (Molyneux, 2006).

16.5.1 MOLECULAR MECHANISM OF NUTRITION ON THE ONSET OF INFECTIOUS DISEASES

Nutritional status of an organism affects its defense mechanisms and susceptibility to disease. As a result, infectious diseases, including cancer, can be prevented, in part, by processes that help maintain the stability and genomic integrity of organisms. The immune system of a living thing serves as a vital defense against both internal and external dangers. Nutrition is not only necessary for the survival of living things; it also affects how well and how long different biological systems function, how accurate they are, how long they last, and how long living things live overall. The immune system of the body triggers the inflammatory process in reaction to injuries, infections, and/or any tissue damage. Malnutrition poses a major threat to an immune system that is functioning properly. In this section, the emphasis is on the molecular mechanism underpinning the impact of nutrition on the development of infectious diseases. Among the mechanisms are malnutrition deficiency and immunodeficiency complex, antioxidant interventional role, and leptin-receptor activation and immunity.

16.5.1.1 Malnutrition Deficiency and Immunodeficiency Complex

Immunodeficiency is a disorder where the capacity of immune system to fight off infectious diseases or cancer is severely compromised or non-existent. Immunodeficiency happens when immune system elements such lymphocytes, phagocytic cells, and the complement system are absent. Immunodeficiency can be a primary condition, like Bruton's disease, or a secondary condition brought on by HIV infection. Intrinsic flaws in immune cells, such as T-cells, complement component, and phagocytic cells, are the root cause of primary immunodeficiency illness. Recurrent pneumonia is caused by extracellular bacteria and is a sign of an antibody deficiency.

T-lymphocyte deficiencies may also have a role in the recurrence of fungal infections (Murata *et al.*, 2015). Drugs that interfere with T and B lymphocyte function can result in secondary immunodeficiency. Acquired immunodeficiency syndrome (AIDS), which has varying prevalence rates around the world, is the most common secondary immunodeficiency and it is caused by HIV. AIDS predominantly damages $CD4^+$ T cells, and this down-regulation of the cell-mediated immune response results in sneaky infections and malignancies that are dangerous to human health (Vaillant & Qurie, 2018). Reduced levels of leptin during malnutrition or starvation have been linked to both immunodeficiencies, at least in part (Ahima *et al.*, 1996). Most immunodeficiencies are congenital, and X-linked autosomal recessive inheritance patterns, including immunodeficiency with ataxia-telangiectasia, are autosomal recessive disorders brought on by mutations in genes encoding DNA repair enzymes. On chromosome 14, abnormalities are caused by cleavage of the T-cell receptor (TCR) and Ig-heavy chain gene loci (Routes *et al.*, 2014). According to Mora *et al.* (2008), there is a mechanism through which retinol (vitamin A) influences immunity to infectious diseases and this is shown in Figure. The intestinal system produces a significant amount of retinoic acid, which affects intestinal immune defense and homeostasis. This partly explains why deficiency of vitamin A is linked to decreased effector T-cell responses, inadequate immunological responses to particular vaccines, and a higher risk for specific infections (Sudfeld *et al.*, 2010; Ibrahim *et al.*, 2017).

The fat-soluble vitamin A is present in foods that include beta-carotene, retinyl esters, or all-trans-retinol. These forms are dissolved in the byproducts of fat digestion and taken up as micelles by the membrane of the enterocyte. Retinol circulates in the bloodstream along with transthyretin (TTR) and retinol-binding protein (RBP). Retinol is oxidized to all-trans-retinal, which is further converted to all-trans-retinoic acid (RA) by retinal dehydrogenases found in intestinal epithelial cells and dendritic cells associated with the gut. Retinoic acid is exported from the cell and exerts autocrine and paracrine effects on immune cells through binding to nuclear receptors of the retinoic acid receptor (RAR) family, which heterodimerize with receptors of the retinoic X receptor (RXR) family. These forms, together, bind to retinoic acid response elements found in the promoters of retinoic acid response genes. In response to inflammatory stimuli, RA speeds up dendritic cell maturation and antigen-presenting capacity. Additionally, RA that affects other immune cells is stored and secreted by dendritic cells. The effects of RA on naive T lymphocytes result in an upregulation of the expression of gut-homing receptors. It reduces Th1 differentiation by blocking the expression of the transcription factor Tbet, Th1 cytokines, and IL-12 on dendritic cells. Additionally, it suppresses the synthesis of the transcription factor retinoic acid receptor-related orphan receptor γt (RORγt) as well as Th17 cell development. In contrast, RA increases the expression of GATA3 and IL-4, which enhances Th2 differentiation. It also encourages intestinal-tissue-naive T-cells to differentiate into $FoxP3^+$ regulatory T-cells. When exposed to RA, B-cells in the mucosa as well as gut-associated lymphoid organs become IgA^+ antibody-secreting cells (Mora *et al.*, 2008).

Protein deficiency impairs not only phagocytosis and cell-mediated immunity against microorganisms but it also impairs the capacity of phagocytic cells to eliminate intracellular organisms. Malnutrition deficit is the source of secondary deficiency. Cancer, chronic renal disease, numerous injuries, and chronic infections can all be caused by nutritional inadequacies. A delayed reduction in cutaneous hypersensitivity is one of the consequences of zinc and iron deficiency on immunity. Supplemental vitamin B_6, B_{12}, selenium, and copper are essential for the immune system and are all linked to scavenging free radicals. According to Stefanis *et al.* (1997), oxidative stress is now understood to be a contributor to all major diseases, including ischemic diseases, AIDS, emphysema, organ transplantation, stomach ulcers, high blood pressure, and neurological conditions including Alzheimer's, Parkinson's, and muscular dystrophy. Oxidative stress is initiated by an imbalance between the production of free radicals and antioxidant defense. According to McCord (2000), increased ROS production in the body can alter DNA structure, which, in turn, can modify proteins and lipids, activate transcription factors, and produce pro- and anti-inflammatory cytokines.

16.5.1.2 Antioxidant Interventional Roles

It has been postulated that antioxidants aid the immune system in the body, at least in part, to explain this fact that consuming a diet high in antioxidant elements is strongly linked to a lower risk of infectious diseases and cancer. It is unquestionably essential to work toward maintaining a steady ratio of reactive oxygen species (ROS) to antioxidants as early as possible, ideally through dietary rather than supplemental means, in order to postpone, if not completely prevent, the onset of many age-related disorders. The immune system suffers from oxidative stress. To function efficiently, immune cells, in particular, rely heavily on cell-to-cell communication, particularly through membrane-bound receptors. Since polyunsaturated fatty acids make up a large portion of cell membranes, when they are peroxidized, they can affect intracellular signaling, alter membrane fluidity, and impair cell function (Khadim & Al-Fartusie, 2021). Reduced cell-membrane receptor expression has been connected to exposure to ROS (Gruner et al., 1986). Cells that are therefore undersupplied with antioxidants may be harmed by phagocytic immune cells that release ROS.

16.5.1.3 Leptin-Receptor Activation and Immunity

Leptin is one mechanism through which the metabolic state of immune cells is linked to systemic nutritional condition. As previously stated, adipocytes release leptin in proportion to adipocyte mass and leptin levels, which correspond with nutritional status (Maffei et al., 1995).

Circulating levels of leptin fall during periods of malnutrition or after fasting. Through the LepR, leptin directly affects CD4+ T lymphocytes, changing the metabolism and functionality of these cells (De Rosa et al., 2006; Saucillo et al., 2014; Gerriets et al., 2016). Given the close relationship between T-cell metabolism and its function, any modification to the metabolism of the cell can affect its ability to proliferate, differentiate, and produce cytokines. It has been demonstrated that leptin stimulates glucose metabolism and CD4+ T-cell production of inflammatory cytokines.

A key mediator between dietary intake and immune function is leptin. Leptin, a pleiotropic hormone that controls satiety, has lower levels in PEM patients. Fasting causes a rapid drop in leptin levels, which are correlated with body-fat mass (Matarese et al., 2005). Leptin, a 16 kDa protein of the A-helix type that is similar to the cytokines IL-6 and IL-12, is mostly produced by adipose tissue. There are at least six receptors on different types of cells, each of which represents a different splice variation expressed by the same gene. In addition to the hypothalamus, the full-length ObRb isoform is broadly expressed on lymphocytes and macrophages (Matarese et al., 2002; Matarese et al., 2005). Leptin binding to ObRb triggers the JAK-2/STAT-3 and MAPK pathways, which also stimulates macrophages to release IL-6, IL-12, and TNF-a. Leptin promotes the development of naive T-cells (CD45RA+), while it inhibits the formation of memory T-cells (CD45RO+).

According to Lord et al. (1998, 2002), leptin simultaneously increases the activation markers CD69, CD25, and CD71, suppresses Th2 responses, and promotes the generation of IFN-γ by memory T-cells. In addition to promoting lymphopoiesis, leptin appears to boost the anti-apoptotic proteins Bcl-xL and Tbet, which provide T-cells with survival signals (Matarese et al., 2005). According to Cakir et al. (1999), active TB can cause cachexia, weight loss, and low leptin serum concentrations. The fact that leptin-deficient animals are more susceptible to *M. tuberculosis* than wild-type mice and that the number of T-cells, particularly those that produce IFN-γ, is reduced in infected lungs further supports the idea that leptin aids in TB defense (Wieland et al., 2005).

A causal link between the severity of tuberculosis and leptin has not yet been fully established, and leptin concentrations do not predict wasting in people with tuberculosis (Van Lettow *et al.*, 2005).

Leptin as well as hypothalamic-pituitary-adrenal axis are two of the many mechanisms by which malnutrition suppresses the immune system. PEM lowers leptin levels while raising glucocorticoid levels in the blood, which are stress hormones (Alleyne & Young, 1967; Scimshaw & SanGiovami, 1997; Woodward, 1998; Jacobson, 2005; Monk *et al.*, 2006). It follows that the hypothalamic-pituitary-adrenal axis probably contributes significantly to the immunological deficit caused by starvation. In well-nourished individuals, infection and inflammation promote leptin levels in an IL-1-dependent way and raise glucocorticoid concentrations, which ultimately reduces inflammation (Auphan *et al.*, 1997; Tanaka *et al.*, 2000; Faggioni *et al.*, 2001). Glucocorticoids reduce the translocation of NF-kB into the nucleus when PEM and low leptin concentrations are present, impairing macrophage performance (Auphan *et al.*, 1997).

Microbial cell disorders result in alarming response, which activates the recognition by receptors. Congenital pattern recognition receptors (PRRs), comprising of Toll-like receptors (TLRs), NOD-like receptors (NLRs), RIG-like receptors (RLRs), and C-type lectin receptors (CLRs), are thought to be the primary mediators of the underlying perception of disease. These PRRs cause expression of the transcription, which leads to elimination of the pathogens as well as infected cells by activating a cascade of intracellular signaling. However, the development of autoimmunity, immunodeficiency, and ultimately, the initiation of infectious diseases causes this system to become abnormally activated (Tanaka *et al.*, 2000).

16.6   CONCLUSION AND PERSPECTIVES

Nutrition, indeed, plays a significant role in the onset of infectious diseases due to a compromised immune response, which fails to offer expected protection to the living organism. Malnutrition (under-nutrition) encompasses poor nutrition, digestion, and absorption of food components. This abnormal nutrition intricately leads to immunodeficiency in cascades of mechanisms, which increase the chances of infections. Deficiencies of nutrients remain predisposing factors to the onset and progression of infectious diseases.

REFERENCES

Ahima, R. S, Prabakaran, D., Mantzoros, C., Qu, D., Lowell, B., Maratos-Flier, E., Flier, J. S. (**1996**). Role of leptin in the neuroendocrine response to fasting. Nature 382(6588): 250–252.
Alleyne, G. A., Young, V. H. (**1967**). Adrenocortical function in children with severe protein-calorie malnutrition. Clin Sci 33: 189–200.
Arroyave, G., Calcano, M. (**1979**). Descenso de los niveles de retinol y suproteina de enlace (RBP) durance las infecciones. Arch Latinoamer Nutr 29: 233–260.
Auphan, N., Didonato, J. A., Helmberg, A., Rosette, C., Karin, M. (**1997**). Immunoregulatory genes and immunosuppression by glucocorticoids. Arch Toxicol Suppl 19: 87–95.
Cakir, B., Yonem, A., Guler, S., Odabasi, E., Demirbas, B., et al. (**1999**). Relation of leptin and tumor necrosis factor alpha to body weight changes in patients with pulmonary tuberculosis. Horm Res 52: 279–283.
Chandra, R. K., Newbeme, P. M. (**1977**). Nutrition, Immunity and Infection. Mechanisms of Interactions. New York. Plenum, 246 pp.
Chatterjee, A., Abraham, J. (**2017**). Microbial contamination, prevention, and early detection in food industry. Microb Contam Food Degrad 10: 21.
Chen, L. C., Alauddin-Chowdhury, A. K. M., Huffman, S. L. (**1980**). Anthropometric assessment of energy-protein malnutrition and subsequent risk of mortality among preschool aged children. Am J Clin Nutr 33: 1836–1845.
Davies, H. G, Bowman C, Luby S. P. (**2017**). Cholera-management and prevention. J Infect 74: 66–73.
De Rosa, V., Procaccini, C., La Cava, A., Chieffi, P., Nicoletti, G. F., Fontana, S., et al. (**2006**). Leptin neutralization interferes with pathogenic T cell autoreactivity in autoimmune encephalomyelitis. J Clin Invest 116(2): 447–55. doi:10.1172/JCI26523

Faggioni, R., Feingold, K. R., Grunfeld, C. (**2001**). Leptin regulation of the immune response and the immunodeficiency of malnutrition. Faseb J 15: 2565–2571.

Farhadi, S., Ovchinnikov, R. S. (**2018**). The relationship between nutrition and infection. Biomed Biotechnol Res J 2(3) July–September.

Farhadi, T., Hashemian S. M. (**2017**). Constructing novel chimeric DNA vaccine against *Salmonella enterica* based on SopB and GroEL proteins: An *in silico* approach. J Pharm Investig. [In press]. doi:10.1007/s40005-017-0360-6.

Gerriets, V. A., Danzaki, K., Kishton, R. J., Eisner, W., Nichols, A. G., Saucillo, D. C., et al. (**2016**). Leptin directly promotes T-cell glycolytic metabolism to drive effector T-cell differentiation in a mouse model of autoimmunity. Eur J Immunol 46(8): 1970–1983. doi:10.1002/eji.201545861

Good, R. A., Fernandes, G. (**1980**). Zinc and immunity, in Isliker, H., Schurch, B. (eds): The Impact of malnutrition on immune defense in parasitic infestation. Bern, Hans Huber Pub., Switzerland, pp. 136–139.

Greenwood, D. (**2012**). Protozoa: Malaria; toxoplasmosis; cryptosporidiosis; amoebiasis; trypanosomiasis; leishmaniasis; giardiasis; trichomoniasis, in Greenwood, D., Barer, M., Slack, R., Irving, W. (eds): Medical Microbiology (Eighteenth Edition). Elsevier Pub., Churchill Livingstone, London, United Kingdom. pp. 642–654.

Gruner, S., Volk, H-D., Falck, P., Baehr, R. V. (**1986**). The influence of phagocytic stimuli on the expression of HLA-DR antigens; role of reactive oxygen intermediates. Eur J Immunol 16: 212–215.

Ibrahim, M. K., Zambruni, M., Melby, C. L., Melby, P. C. (**2017**). Impact of childhood malnutrition on host defense and infection. Clin Microbiol Rev 30: 919–971. doi:10.1128/CMR.00119–16

Jacobson, L. (**2005**). Hypothalamic-pituitary adrenocortical axis regulation. Endocrinol Metab Clin North Am 34: 271–292.

Katona, P., Katona-Apte, J. (**2008**). The interaction between nutrition and infection. Clin Infect Dis: An Official Publication of the Infectious Diseases Society of America 46. doi:10.1086/587658

Keusch, G. T. (**2003**). Symposium: Nutrition and infection, prologue and progress since 1968: The history of nutrition—malnutrition, infection and immunity. J Nutr 133: 336S–40S.

Khadim, R. M., Al-Fartusie, F. S. (**2021**). Antioxidant vitamins and their effect on immune system. J Phys: Conf Ser 1853 012065

Lord, G. M., Matarese, G., Howard, J. K., Baker, R. J., Bloom, S. R., et al. (**1998**). Leptin modulates the T-cell immune response and reverses starvation-induced immunosuppression. Nature 394: 897–901.

Lord, G. M., Matarese, G., Howard, J. K., Bloom, S. R., Lechler, R. I. (**2002**). Leptin inhibits the anti-CD3-driven proliferation of peripheral blood T cells but enhances the production of proinflammatory cytokines. J Leukoc Biol 72: 330–338.

Maffei, M., Halaas, J., Ravussin, E., Pratley, R. E., Lee, G. H., Zhang, Y., et al. (**1995**). Leptin levels in human and rodent: Measurement of plasma leptin and ob RNA in obese and weight-reduced subjects. Nat Med 1(11): 1155–1161. doi:10.1038/nm1195-1155

Mata, L. J, (**1978**). The Children of Santa Maria Cauque. A Prospective Field of Health and Growth. Cambridge, MIT Press, 395 pp.

Matarese, G., La Cava, A., Sanna, V., Lord, G. M., Lechler, R. I., et al. (**2002**). Balancing susceptibility to infection and autoimmunity: A role for leptin? Trends Immunol 23: 182–187.

Matarese, G., Moschos, S., Mantzoros, C. S. (**2005**) Leptin in immunology. J Immunol 174: 3137–3142.37.

McCord, J. M. (**2000**). The evolution of free radicals and oxidative stress Am J Med 108: 652–659.

Molyneux, D. H. (**2006**). Control of human parasitic diseases: Context and overview. Advances in Parasitology 61: 1–45.

Monk, J. M., Makinen, K., Shrum, B., Woodward, B. (**2006**) Blood corticosterone concentration reaches critical illness levels early during acute malnutrition in the weanling mouse. Exp Biol Med (Maywood) 231: 264–268.

Mora, J. R., Iwata, M., and von Andrian, U. H. (**2008**). Vitamin effects on the immune system: Vitamins A and D take centre stage. Nat Rev Immunol 8: 685–698.

Murata, C., Ramírez, A. B., Ramírez, G., et al. (**2015**). Discriminant analysis to predict the clinical diagnosis of primary immunodeficiencies: A preliminary report. Revista Alergia México 62: 125–133.

Murray, M. I., Murray, A. B. (**1977**). Starvation suppression and refeeding activation of infection. *Lancet* 1: 123–125.

Rodriguez-Morales, A. J., Bolivar-Mejía, A., Alarcón-Olave, C., Calvo-Betancourt, L. S. (**2016**). Nutrition and Infection in Encyclopedia of Food and Health. Amsterdam: Elsevier Ltd, 98–103.10.1016/B978-0-12-384947-2.00491–8

Routes, J., Abinun, M., Al-Herz, W., et al. (**2014**). ICON: The early diagnosis of congenital immunodeficiencies. J Clin Immunol 34: 398–424.

Sanson, G., Bertocchi, L., Dal Bo E., Di Pasquale, C. L., Zanetti, M. **(2018).** Identifying reliable predictors of protein-energy malnutrition in hospitalized frail older adults: A prospective longitudinal study. Int J Nurs Stud 82: 40–48.

Saucillo, D. C., Gerriets, V. A., Sheng, J., Rathmell, J. C., Maciver, N. J., **(2014).** Leptin metabolically licenses T cells for activation to link nutrition and immunity. J Immunol 192(1): 136–144. doi:10.4049/jimmunol.1301158

Scrimshaw, N. S., SanGiovanni, J. P. **(1997).** Synergism of nutrition, infection, and immunity: An overview. Am J Clin Nutr 66: 464S–477S.

Scrimshaw, N. S., Taylor, C. E., Gordon, J. E. **(1968).** Interactions of Nutrition and Infection. WHO Monog Ser 57.329 pp

Singh, B. B, Khatkar M. S, Aulakh R. S, Gill J. P. S, Dhand N. K. **(2018).** Estimation of the health and economic burden of human brucellosis in India. Prev Vet Med 154: 148–155.

Stefanis, L., Burke, R. E., Greene, L. A. **(1997).** Apoptosis in neurodegenerative disorders. Curr Opin Neurol 10: 299–305.

Sudfeld, C. R., Navar, A. M., Halsey, N. A. **(2010).** Effectiveness of measles vaccination and vitamin A treatment. Int J Epidemiol 39(Suppl 1): i48–ii55.

Suskind, R. M. (ed) **(1977).** Malnutrition and the immune Response. New York: Raven, 468 pp.

Tanaka, S., Isoda, F., Kiuchi, Y., Ikeda, H., Mobbs, C. V, et al. **(2000).** T lymphopenia in genetically obese-diabetic Wistar fatty rats: Effects of body weight reduction on T cells. Metabolism 49: 1261–1266.

Targett, G. A. T. **(1980).** Malnutrition and immunity to protozoan parasites, in Isliker, H., Schurch, B. (eds): The Impact of Malnutrition on Immune Defense in Parasitic Infestation. Bern: Has Huber Pub, pp. 158–179.

Vaillant, A. A. J., Qurie, A. **(2018).** Immunodeficiency. StatPearls [Internet]. StatPearls Publishing.

van Lettow, M., van der Meer, J. W., West, C. E., van Crevel, R., Semba, R. D. (2005) Interleukin-6 and human immunodeficiency virus load, but not plasma leptin concentration, predict anorexia and wasting in adults with pulmonary tuberculosis in Malawi. *J Clin Endocrinol Metab* 90: 4771–4776.

Warren, K. S., Mahmoud, A. A. F. (eds) **(1984).** Tropical and Geographical Medicine. New York, McGraw Hill, pp. 206–211.

Wieland, C. W., Florquin, S., Chan, E. D., Leemans, J. C., Weijer, S., et al. **(2005).** Pulmonary Mycobacterium tuberculosis infection in leptin-deficient ob/ob mice. Int Immunol 17: 1399–1408.

Woodward, B. **(1998).** Protein, Calories, and Immune Defenses. Nutr Rev 56: S84–S92.

17 Therapeutic Potentials of Dietary Phytochemicals in Neurodegenerative Diseases

Johnson Olaleye Oladele, Omowumi
O. Adewale, and Adenike Temidayo Oladiji

17.1 INTRODUCTION

There exist a number of risk factors that impact brain vulnerability. These include non-modifiable risk factors such as genetics, family history, and age; and modifiable factors, including stress, drug intake, alcohol/tobacco consumption, physical activity, sleep apnea, preventable diabetes, obesity, and cardiovascular risk-factors (Flanagan et al., 2020; Vauzour et al., 2017). Diet represents one of the most critical lifestyle variables that might affect brain susceptibility. Increasing data from clinical and scientific research suggest that food is as critical to brain functioning and mental welling as it is to the maintenance of other biological functions such as the digestive, endocrine, and cardiovascular systems (Sarris et al., 2015). Almost all cellular/biochemical activities require micronutrients, including trace mineral elements and vitamins, which are also crucial for the health of the neurological, cardiovascular, immune as well as the antioxidant defense systems in the body. Low concentrations of micronutrients decrease the function of enzymatic antioxidants, which may cause fatty acid, protein, and DNA oxidation and crosslinking as well as mitochondrial ATP deficiency, which may exacerbate the pathogenesis of neurodegeneration and neurological illnesses (Kazmierczak-Baranska et al., 2020).

It is currently impossible to overemphasize the importance of dietary phytochemicals in maintaining the integrity of the structure of nerve cells and tissues, neuronal homeostasis, and disease protection. Dietary polyphenols, which are more substantial polymeric hydroxyl-containing substances that serve as secondary metabolites, are the most noteworthy phytochemicals. Dietary polyphenols are abundant in plant products such as fruit and vegetables. They are primarily categorized as polypohenols based on flavonoids and non-flavonoids that selectively cross the blood–brain barrier to carry out their therapeutic functions in neuronal detoxification and the healing process in order to improve memory, learning, and cognitive abilities. Numerous cellular and neuronal oxidative damages, as well as inflammation, which all contribute to the formation of neurodegenerative diseases, are combated by dietary phytochemicals in a variety of therapeutic strategies.

Research on dietary phytochemicals reveals their ability to chelate metals and act as antioxidants by scavenging free radicals. However, some subclasses of polyphenols are not naturally bioactive polyphenols and are therefore regarded as xenobiotics because they are subjected to biological transformation by the gut microbiota before becoming biologically, therapeutically, and pharmacologically active. Flavonoids are biologically active phytochemicals (Deprez et al., 2001).

Due to their identified neuroprotective therapeutic role in the prevention of neurological and cognitive decline disorders as well as age-related cognitive malignancies, phytochemicals are presently the subject of significant debate among the population of researchers. Through downstream modulation of oxidative stress, inflammatory, and necrosis signaling pathways as well as transcription, translation, amyloid congestion, and neuronal disruption pathways within the nerve cells,

DOI: 10.1201/9781003361497-19

phytochemicals' molecular mechanism in neuronal damage and disorder prevention and treatment occurs (Smolensky et al., 2018; Oladele et al., 2020, 2021b, 2021c, 2022).

The molecular mechanism related to polyphenols involves the inhibition of the expression of pro-oxidant biological catalyst as well as some molecules linked to and vulnerable to oxidative attacks, such as nuclear factor kB, direct ROS scavenging, touch down-regulation of Bcl-2, and other molecules linked to apoptotic pathways. Developmental protective mechanisms against neuronal damage processes include modulation of MAPK (mitogen-activated protein kinase) activity, dissociation of nuclear factor erythroid 2-related factor 2 (Nrf2) linked complexes, and other signaling pathways (Bhakkiyalakshmi et al., 2016; Gupta et al., 2004; Oladele et al., 2020, 2021c, 2022).

Developmental neuronal losses of functions and structure that result in deteriorating conditions like Parkinson's disease, Alzheimer's disease, Huntington's disease, and other neurodegenerative diseases are primarily caused by neuronal damages, amyloid congestion within nerve cells, and impairment of nerve cells (Oladele et al., 2020, 2021). Over 50 million people globally currently have one of these diseases, and statistics have shown that, by 2025, that number could rise to 115 million. The prevalence of these diseases has been rising each year (Livingston et al., 2020; Oladele et al., 2020, 2022). Thus, this chapter gives a comprehensive account of the therapeutic role of dietary phytochemicals in neurodegenerative diseases.

17.2 NEURODEGENERATIVE DISEASES

Neurodegenerative diseases are a detrimental group of human diseases that impair motor or cognitive functions. They are speedily becoming a worldwide societal disease, with over 46.8 million people around the world diagnosed with dementia. Neuronal loss and progressive damage in neural cells are two of their major pathophysiological characteristics. Parkinson's disease (PD), Spinocerebellar Ataxia, Alzheimer's disease (AD), Amyotrophic lateral sclerosis (ALS), and Huntington's disease (HD) are examples of neurodegenerative disorders (SCA) (Matilla-Duenas et al., 2014). More than 10 million people with these illnesses are expected to live in the top ten most densely populated nations by 2030. Neurodegenerative disease cases have a major influence on the total hospital frequency of neurological illnesses reported in Nigeria (Okubadejo et al., 2010; Parkinson Disease Foundation, 2016).

Delayed reaction times, resting tremor, stiffness, postural instability, bradykinesia, and freezing of gait are some of the clinical symptoms of these illnesses, which can progress to inflexible facial expression and unconscious facial movement (Blandini, 2013). Pathogenetic investigations have revealed that persons who are subjected to agricultural, occupational, and environmental hazardous substances that might interact with and degrade dopaminergic neurons are more likely to acquire neurodegenerative disorders like Parkinson's (Costello et al., 2009; Oladele et al., 2021).

The complicated pathophysiology of neurodegenerative diseases has not been fully understood; nevertheless, existing data and evidence from experimental and clinical investigations demonstrated that the diseases are characterized by neuroinflammation, oxidative stress, cell death, and protein misfolding. As high levels of oxidative stress are commonly documented in the brain areas of individuals suffering from various types of neurodegenerations, reactive oxygen species (ROS) may play an important role in disease etiology (Dias et al., 2013).

ROS are chemically reactive molecules that are spontaneously produced within the biological system and play important roles in modulating cellular processes such as stressor responses, cell survival, and inflammation. Nevertheless, if their levels are not effectively controlled or managed, they can be harmful to health and contribute to the pathogenesis of a variety of illnesses, including neurological diseases, cancer, allergies, muscle dysfunction, and cardiovascular problems (Zuo et al., 2015; He and Zuo, 2015). Because of their reactivity, the presence of large levels of ROS may result in oxidative stress (OS) and, eventually, cell death, if not managed or treated. Oxidative stress is defined as a disruption in the equilibrium of antioxidant and pro-oxidant levels in biological systems (Zuo et al., 2015).

Neuroinflammation is another important factor in the etiology of neurodegenerative disorders. On a molecular level, the existence of neuroinflammatory processes at post-mortem has also been demonstrated. Interleukins 1, 6, 2, interferon, transforming growth factor (TGF), TGF1, epidermal growth factor (EGF), 2-microglobulin, and TNF-alpha were found in the striatum of Parkinson's disease patients (Mogi et al., 1994a, 1994b, 1995a, 1995b). The key process involved in the increasing neuronal cell death/loss found in neurodegenerative disorders has been identified as apoptosis. The disintegration of one or more neuronal cells is a common feature of neurological illnesses. Many neurodegenerative illnesses exhibit several criteria for apoptotic cell death.

Several indications from cellular, genetic, neuropathological, and biochemical investigations have demonstrated that monomeric proteins can misfold, oligomerize, form aggregates, and become accumulated in the brain, which is the major cascade of processes that activate pathological abnormalities associated with neurodegenerative diseases (Goedert, 2015). The following proteins in neurodegenerative diseases have been reported to involve cerebral misfolded aggregates accumulation: prion proteins in chronic wasting disease, prion diseases (PrDs) (i.e., Creutzfeldt–Jakob disease (CJD), scrapie, and bovine spongiform encephalopathy; and TAR DNA-binding protein 43 (TDP-43) in frontotemporal dementia and amyotrophic lateral sclerosis; dementia with Lewy bodies and multiple system atrophy, alpha-synuclein (A-Syn) in PD; amyloid-beta (Aβ) in AD; tau in chronic traumatic encephalopathy, frontotemporal dementia, corticobasal degeneration, progressive supranuclear palsy, argyrophilic grain disease, and AD). Although, the formation of protein aggregates differs amongst neurodegenerative illnesses, the pathogenic process of protein misfolding, intermediates, end-products, and key features are clearly similar (Soto et al., 2006).

The prophylactic use of dietary phytochemicals in the treatment and management of human diseases such as neurodegenerative diseases have continuously been discovered. Given the critical roles of apoptosis, neuroinflammation, protein misfolding, and oxidative stress in neurodegenerative diseases, modulating important mediators in each of the pathological mechanisms may provide a promising intervention option to halt, retard, or slow the progression of neurodegeneration and alleviate associated symptoms. Preclinical trials identified several mechanisms underlying the observed neuroprotective effects of medicinal plants, including antioxidant, anti-inflammatory, antiapoptotic, and neurotrophic mechanisms (Oladele et al., 2021, 2022). Understanding these mechanisms at the molecular level will enhance the discovery and development of novel neuroprotective agents for neurodegenerative diseases.

17.3 MOLECULAR MECHANISMS UNDERLYING THE NEUROPROTECTION OF DIETARY PHYTOCHEMICALS

Among the most notable ways by which dietary phytochemicals exhibit neuronal protection against neurological diseases and aging are neurotropic pathways, p53 pathway, anti-apoptotic pathway, anti neuro-inflammatory pathway, NF-kB/MAPK pathways, and Nrf-2 pathway (Kim et al., 2010; Oladele et al., 2020). These mechanisms are via modulation of signaling pathways that are directly or indirectly involved with the molecular and pathological factors of these disorders. The pathogenic mechanisms in neurodegenerative diseases include neuronal oxidative damage, neuroinflammation, protein aggregation and mis-folding, mitochondria dysfunction, and an impaired energy process. Studies have elucidated the molecular mechanisms of dietary phytochemicals in modulating these pathways; some of these mechanisms are discussed in this chapter.

17.3.1 Dietary Phytochemicals Demonstrated Neuroprotection via Suppression of NF-κB

NF-κB is a ubiquitous transcriptional factor hosted in nearly all types of animal cells. The NF-kB, in full, signifies nuclear factor kappa-light-chain-enhancer of activated B-cells. NF-κB's major role involves modulating the genetic expression of cytokines and chemokines, which includes interferons, interleukins, lymphokines, and tumor necrosis factors (Niloo et al., 2015). These factors play wide roles in inflammatory and immune responses, survival of cells, as well as promoting the integrity of signaling pathways in nervous system involved in learning, plasticity, and memory (Mattson et al., 2006). Likewise, its role in management of cancerous cells has been linked with down-line suppression of tumor necrosis factors' cellular cytosol toxicity via the apoptotic route and suppression of c-Jun pathway via the N-terminal enzymatic kinase activities (Papa et al., 2006)

NF-kB undergoes either the canonical or non-canonical route, both of which are dependent on the structural oligomeric dimerized components. The p50 and p65 (RelA) subunits play role in the canonical route while RelB and p52 play role in the non-canonical route.

In a homeostatic state, the NF-kB exit as an inactive hetero-dimer forms, composed of p50 and p65 (RelA) subunits, complexing with inhibitory proteins IkB-A or IkB-β and mask with the cytoplasm, but upon stimulation by microglia, expression of the membranes' receptor-like toll-like receptors (TLRs) and their associates recognize the pathogen-associated molecules and damage-associated molecules of bacteria, virus, fungal, and other parasites as pro-inflammatory ligands (Figuera-Losada et al., 2014; Mogensen, 2009). The signaling response results in the activation of the IκB protein kinases, which phosphorylation inhibits protein and dissociates from the complexes to free NF-kB for nuclear transport in order to bind with its nuclear receptor for expression and recruitment of expression of chemokines, inflammatory enzymes COX-2 and iNOS, pro-inflammatory cytokines, and tissues' adhesion-cytokine molecules (Ghosh and Karin, 2002; Perkins, 2007). These molecules are collectively markers for cellular or tissues or neuronal inflammatory responses.

Suppression of the active level of NF-KB should be a therapeutic tool in the prevention of cancer and cardiovascular and degenerative diseases. Research has shown that dietary phytochemicals such as flavonoids, tannins, and polyphenols exhibit anti-inflammatory potential in neuronal cells via these mechanisms:

(i) by inhibiting the activity of the enzyme IκB protein kinases, thereby halting the phosphorylation and ubiquitination processes, which are essential for liberation of IkB moiety from the NF-IkB complexes (Ruiz and Haller, 2006);

(ii) by inhibiting the productive interaction of the NF-κB subunits, even after translocation into the nucleus with the targeted DNA (Ruiz and Haller, 2006);

(iii) dietary phytochemicals also interfere directly with arachidonic acid (AA) dependent pathways by inhibiting the expression of the enzyme that promotes the progression of the inflammatory process cyclooxygenase-2 and AA independent pathways indirectly, as this depends on its counterpart pathway (Yoon and Baek, 2005).

Among the reported dietary phytochemicals that have been shown to exhibit these neuronal anti-inflammatory mechanisms are curcumin, quercetin, epigallocate catechin, and resveratrol (Endale et al., 2013; Kundu and Surh, 2007; Oladele et al., 2021). Dietary phytochemicals such as flavonoids have been shown to exhibit neuroprotective effects via the lowering of amyloid protein (Aβ) production in Alzheimer's via a dependent NF-κB mechanism. Accumulated amyloid (Aβ) protein is an integral disease pathology of most degenerative diseases. Daidzein, A- and β-napthofalvone, apigenin, genistein, luteolin, and kaemferol were most notable dietary flavonoids proven to exhibit such beneficial effects. The β-active site cleavage enzyme-1 (BACE-1), which is the rate-limiting enzyme responsible for the generation of Aβ-peptides, is the major target of these flavonoids, as they directly inhibit this site in order to lower the effects of their operation (Paris et al., 2011). Aside from this route, these dietary flavonoids can also inhibit transcription of the gene of BACE-1(Shimmyo et al., 2008)

17.3.2 DIETARY PHYTOCHEMICALS DEMONSTRATED NEUROPROTECTION VIA ENHANCEMENT OF NRF2

Many dietary phytochemicals have been identified to play significant roles in the heterodimers' transcription factor, nuclear-factor-erythroid factor-2-related factor 2 (Nrf2) in mediating neuronal protection against oxidative destruction/stress and inflammation (Nakatani, 2000; Van Dyk and Sano, 2007). Nrf2 is a transcription factor that belongs to the Cap "n" Collar family of basic leucine zippers (bZip) that wallow in the cytoplasm to regulate the main genes for antioxidant and cellular protection (Sun et al., 2007). It interacts under physiological conditions with Kelch-like ECH-associated protein 1 (Keap 1) to enhance proteosomal degradation via interaction with ubiquitin ligase. This complex, Nrf2-Keap1, is essential for passage of Nrf2 into the nucleus for associative interaction other leucine zipper (bZip) transcription factors and to the non-coding region of DNA, which plays a role in the pleiotropy of many neighboring genes, called Cis-acting elements – specifically, the antioxidant response element (ARE).

Under cellular oxidative stress, the condition serves as a signal for the Nrf2 to dissociate from the complexes and for its activation, which further translocates into the nucleus through E3 ubiquitin ligase catalytic action. The ARE responses give rise to induction of inducible cytoprotective biological catalysts like Hemeoxygenase 1(HO-1), glutathione-s-Transferase, and other associated enzyme complexes, which all play roles in the detoxification of xenobiotics and removal of some endogenously generated molecules (Ma, 2008). The Nrf2-ARE interaction is the major target for dietary phytochemicals signaling neuroprotective roles; dietary phytochemicals promote NrF2 and ARE interaction, as this associate activates HO-1 (regulatory enzymes) and activates xenobiotics/drug detoxifying enzymes complexes. Likewise, the end products of HO-1 catabolic action result in generation of carbon monoxide and bilirubin (Pamplona et al., 2007). These end products enable the HO-1 to exact its immuno-modulatory role and neuronal anti-inflammation role via end products' regulatory actions, which include regulation of neuronal vessel tone, platelet-aggregation prevention, neuronal tissue injury prevention, neuronal tissue congestion, and neuro-inflammation prevention (Pamplona et al., 2007; Scapagnini et al., 2002).

Aside from the direct free radicals' and lipid peroxides' quenching potentials, dietary phytochemicals also exhibit neuroprotective properties through the phase II detoxifying enzymes system via HO-1 expression and Nrf2-ARE signaling complex activation. Curcumin, caffeic acid, phenethylester, and the green tea catechins have been shown to exhibit this neuroprotective role via HO-1 expression and Nrf2-ARE signaling routes (Scapagnini et al., 2002; Yang et al., 2009). Curcumin-rich diets have been reported to enhance memory, learning, and cognitive functions through decreased amyloid protein aggregation, suppression of inflammation responses, reversing of brain lipid peroxidation, and lipid modifications and via increased glutathione levels in Alzheimer's and Parkinson's patients. Likewise, the green tea catechins have been shown to possess anti-inflammation properties, in addition to their neuroprotective actions; daily intake has been reported to help delay the occurrence of aging and age-related diseases. Aside from these, cancer cell line invasion, neuronal vessel formation, and inhibition of the spread of cancer were other beneficial roles that accounted for the intake of dietary phytochemicals (Khan and Mukhtar, 2007).

The health benefits of dietary phytochemicals have accounted for direct antioxidant and anti-inflammatory roles due to their ability to scavenge free radicals through the hydroxyl functional group they possess in their structure (Oladele et al., 2020, 2021, 2022), but an underlined, indirect neuroprotective mechanism not well studied is their role in the modulation of signaling pathways within the cells. Curcumin, green tea catechins, cinnamic acid, ferulic acid, and caffeic acid phenethyl ester are all dietary polyphenols that modulate the Nrf2 signaling pathway; specifically, enhancing Nrf2-ARE interaction, which activates and promotes the expression of the phase II detoxifying and expression of the HO-1 gene, accounts for their powerful antioxidant, neuroprotective, and anti-inflammatory capacities (Scapagnini et al., 2002). Additionally, the NrF2 pathway helps in moderating the levels and affects principal neurotransmitters, including norepinephrine, dopamine, and glutamate. This underlined mechanism of action could be another significant therapeutic tool for the treatment of cancer and neurodegenerative diseases.

Dietary phytochemicals also exhibit neuroprotective protective effects on stroke and neurodegenerative disease pathology via the Nrf2 pathway. Flavonoids facilitate, mediate, and cause nuclear translocation of Nrf2 (nuclear factor erythroid 2-related factor 2) and bind to anti-oxidant response elements (AREs) to promote transcription of genes responsible for production phase II detoxifying enzymes and other cytoprotective proteins. Also, they act as potent regulators of the peripheral inflammatory-response genes.

The AREs genes are encoding genes for the transcription and production of detoxifying enzymes. Nrf2 actuates the expression of qualities (AREs) that give cellular detoxification through the glutathione (glutathione [GSH], glutathione S-transferase [GST], glutamate cysteine ligase catalytic, and modulatory subunits [Gclc, Gclm]), and thioredoxin (thioredoxin reductase [TrxR], peroxiredoxin 1 [Prx1]) frameworks help in the NAD(P)H generation and catabolism of pro-oxidant heme (heme oxygenase 1 [HO1]), free press, and copper/zinc sequestration (ferritin light chain 1, metallothionein 1 [MT1]), security from superoxide radicals (superoxide dismutase 1 [SOD1]), and avoidance of unusual intracellular protein aggregation (warm stun protein 40), and proteasomal subunits (19S, 20S). Evidence of these were reported by Shin et al. (2010), Sinha et al. (2002), and Niture and Jaiswal (2010).

17.3.3 Dietary Phytochemicals Demonstrated Neuroprotection via Inhibition of MAPK Pathway

Among the important pathways that help in signal transduction from the extracellular components of the cell to the intracellular or target region is the MAPK pathway. The mitogen-activated protein kinase (MAPK) pathway is comprised of a cascade of events that plays a role in modulating the signaling event, which is vital for mammalian cell proliferation, development and differentiation, inflammatory responses, and apoptosis (Behl et al., 2022). The pathway is comprised of many proteins that transfer a signal via phosphorylation of their tyrosine, serine, or threonine amino acids containing moiety in their structure of the neighboring proteins in order to send a signal to the DNA for transcription purposes. The phosphorylation process causes conformational changes in their protein structure, enabling them to activate neighboring proteins. Mutation is the gene expression of any of these proteins, and it results in the development of cancer (Yu et al., 2020). C-Jun N-terminal kinases (JNK), extracellular signal-regulated kinases (ERKs), and p38 mitogen-activated protein kinases are major MAPK subfamilies of popular discussions, although other subfamilies, like Nemo-like kinase, exist (Yu et al., 2020). In general, each cascade event is activated by the binding of ligands to the extracellular receptor sites, which pronounce three sequential kinase events, where MAPK kinase kinase (MAPKKK) stimulates MAPK kinase (MAPKK), which finally turns on MAP kinase (MAPK).

Although the ligand type determines which cascade among the subfamilies will be activated within the enzymatic complexes, the canonical ERKs is activated by growth factor and cytokines, while oxidative stress, cytokines, lipopolysaccharide, and infections turn on the p38 and JNK signaling routes (Behl et al., 2022).

The MAPK pathway plays a crucial role in response to oxidative stress and oxidative damage that occurs as a result of the destructive effect of free radicals and reactive nitric oxides species. This occurs via activation and expression of transcriptional factors for the regulation of apoptosis and inflammatory processes. When the cell is under oxidative stress, irrespective of the causative agent, either ROS or iNOS, this serves as an effector ligand that binds the extracellular receptor components causing activation of the MAPK upstream regulatory protein thioredoxin, which is a classical component of apoptosis signal-regulating kinase 1 (ASK1) (Matsuzawa et al., 2005). The ROS causes dissociation of the thioredoxin from the complexes, converting it to active form, where its kinase activity catalyzes phosphorylation of the MEKs component – i.e., MAPKs – and proceeds, further, to the phosphorylate JNK and p38 of MAPK. Likewise, the causative agent, ROS, can also directly activate MAPK via inhibition of its phosphatase components. This cascade event causes expression of the transcriptional factor that regulates apoptosis and inflammation (Behl et al., 2022; Matsuzawa et al., 2005). With respect to inflammation, the MAPK pathway plays roles in turning on the transcriptional factor gene NFκB, which is crucial for induction of pro-inflammatory cytokines, cyclooxygenase-2, and the inducible nitric oxide synthase, which are all promoters of the inflammation response (Behl et al., 2022).

From this point of view, inhibition of the signal transduction of MAPK vis ERKs, JNK, and p38 pathways at the transcriptional level should be the major target of therapeutic drugs for promoting neuroprotection against oxidation and inflammation. Many reports have shown that dietary phytochemicals exhibit a neuroprotective role via this mechanism. Dietary phytochemicals regulate the MAPK pathway by inhibiting the activation processes at each step. For example, a scientific study has documented that using activated human THP1 monocyte cell line shows that dietary phytochemicals (catechins) regulate the MAPK pathway by inhibiting activity of the p38 and JNK of MAPK and their phosphorylated form, while quercetin exacts its inhibition on ERK, JNK, and their phosphorylated forms, thereby preventing further signaling transduction via phosphorylation processes catalyzed by kinases (Huang et al., 2006). Likewise, a study on lipopolysaccharide activated macrophages in mice shows that the dietary phytochemicals (quercetin) display a regulatory role against expression of TNF-A by inhibiting the prevention production of TNF-A protein synthesis via inhibiting the phosphorylation ERK1/2 and activity of p38 MAPK as well as TNF-A expression by halting phosphorylation (Wadsworth et al., 2001).

Green tea catechins display their neuroprotective mechanism by inhibiting the expression of the gene for cyclooxygenase-2, an enzyme that promotes the inflammatory response by inhibiting the activation via phosphorylation of the p38 MAPK pathway and binding it to the DNA of NFκB (Kundu et al., 2007).

Dietary flavonoids exact modulatory effects on MAPK's signaling pathway, specifically through inhibitory action on their kinase cascades. Flavonoids do this by binding to the ATP binding site of the protein kinase moiety. Naringenin, hesperetin, and flavanone, which are citrus flavonoids, and resverastol of stilbene are classical examples of dietary flavonoids that have been reported to exhibit such actions in order to arrest cumulated neuronal cell death via apoptosis (Williams et al., 2004). Flavonoids also exact their neuronal protection role via the extracellular signal-regulated protein kinase (ERK) and c-Jun N-terminal kinase (JNK) pathways. The flavone luteolin suppresses IL-6 production in activated microglia by blocking the JNK-signaling pathway, and fisetin inhibits p38 MAP kinase activation in LPS-stimulated BV-2 microglial cells (Zheng et al., 2008). Likewise, quercetin has been shown to act by controlling apoptotic gene expression, avoiding apoptosis, and encouraging cell survival through inhibiting p38 MAPK and JNK; phosphorylation is caused by caspases-3 activation via hydrogen peroxide (Choi et al., 2005).

17.3.4 DIETARY PHYTOCHEMICALS DEMONSTRATED NEUROPROTECTION VIA MODULATION OF P53 PATHWAY

The P53 pathway is another signaling pathway of great significance to the biological cells, including neuronal cells. This pathway and its transcriptional products participate in stress-response-signaling processes like cell cycle arrest, senescence, and apoptosis. Most importantly, the pathway helps in expression and synthesis of the p53 protein, which act as tumor-suppressor protein preventing the development of cancer (Levin et al., 2006). Additionally, the p53 helps in the process of inhibition of angiogenesis, metastasis, and IGF-1/mTOR pathway, facilitating exosome secretion and DNA damage repair.

Damaged DNA via ROS and radiation, activated oncogenes, nitric oxide, cold and heat shock, hypoxia, and damage spindle are stress signals that activate p53 genes, which results in expression of p53 in the same way the Murine double minute 2 (MDM-2) are degraded in response to these stress signals via MDM-2 ubiquitin ligase (Vogelstein et al., 2000; Zhao et al., 2000). P53 response genes' upstream mediating follows, and the activated p53 proteins cause transcription of many genes, among which are GADD-45, MDM-2, cycling G, and p21, which play a role in cell cycle arrest; secreted protein fas and killer/DR5, which works in conjunction with PIDD to activate caspases 8 and Bid to release cytochrome c in the extrinsic apoptotic pathway; Bax, p53AIP and PIGs in the intrinsic apoptotic pathway; p48, GADD-45, and p53R2, which play a role in the DNA damage-repair mechanism; BAI-1, KAI, Maspin, which play a role as inhibitors of protease, which degrades the extracellular matrix and surface and PTEN/IGF-BP3 genes, which gene products IGF-1R, IGF 1, and others inhibit the activation of growth response signal transduction routes, thereby regulating cell growth negatively after stress signals are triggered with cells (Chipuk et al., 2004; Moll et al., 2005)

Available evidence proves that the p53 passes out of the nucleus itself, acting directly on mitochondria and its protein components, BCL-2, to enhance the liberation of cytochrome c and apoptosis. p53 also plays a role in communication between neighboring cells by inducing the TSAP-6 gene, which enhances production of exosomes for cell-cell communication. However, the p53 protein level is regulated by MDM-2 via ubiquitin ligase enzymes like COP1 (constitutively photomorphogenic 1) and Pirh2 (p53-induced RING-H2 domain protein) and catalytic turn-over (Levin et al., 2006).

Dietary phytochemicals help in activation of p53 transcriptional activity in order to mediate increased synthesis of p53 protein, which suppresses neuronal tumors and neurological cancer via initiation of apoptosis, cell arrest, ROS generation, and cell senescence with the neurological tumor (Khan et al., 2020; Sheikh and Fornace, 2000). Dietary phytochemicals such as polyphenols cause up-regulation of p53-dependent targets like p21, Bax, and DR5 (Khan et al., 2020).

A report on the neuroprotective effect of flavonoids on neuronal acute and chronic inflammation has been linked to its ability to suppress inflammatory processes by modulating the expression of the P53 response gene. Dietary flavonoids such as luteolin modulate the P53 gene by increasing its expression and enhance its translocation into the mitochondria in order to regulate its apoptosis. A report on the neuroprotective effect of Naringenin via p53 shows reverses in memory damage and decreased cognitive and learning ability as well as memory caused by exposure to Aβ25–35 as well as decreasing the anxiety and inflammation response (Song et al., 2017).

17.4   CONCLUSION AND FUTURE PROSPECTS

Dietary phytochemicals are naturally occurring compounds found in fruits, vegetables, herbs, and spices. They have a variety of health benefits, including antioxidant, anti-inflammatory, and neuroprotective effects. Neurodegenerative diseases are a group of conditions that cause progressive damage to the brain and nervous system. They include Alzheimer's disease, Parkinson's disease, and amyotrophic lateral sclerosis (ALS). These diseases are characterized by the death of neurons, which can lead to cognitive decline, movement disorders, and other symptoms. There is growing evidence that dietary phytochemicals may have therapeutic potential in neurodegenerative diseases. These compounds have been shown to protect neurons from damage, promote neuronal regeneration, and reduce inflammation.

Some of the most promising phytochemicals for neurodegenerative diseases include flavonoids, a type of antioxidant that is found in many fruits and vegetables. They have been shown to protect neurons from damage caused by free radicals, and they may also help to reduce inflammation. Curcumin, a compound found in turmeric, has strong antioxidant and anti-inflammatory properties, and it has been shown to improve cognitive function in people with Alzheimer's disease. Also, resveratrol is a compound found in grapes, red wine, and peanuts. It has been shown to protect neurons from damage, and it may also help to slow down the progression of Alzheimer's disease.

EGCG is a compound found in green tea. It has strong antioxidant and anti-inflammatory properties, and it has been shown to protect neurons from damage caused by beta-amyloid plaques, which are a hallmark of Alzheimer's disease. Omega-3 fatty acids are found in fish, walnuts, and flaxseed. They have anti-inflammatory properties, and they may help to protect neurons from damage. The molecular mechanisms governing the neuroprotective effects of these dietary phytochemicals include neurotropic pathways, the p53 pathway, the anti-apoptotic pathway, the anti-neuro-inflammatory pathway, NF-kB/MAPK pathways, the Nrf-2 pathway, and so on.

Taken together, more research is still needed to fully understand the role of dietary phytochemicals in neurodegenerative diseases. However, the available evidence suggests that these compounds may have a beneficial effect on brain health and may help to delay or prevent the onset of these diseases. In addition to eating a diet rich in fruits, vegetables, herbs, and spices, there are other lifestyle changes that can help to reduce the risk of neurodegenerative diseases.

REFERENCES

Behl T, Rana T, Alotaibi GH, Shamsuzzaman M, Naqvi M, Sehgal A, Singh S, Sharma N, Almoshari Y, Abdellatif AAH, Iqbal MS, Bhatia S, Al-Harrasi A, Bungau S (2022) Polyphenols inhibiting MAPK signalling pathway mediated oxidative stress and inflammation in depression. Biomed Pharmacother. 146: 112545, Feb. Doi: 10.1016/j.biopha.2021.112545.

Bhakkiyalakshmi E, Dineshkumar K, Karthik S, Sireesh D, Hopper W, Paulmurugan R, Ramkumar KM (2016) Pterostilbene-mediated Nrf2 activation: Mechanistic insights on Keap1: Nrf2 interface. Bioorg Med Chem. 24: 3378–3386.

Blandini F (2013) Neural and immune mechanisms in the pathogenesis of Parkinson's disease. J Neuroimmune Pharmacol. 8: 189–201.

Chipuk JE, Kuwana T, Bouchier-Hayes L, Droin NM, Newmeyer DD, Schuler M, Green DR (2004) Direct activation of Bax by p53 mediates mitochondrial membrane permeabilization and apoptosis. Sciencem. 303: 1010–1014.

Choi YJ, Jeong YJ, Lee YJ, Kwon HM, Kang YH (2005) (–)Epigallocatechin gallate and quercetin enhance survival signalling in response to oxidant-induced human endothelial apoptosis. J Nutr. 135: 707–713.

Costello S, Cockburn M, Bronstein J, Zhang X, Ritz B (2009) Parkinson's disease and residential exposure to Maneb and paraquat from agricultural applications in the central valley of California. Am J Epidemiol. 169: 919–926.

Deprez S, Mila I, Huneau JF, Tome D, Scalbert A (2001) Transport of proanthocyanidin dimer, trimer, and polymer across monolayers of human intestinal epithelial Caco-2 cells. Antioxid Redox Signal. 3: 957–967.

Dias V, Junn E, Mouradian MM (2013) The role of oxidative stress in Parkinson's disease. J Parkinson Dis. 3: 461–491.

Endale M, Park SC, Kim S, Kim SH, Yang Y, Cho JY, et al. (2013) Quercetin disrupts tyrosine-phosphorylated phosphatidylinositol 3-kinase and myeloid differentiation factor-88 association, and inhibits MAPK/AP-1 and IKK/NF-kappa B-induced inflammatory mediators production in RAW 264.7 cells. Immunobiol. 218: 1452–1467. DOI: 10.1016/j.imbio.2013.04.019.

Figuera-Losada M, Rojas C, Slusher BS (2014) Inhibition of microglia activation as a phenotypic assay in early drug discovery. J Biomol Screen. 19: 17–31. DOI: 10.1177/1087057113499406.

Flanagan E, Lamport D, Brennan L, Burnet P, Calabrese V, Cunnane SC, et al. (2020) Nutrition and the ageing brain: Moving towards clinical applications. Ageing Res Rev. 62: 101079. DOI: 10.1016/j.arr.2020.101079.

Ghosh S, Karin M (2002) Missing pieces in the NF-kappa B puzzle. Cell. 109(Suppl.): S81–S96. DOI: 10.1016/S0092-8674(02)00703-1.

Goedert M (2015) Neurodegeneration. Alzheimer's and Parkinson's diseases: The prion concept in relation to assembled Aβ, tau, and A-synuclein. Science. 349: 1255555.

Gupta S, Hastak K, Afaq F, Ahmad N, Mukhtar H (2004) Essential role of caspases in epigallocatechin-3-gallate-mediated inhibition of nuclear factor kappa B and induction of apoptosis. Oncogene. 23: 2507–2522.

He F, Zuo L (2015) Redox roles of reactive oxygen species in cardiovascular diseases. Int J Mol Sci. 16: 27770–27780.

Huang SM, Wu CH, Yen GC (2006) Effects of flavonoids on the expression of the pro-inflammatory response in human monocytes induced by ligation of the receptor. For AGEs, Mol Nutr Food Res. 50: 1129–1139.

Kazmierczak-Baranska J, Boguszewska K, Karwowski BT (2020) Nutrition can help DNA repair in the case of aging. Nutrients. 12: 3364. DOI: 10.3390/nu12113364.

Khan H, Reale M, Ullah H, Sureda A, Tejada S, Wang Y, Zhang ZJ, Xiao J (2020) Anti-cancer effects of polyphenols via targeting p53 signaling pathway: Updates and future directions. Biotechnol Adv. 38: 107385. DOI: 10.1016/j.biotechadv.2019.04.007.

Khan N, Mukhtar H (2007) Tea polyphenols for health Promotion. Life Sci. 81: 519–553.

Kim J, Lee HJ, Lee KW (2010) Naturally occurring phytochemicals for the prevention of Alzheimer's disease. J Neurochem. 112(6): 1415–1430.

Kundu JK, Surh YJ (2007) Epigallocatechingallate inhibits phorbol ester-induced activation of NF-kappa B and CREB in mouse skin: Role of p38 MAPK. Ann N Y Acad Sci. 1095: 504–512.

Levin AJ, Hu W, Feng Z (2006) The P53 pathway: What questions remain to be explored? Cell Death Differ 13: 1027–1036. DOI: 10.1038/sj.cdd.4401910; published online 24 March 2006.

Livingston G, Huntley J, Sommerlad A (8 August 2020) Dementia prevention, intervention, and care: 2020 report of the Lancet commission. Lancet. 396(10248): 413–446.

Ma Q (2008) Xenobiotic-activated receptors: From transcription to drug metabolism to disease. Chem Res Toxicol. 21: 1651–1671.

Matilla-Duenas A, Ashizawa T, Brice A (2014) Consensus paper: Pathological mechanisms underlying neuro-degeneration in spinocerebellar ataxias. Cerebellum. 13: 269–302.

Matsuzawa A, Saegusa K, Noguchi T, Sadamitsu C, Nishitoh H, Nagai S, Koyasu S, Matsumoto K, Takeda K, Ichijo H (2005) ROS-dependent activation of the TRAF6-ASK1-p38 pathway is selectively required for TLR4-mediated innate immunity. Nat Immunol. 6: 587–592.

Mattson MP, Meffert MK (2006) Roles for NF-kappa B in nerve cell survival, plasticity, and disease. Cell Death Differ. 13(5): 852–860. DOI: 10.1038/sj.cdd.4401837. PMID 16397579.

Mogensen TH (2009) Pathogen recognition and inflammatory signaling in innate immune defenses. Clin Microbiol Rev. 22: 240–273. DOI: 10.1128/CMR.00046-08

Mogi M, Harada M, Kondo J (1994a) Interleukin-1 beta, interleukin-6, epidermal growth factor and trans-forming growth factor-alpha are elevated in the brain from parkinsonian patients. Neurosci Lett. 180: 147–150.

Mogi M, Harada M, Kondo T, Narabayashi H, Riederer P, Nagatsu T (1995a) Transforming growth factor-beta 1 levels are elevated in the striatum and in ventricular cerebrospinal fluid in Parkinson's disease. Neurosci Lett. 193: 129–132.

Mogi M, Harada M, Kondo T, Riederer P, Nagatsu T (1995b) Brain beta 2-microglobulin levels are elevated in the striatum in Parkinson's disease. J Neural Transm Park Dis Dement Sect. 9: 87–92.

Mogi M, Harada M, Riederer P, Narabayashi H, Fujita K, Nagatsu T (1994b) Tumor necrosis factor-alpha (TNF-alpha) increases both in the brain and in the cerebrospinal fluid from parkinsonian patients. Neurosci Lett. 165: 208–210.

Moll UM, Wolff S, Speidel D and Deppert W (2005) Transcription-independent pro-apoptotic functions of p53. Curr Opin Cell Biol. 17: 631–636.

Nakatani N (2000) Phenolic antioxidants from herbs and spices. Biofactors. 13: 141–146.

Niloo K, Raju R, Gyengesi E, Münch G (2015) Plant polyphenols as inhibitors of NF-κB induced cytokine production – a potential anti-inflammatory treatment for Alzheimer's disease? Mol Neurosci. 8: 24.

Niture SK, Jaiswal AK. (2010) Hsp90 interaction with INrf2 (Keap1) mediates stress-induced Nrf2 activation. J Biol Chem. 285(47): 36865–36875.

Okubadejo NU, Ojo OO, Oshinaike OO (2010) Clinical profile of Parkinsonism and Parkinson's disease in Lagos, South Western Nigeria. BMC Neurol. 10: 1.

Oladele JO, Oladele OT, Adewole TS, Oyeleke OM, Oladiji AT (2022) Phytochemicals and natural prod-ucts: Efficacy in the management/treatment of neurodegenerative diseases. Chapter 10. In *Handbook of Research on Advanced Phytochemicals and Plant-Based Drug Discovery*. Hershey, PA: IGI Global. DOI: 10.4018/978-1-6684-5129-8.ch010.

Oladele JO, Oyeleke OM, Oladele OT, Olaniyan MD (2020) Neuroprotective mechanism of *Vernonia amygda-lina* in a rat model of neurodegenerative diseases. Toxicol Rep. 7: 1223–1232.

Oladele JO, Oladele OT, Oyeleke OM (2021c) Possible health benefits of polyphenols in neurological compli-cations associated with COVID-19. Acta Fac Medicae Naissensis. 38: 294–309.

Oladele JO, Oladele OT, Oyeleke OM, Oladiji AT (2021b) Neurological complications in COVID-19: Implications on international health security and possible interventions of phytochemicals. In *Contemporary Developments and Perspectives in International Health Security*, vol. 2. Londo: Intechopen. DOI: 10.5772/intechopen.96039.

Oladele JO, Oladiji AT, Oladele OT, Oyeleke OM (2021) *Reactive Oxygen Species in Neurodegenerative Diseases: Implications in Pathogenesis and Treatment Strategies* [Online First]. London: IntechOpen. DOI: 10.5772/intechopen.99976.

Pamplona A et al. (2007) Heme oxygenase-1 and carbon monoxide suppress the pathogenesis of experimental cerebral Malaria. Nat Med. 13(6): 703–710.

Papa S, Bubici C, Knabb JR, Dean K, Franzoso G (2006) The NF-kappa B-mediated control of the JNK cascade in the antagonism of programmed cell death in health and disease. Cell Death Differ. 13 (5): 712–729. DOI: 10.1038/sj.cdd.4401865. PMID 16456579.

Paris D, Mathura V, Ghezala G et al. (2011) Flavonoids lower Alzheimer's Aβ production via an NFκB depen-dent mechanism. Bioinformation 6: 229–236.

Parkinson Disease Foundation (PDF) (2016) Statistics on Parkinson's [WWW Document]. www.pdf.org/symptoms_statistics.

Perkins ND (2007) Integrating cell-signalling pathways with NF-kappa B and IKK function. Nat Rev Mol Cell Biol. 8: 49–62. DOI: 10.1038/nrm2083.

Ruiz PA, Haller D (2006). Functional diversity of flavonoids in the inhibition of the proinflammatory NF-kappa B, IRF, and Akt signaling pathways in murine intestinal epithelial cells. J Nutr. 136: 664–671.

Sarris J, Logan AC, Akbaraly TN, Amminger GP, Balanzá-Martínez V, Freeman MP et al. (2015) Nutritional medicine as mainstream in psychiatry. Lancet Psychiatry. 2: 271–274. DOI: 10.1016/S2215-0366(14)00051-0.

Scapagnini G, Foresti R, Calabrese V, Giuffrida Stella AM, Green CJ, Motterlini R (2002) Caffeic acid phenethyl ester and curcumin: A novel class of heme oxygenase-1 inducers. Mol Pharmacol. 61(3): 554–561, Mar. DOI: 10.1124/mol.61.3.554.

Sheikh MS, Fornace AJ, Jr (2000) Death and decoy receptors and p53-mediated apoptosis. Leukemia. 14: 1509–1513. DOI: 10.1038/sj.leu.2401865.

Shimmyo Y, Kihara T, Akaike A et al. (2008) Flavonols and flavones as BACE-1 inhibitors: Structure–activity relationship in cell-free, cell-based and in-silico studies reveal novel pharmacophore features. Biochem Biophy Acta. 1780: 819–825.

Shin JA, Lee H, Lim YK, Koh Y, Choi JH, Park EM (2010) Therapeutic effects of resveratrol during acute periods following experimental ischemic stroke. J Neuroimmunol. 227(1–2): 93–100.

Sinha K, Chaudhary G, Gupta YK (2002) Protective effect of resveratrol against oxidative stress in middle cerebral artery occlusion model of stroke in rats. Life Sci. 71(6): 655–665.

Smolensky D, Rhodes D, McVey DS, Fawver Z, Perumal R, Herald T, Noronha L (2018) High-polyphenol sorghum bran extract inhibits cancer cell growth through ROS induction, cell cycle arrest, and apoptosis. J Med Food. 21: 990–998.

Song X, Zhou B, Cui L (2017) Silibinin ameliorates Aβ25–35-Induced memory deficits in rats by modulating autophagy And attenuating neuroinflammation as well as oxidative stress. Neurochem Res. 42(4): 1073–1083.

Soto C, Estrada L, Castilla J (2006) Amyloids, prions and the inherent infectious nature of misfolded protein aggregates. Trends Biochem Sci. 31: 150–155.

Sun Z, Zhang S, Chan JY, Zhang DD (2007) Keap1 controls postinduction repression of the Nrf2-mediated antioxidant response by escorting nuclear export of Nrf2. Mol Cell Biol. 27(18): 6334–6349, Sep. DOI: 10.1128/MCB.00630-07.

Van Dyk K, Sano M (2007) The impact of nutrition on cognition in the elderly. Neurochem Res 32: 893–904.

Vauzour D, Camprubi-Robles M, Miquel-Kergoat S, Andres-Lacueva C, Bánáti D, Barberger-Gateau P et al. (2017) Nutrition for the ageing brain: Towards evidence for an optimal diet. Ageing Res Rev. 35: 222–240. DOI: 10.1016/j.arr.2016.09.010.

Vogelstein B, Lane D and Levine AJ (2000) Surfing the p53 network. Nature. 408: 307–310.

Wadsworth TL, McDonald TL, Koop DR (2001) Effects of Ginkgo biloba extract (EGb 761) and quercetin on lipopolysaccharide-induced signaling pathways involved in the release of tumor necrosis factor-alpha. Biochem Pharm. 62: 963–974.

Williams RJ, Spencer JP, Rice-Evans C (2004) Flavonoids: Antioxidants or signalling molecules? Free Radic Biol Med. 36: 838–849.

Yang C, Zhang X, Fan H, Liu Y (2009) Curcumin upregulates transcription factor Nrf2, HO-1 expression and protects rat brains against focal ischemia. Brain Res. 1282: 133–141.

Yoon JH, Baek SJ (2005) Molecular targets of dietary polyphenols with anti-inflammatory properties. Yonsei Med J. 46: 585–596. DOI: 10.3349/ymj.2005.46.5.585.

Yu J, Sun X, Goie J, Zhang Y (2020) Regulation of host immune responses against influenza A virus infection by mitogen-activated protein kinases (MAPKs). Microorganisms. 8(7): 1067. DOI: 10.3390/microorganisms8071067. PMC 7409222. PMID 32709.

Zhao R, Gish K, Murphy M, Yin Y, Notterman D, Hoffman WH, Tom E, Mack DH and Levine AJ (2000) The transcriptional program following p53 activation. Cold Spring Harb. Symp Quant Biol. 65: 475–482.

Zheng LT, Ock J, Kwon BM et al. (2008) Suppressive effects of flavonoid fisetin on lipopolysaccharide-induced microglial activation and neurotoxicity. Int Immunopharmacol. 8: 484–494.

Zuo L, Hemmelgarn BT, Chuang CC, Best TM (2015) The role of oxidative stress-induced epigenetic alterations in amyloid-beta production in Alzheimer's disease. Oxid Med Cell Longev. 604658: 13.

18 Chrono-Nutrition
Circadian Rhythms and Diet

John Adeolu Falode

18.1 INTRODUCTION

Chrono-nutrition: Chrono- refers to the passage of time, while nutrition refers to the act of absorbing nutrients from food and processing them in the body in order to maintain health. As a result, chrono-nutrition can be defined as the science of time-controlled eating for maximum dietary benefits. The art of well-controlled eating habits is thought to be beneficial to one's health. This eating habit normalizes blood cholesterol concentrations as a result of making the liver clock gene and rhythm of the CYP7A1 gene more stable, frequently through insulin formation. The internal processes (from the heart blood-pumping rhythm to the blinking of the eyes and subsequent responses to these rhythms) are filled with rhythm (the regular pattern of flow of matter in the space). Circadian rhythms are named for the fact that they come about on a 24-hour cycle (circa = around, and dia = day). Changes in dietary habits frequently have an impact on metabolism and other bodily functions, such as sleep. Changing one's sleeping time may potentially have physiological consequences. Nutrition experts have been incorporating chrono-biology, or biological chronological rhythms, into their research for the past decade, and this unique part of diet investigation is known as chrono-nutrition (Garaulet & Gómez-Abellán, 2014; St-Onge et al., 2017; Tahara & Shibata, 2013). Chrono-nutrition deals with meal frequency and regularity, energy intake and transmission, eating and fasting intervals, and the comparative significance of these parameters for metabolic healthiness and chronic disease pathogenesis (Flanagan et al., 2020; Pot et al., 2016). Various scholars have published papers on sleep, eating food (breakfast), and time-restricted meals, all of which are important aspects of chrono-nutrition (Clayton et al., 2020; Darzi et al., 2017; Edinburgh et al., 2017; Gibson, 2018; Gibson-Moore & Chambers, 2019; Lynch et al., 2021; Ruddick-Collins et al., 2018). Supplementary aspects of chrono-nutrition, such as meal regularity, frequency, and clock time (eating time) are not included in this basic issue. The following chart (Figure 18.1) can help to illustrate this.

18.2 SYSTEMS OF BIOLOGICAL TIMEPIECE

Our diet has a significant impact on our health, and chrono-nutrition has a significant impact on an individual's health state. Understanding the biological clock, how it operates, and the effect(s) of chrono-nutrition on the biological clock is important because chrono-nutrition has numerous mechanisms that underpin its effects on health. The circadian timing system, in a nutshell, regulates daily biological cycles and synchronizes physiology and behavior with the temporal universe (Flanagan et al., 2020). Two main signals (also known as zeitgebers) entice the central (primary) regulator, which is situated in the hypothalamic suprachiasmatic nuclei (SCN) (Green et al., 2008). Moreover, nearly all of our bodily tissues have peripheral (secondary) clocks that are managed by circadian genes (i.e., clock genes) (Flanagan et al., 2020; Dashti et al., 2015b). This system, which includes both the fundamental and peripheral clocks, imposes a rhythmic control over practically all of our physical function, such as when we are drowsy or hungry. Typically, diurnal or circadian guides influence an organism's feeding patterns; for example, nocturnal rodents like mice and rats guzzle the majority of their calories during their active phase in the dark (Flanagan et al., 2020). When mice are compulsory fed a lot of calories during their resting condition, they gain more weight than

DOI: 10.1201/9781003361497-20

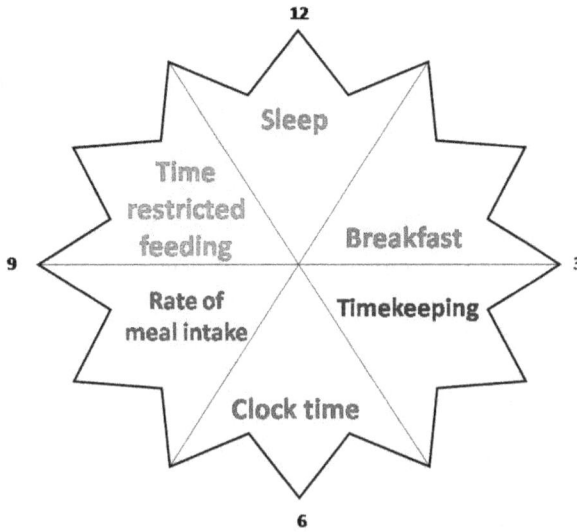

FIGURE 18.1 Components of chrono-nutrition.

when they are fed normally during their active state (Arble et al., 2009). This suggests that calorie consumption may not always have the same metabolic effect and that the metabolic effects observed may be due to the time of day. These findings have also been confirmed in people, with human intervention studies revealing that the time of day at which meals are consumed has a significant impact on metabolic responses (Garaulet et al., 2013; Jakubowicz et al., 2013). Researchers discovered that some women who were seeking to lose weight during a 20-week weight-reduction intervention in 420 obese women ate their primary meal before 3 p.m., whereas others ate it after 3 p.m. The former had a greater weight loss than the latter (Garaulet et al., 2013). In addition, another research study demonstrated similar results in a number of women having overweightness or obesity as a medical condition; the study revealed that a breakfast rich in calories had plentiful implausible advantages on biophysical features such as weight loss, waist perimeter, appetite scores, among others, when compared to taking a high calorie meal as dinner (Jakubowicz et al., 2013).

18.3 THE MANAGEMENT OF FEEDING BY METABOLIC CLOCKS

The body's energy requirements, according to homeostatic control and viewpoint, are in charge of nourishment pattern. This is tightly regulated in order to maintain an equilibrium between energy intake and expenditure and vice versa. On the other hand, homeostatic controls must be able to predict and ease phases of unclear or insufficient food accessibility as well as behavioral prototypes that limit feeding, such as protracted sleep, fasting, or increased energy demand over a lengthy period of time. Consequently, food intake regulation is a complicated network connecting short- and long-term homeostatic organization, food-linked impetus and compensation system, and better cognitive choice-making, particularly in humans. The feeding behavior of mice and rats is substantially diurnal/circadian, with greater than 70% of food taken through the dark/active period daily. Furthermore, rodent experiments demonstrated that diet formulation is important, such as carbohydrates vs. lipids, and that the extent to which fasting stimulates re-feeding varies depending on the moment in time (Rivera-Estrada et al., 2018). SCN injury significantly disrupts the usual feeding–fasting cycle, although there is no significant change in overall food consumption (Challet, 2019; Mistlberger & Antle, 2011). This draws attention to the importance of SCN output in determining the daily food intake model.

The hypothalamus and brainstem primarily houses the orexigenic and anorexigenic neurons, which are regulatory neurons that influence the desire to eat or not eat (Lenard & Berthoud, 2008; Morton et al., 2014). These neurons respond to the concentration of nutrients and hormones flowing in the body, such as glucose, amino acids, ghrelin, insulin, cholecystokinin (CCK), among others. This nutrient and hormone levels reflect the nutritional status and peripheral energy storage of individuals (Coll et al., 2007; Williams & Elmquist, 2012). Furthermore, the hypothalamus is home to a number of nuclei that have been linked to the regulation of feeding behavior and the preservation of energy balance. The SCN communicates with the subparaventricular zone (SPZ), median preoptic nucleus (MPO), and dorsomedial hypothalamus (DMH) at a deep level (Abrahamson & Moore, 2001; Watts et al., 1987; Flanagan et al., 2020). SCN protrusions to the paraventricular nucleus (PVN) have also been verified in rats and humans (Cui & Dyball, 1996; Dai et al., 1997), where SCN clock neurons offer temporal control of pre-autonomic and neuroendocrine pathway activities (Acosta-Galvan et al., 2011; Buijs et al., 2017; Kalsbeek et al., 2006; Paul et al., 2020). Awakening-promoting orexin neurons in the lateral hypothalamus (LH) (Abrahamson et al., 2001), sleep-promoting neurons in the ventrolateral preoptic nucleus (VPN), and energy-sensing neurons in the arcuate nucleus (ARC) (Sun et al., 2001) are all potential targets (Buijs et al., 1994). Behavioral rhythmicity can also be restored by SCN tissue relocation; this means that SCN timing also has a way of getting across through the action of some products (Silver et al., 1996; Flanagan et al., 2020). However, there is an assumption that the local clock-function controls the energy responsive neuronal populations in terms of feeding behavior. Unfortunately, due to SCN's control over behavioral rhythm, which likely masks more changes in food-related behavior, proving this assertion is more said than done. Regardless, evidence suggests that the local clock function and other aspects of energy balance are linked. For instance, the ARC has established strong circadian rhythms in the activity of neurons, clock gene/protein expression, and neuropeptide expression correlated to diet (Guilding et al., 2009; Kalra et al., 2004; Tan et al., 2014). Another study found that the loss of timer role in Agouti-related peptide (AGRP) neurons caused by cell-specific Bmal1 removal affects the cells' shared hormonal (leptin) response (Cedernaes et al., 2019). The RNA expression and modification system in cells revealed that bioenergetics and peptide-dependent neuronic pathways are directed by the day time and energy level. Outside of the hypothalamus, some areas have been shown to be critical for feeding control and to have circadian features. Brainstem locations – for example, the region postrema and nuclei of the solitary tract (NTS) – are crucial for peripheral metabolic status monitoring (Grill et al., 2012). These locations are sensitive to distribution of feeding and non-eating (satiety) hormones like GLP1, CCK, as well as intuitive input from the vagus nerve, which alerts the brain to gastric swelling and nutrition intake. Clock gene(s) have been found to be expressed in the brainstem (Herichová et al., 2006; Kaneko & Sawamoto, 2009), and a current investigation found that both the NTS and AP harbor substantial circadian clock function (Chrobok et al., 2020). On reward-based parts of feeding behavior, the clock is also likely to interrupt (DePoy et al., 2017; Murray et al., 2002). Time-of-day and circadian rhythmicity in recompense and motivational responses have been established in both human and animal research. In brain areas involved in dopamine signaling, such as the ventral tegmental area (VTA) and prefrontal cortex, periodic activity and clock gene expression have also been seen (Ángeles-Castellanos et al., 2008; Chung et al., 2014; DePoy et al., 2017; Verwey et al., 2016). Koch et al. (2020) found that VTA regulates pleasure appetite control and sensitivity to over-delicious food consumption through modifying cycles in this region. A gene referred to as REVERBa has been found to play a role in controlling production of dopamine (through direct control of tyrosine hydroxylase, which is the rate-limiting enzyme in dopamine production) in the VTA, despite its lack of effect on food intake (Chung et al., 2014). Mice missing Reverba expression consume more appealing meals, corroborating the findings (Feillet et al., 2015). Food-related reaction from the periphery reinforces eating rhythms. Circulating metabolic hormones and nutrients as well as sensory input from the gastrointestinal tract (GIT) that follows feeding examples both engage acute homeostatic reactions in a periodic manner (due to the normal feeding/fasting cycle) and directly control central circadian clocks (due to metabolic state sensitivity). The profound behavioral and physiological entrainment observed in experimental animals to constrained feeding regimens exemplifies clockwork's sensitivity to food-related information (Mistlberger & Antle, 2011).

18.4   IMMENSE VALUE OF CHRONO-NUTRITION IN THE POPULATION OF PEOPLE WHO DON'T GET ENOUGH SLEEP

Chrono-nutrition is currently thought to be a modifiable risk factor for a variety of non-communicable diseases. Our modern lifestyles, however, include prolonged exposure to artificial light, long hours at work, particularly jobs that require sedentary daily activities, and irregular eating patterns. All of these muddle with our circadian rhythms and have unintended negative consequences for our health (Cornelissen & Otsuka, 2017). Shift workers, particularly those who work at night, are at an elevated danger of developing persistent non-communicable diseases like type 2 diabetes and metabolic and cardiovascular diseases, according to a growing body of evidence (Depner et al., 2014; Reutrakul & Knutson, 2015). As a result of changes in circadian cycles throughout life, almost everyone (not just sleep-deprived people) in our modern environment requires chrono-nutrition (Van Someren, 2000). As age increases, the change in circadian timing decreases. Sleeping difficulties are more common in people at both ends of the age spectrum – adolescents and older adults. Delayed sleep phase disorder (DSPD) is additionally common in teens, whereas shift work disorder and jet lag disorder are more common in older persons (Duffy et al., 2015). Sleep difficulties in elderly persons is perhaps caused by a higher failure to sleep at an inconvenient natural time as they become older as well as a decreased capacity to phase shift. Some age-related illnesses, such as dementia, are also widespread as a result of changes in circadian rhythm regulation (Van Someren, 2000). Meanwhile, interest in chrono-nutrition for adolescents and older persons as well as night shift workers is expanding. However, in order to ensure public health, this must be passed through a regulatory agency (Gerda, 2021).

18.5   CATEGORY OF CHRONOLOGY

A careful examination of the multifarious connection between the various apparatuses of chrono-nutrition, such as the value of fasting, sleep, working hours, daily distribution of nutrient intake, and its effects on cardiovascular and metabolic health, provides insight into how to develop the health of a noteworthy portion of the populace (Gibson, 2018). While chrono-nutrition is important in the management of diabetes, cardiovascular disease, obesity, and illnesses connected to these diseases, chrono-type must also be carefully examined. A person's favored time of day for an activity/rest cycle is referred to as chrono-type. A person's active time can be classed as morning, middle, or evening (Roenneberg et al., 2007). Chrono-type has been discovered to be a consistent and stable feature that varies only slightly across time (Druiven et al., 2020). Various investigations into the role of chrono-type are still ongoing. New research has found that those with later active time or evening personalities have more unwholesome eating habits linked to obesity (Merikanto & Partonen, 2020) and are less responsive to weight loss therapies (Mazri et al., 2020). These people have a predisposition to eat more energy in the evening (Zerón-Rugerio et al., 2020), which has been linked to an elevated risk of overweightness/obesity (Baron et al., 2011; Martnez-Lozano et al., 2020; Xiao et al., 2019). The answers from these studies may also help to clarify the difference between those obese people who are metabolically healthy and those who are not. When compared to their metabolically unhealthy counterparts, those with metabolically healthy obesity were more physically active and engaged in morning physical activity, had an earlier sleeping time, a complete breakfast, and a larger quantity of meals daily (Torres-Castillo et al., 2020). Additionally, a recent study found that the difference between sleep–wake behavior and circadian inclination was primarily found in youths, implying that the future adult population faces a bigger risk of circadian misalignment if nothing is done to address the problem now (Merikanto & Partonen, 2020). As a result, both observational and interventional chrono-type research will add to the established database of the probable impact of chrono-nutrition on health in real-life settings (Flanagan et al., 2020).

18.6 SLEEPING

Control of sleep at nighttime and waking up and staying awake throughout the day has been linked to the circadian rhythm. Sleep is necessary for human well-being, since it is essential for physi-ological and mental functioning (Van Cauter et al., 2008; Vincent et al., 2017). For instance, sleep is required for appropriate metabolism, cognition, hunger regulation, immunological function, and hormonal balance in humans (Vincent et al., 2017). As a result, interruption of sleep pattern causes metabolic and endocrine changes, such as insulin resistance, among others (Johnston, 2014). Sleep deprivation has also been linked to a higher risk of obesity, among other ailments (Zhou et al., 2019). However, while the impacts of sleep on diet outcomes are likely to be minor, on a long-term basis, it may add to an elevated risk of obesity and associated complications (Dashti et al., 2015a, 2015b). Extending the duration of naps in short sleepers helped enhance appetite hormone regulation, nutri-ent metabolism, body weight, and nutritional intake, according to certain research (Al Khatib et al., 2018; Pizinger et al., 2018). To evaluate whether a good night's sleep will assist in combatting the obesity issue, ingenious, bigger, and longer research employing objective measurements of time and quality of sleep are needed (Gibson-Moore & Chambers, 2019).

18.7 CALORIE COUNTING AND TIME-RESTRICTED EATING ARE TWO WAYS TO LOSE WEIGHT

Fasting is a critical tool for resetting the biological clock in the majority of cases (Tahara & Shibata, 2013). Fasting for a length of time and restricting food consumption during certain times of the day has gained popularity as a way to beat down weight and develop metabolic well-being. Fasting on a regular or irregular basis has also been linked to a healthy aging process (de Cabo & Mattson, 2019). Fasting every other day, 5:2 intermittent fasting (two fasting days per week), and daily time-constrained meal are the three most widely researched intermittent-fasting courses of therapy in humans (de Cabo & Mattson, 2019). Time-constrained meal is a type of irregular fasting that is based on the 24-hour clock (Moon et al., 2020). Human studies on time-restricted eating have been limited to pilot or feasibility studies, with several limitations, ethical difficulties, methods, and individual differences hindering the ability to adapt and convert these findings to real-world situations. An investigation was conducted on the role of early and late time-constrained meals on confirmed type 2 diabetes risk factors (Lynch et al., 2021). It was expected that, during the time of time-restricted feeding intervention, there should be a significant and noticeable reduction in some markers, such as food intake, body weight, and adiposity, while other markers of metabolic illness such as low-density lipoprotein (LDL)-cholesterol and insulin sensitivity should improve. The study also found that early time-restricted food causes more metabolic alterations than late time-restricted feeding (Lynch et al., 2021). Other considerations include the real-world ramifi-cations of eating earlier in the day as well as the effects on social interactions and food choices (Lynch et al., 2021).

18.8 CONCLUSION

The importance of chrono-nutrition cannot be underemphasized; especially in our present world, all the major components of chrono-nutrition such as sleep, time-controlled feeding, and proper breakfast, among others, must be taken with utmost responsibility. This will help improve our daily living and health without necessarily visiting the hospital. Our working-class age group is strongly encouraged to key into this regimen to help improve their life expectancy.

REFERENCES

Abrahamson, E., Leak, R., & Moore, R. (2001). The suprachiasmatic nucleus projects to posterior hypothalamic arousal systems. *Neuro Report*, 12, 435–440.

Abrahamson, E., & Moore, R. (2001). Suprachiasmatic nucleus in the mouse: Retinal innervation, intrinsic organization and efferent projections. *Brain Research*, 916, 172–191.

Acosta-Galvan, G., Yi, C., van der Vliet, J., Jhamandas, J., Panula, P., Angeles-Castellanos, M., del Carmen Basualdo, M., Escobar, C., & Buijs, R. (2011). Interaction between hypothalamic dorsomedial nucleus and the suprachiasmatic nucleus determines intensity of food anticipatory behavior. *Proceedings of the National Academy of Sciences*, 108, 5813–5818.

Al Khatib, H.K., Hall, W.L., Creedon, A. Ooi E. Masri T., McGowan L. et al. (2018). Sleep extension is a feasible lifestyle intervention in free-living adults who are habitually short sleepers: A potential strategy for decreasing intake of free sugars? A randomized controlled pilot study. *American Journal of Clinical Nutrition*, 107(1), 43–53.

Ángeles-Castellanos, M., Salgado-Delgado, R., Rodríguez, K., Buijs, R., & Escobar, C. (2008). Expectancy for food or expectancy for chocolate reveals timing systems for metabolism and reward. *Neuroscience*, 155, 297–307.

Arble, D.M., Bass, J., Laposky, A.D., Vitaterna, M.H., & Turek, F.W. (2009). Circadian timing of food intake contributes to weight gain. *Obesity*, 17(11), 2100–2102.

Baron, K.G., Reid, K.J., Kern, A.S., & Zee, P.C. (2011). Role of sleep timing in caloric intake and BMI. *Obesity*, 19(7), 1374–1381.

Buijs, F., Guzmán-Ruiz, M., León-Mercado, L., Basualdo, M., Escobar, C., Kalsbeek, A., & Buijs, R. (2017). Suprachiasmatic nucleus interaction with the arcuate nucleus; essential for organizing physiological-rhythms. *Eneuro*, 4(2). https://doi.org/10.1523/ENEURO.0028-17.2017

Buijs, R., Hou, Y., Shinn, S., & Renaud, L. (1994). Ultrastructural evidence for intra- and extranuclear projections of GABAergic neurons of the suprachiasmatic nucleus. *The Journal of Comparative Neurology*, 340, 381–391. https://doi.org/10.1002/cne.903400308

Cedernaes, J., Waldeck, N., & Bass, J. (2019). Neurogenetic basis for circadian regulation of metabolism by the hypothalamus. *Genes & Development*, 33, 1136–1158. https://doi.org/10.1101/gad.328633.119

Challet, E. (2019). The circadian regulation of food intake. *Nature Reviews Endocrinology*, 15, 393–405. https://doi.org/10.1038/s41574-019-0210-x

Chrobok, L., Northeast, R., Myung, J., Cunningham, P., Petit, C., & Piggins, H. (2020). Timekeeping in the hindbrain: A multi-oscillatory circadian centre in the mouse dorsal vagal complex. *Communications Biology*, 3, 225. https://doi.org/10.1038/s42003-020-0960-y

Chung, S., Lee, E., Yun, S., Choe, H., Park, S., Son, H., Kim, K., Dluzen, D., Lee, I., Hwang, O., Son, G., & Kim, K. (2014). Impact of circadian nuclear receptor REV-ERBA on midbrain dopamine production and mood regulation. *Cell*, 157, 858–868.

Clayton, D.J., Mode, W.J.A., & Slater, T. (2020) Optimising intermittent fasting: Evaluating the behavioural and metabolic effects of extended morning and evening fasting. *Nutrition Bulletin*, 45(4), 444–455.

Coll, A., Farooqi, I., & O'Rahilly, S. (2007). The hormonal control of food intake. *Cell*, 129, 251–262.

Cornelissen, G., & Otsuka, K. (2017). Chronobiology of aging: A minireview. *Gerontology*, 63(2), 118–128.

Cui, L., & Dyball, R. (1996). Synaptic input from the retina to the suprachiasmatic nucleus changes with the light-dark cycle in the Syrian hamster. *Journal of Physiology*, 497, 483–493.

Dai, J., Swaab, D., & Buijs, R. (1997). Distribution of vasopressin and vasoactive intestinal polypeptide (VIP) fibres in the human hypothalamus with special emphasis on suprachiasmatic nucleus efferent projections. *The Journal of Comparative Neurology*, 383, 397–414.

Darzi, J., Al Khatib, H., & Pot, G.K. (2017). Sleep patterns in relation to dietary patterns and cardio-metabolic risk: An update from Drummond pump priming award recipients. *Nutrition Bulletin*, 42(2), 148–152.

Dashti, H.S., Follis, J.L., Smith, C.E., Tanaka, T., Garaulet, M., Gottlieb, D.J. et al. (2015a). Gene-environment interactions of circadian-related genes for cardiometabolic traits. *Diabetes Care*, 38(8), 1456–1466.

Dashti, H.S., Scheer, F.A., Jacques, P.F., Lamon-Fava, S., & Ordovás, J.M. (2015b). Short sleep duration and dietary intake: Epidemiologic evidence, mechanisms, and health implications. *Advances in Nutrition*, 6(6), 648–659.

de Cabo, R., & Mattson, M.P. (2019) Effects of intermittent fasting on health, aging, and disease. *New England Journal of Medicine*, 381(26), 2541–2551.

Depner, C.M., Stothard, E.R., & Wright, K.P. (2014). Metabolic consequences of sleep and circadian disorders. *Current Diabetes Reports*, 14(7), 507.

DePoy, L., McClung, C., & Logan, R. (2017). Neural mechanisms of circadian regulation of natural and drug reward. *Neural Plasticity*, 1–14. https://doi.org/10.1155/2017/5720842

Druiven, S.J.M., Hovenkamp-Hermelink, J.H.M., Knapen, S.E., Kamphuis, J., Haarman, B.C.M., Penninx, B.W.J.H. et al. (2020). Stability of chronotype over a 7-year follow-up period and its association with severity of depressive and anxiety symptoms. *Depression and Anxiety*, 37(5), 466–474.

Duffy, J.F., Zitting, K.M., & Chinoy, E.D. (2015). Aging and circadian rhythms. *Sleep Medicine Clinics*, 10, 423–434.

Edinburgh, R.M., Betts, J.A., Burns, S.F., & Gonzalez, J.T. (2017). Concordant and divergent strategies to improve postprandial glucose and lipid metabolism. *Nutrition Bulletin*, 42(2), 113–122.

Feillet, C., Bainier, C., Mateo, M., Blancas-Velázquez, A., Salaberry, N., Ripperger, J., Albrecht, U., & Mendoza, J. (2015). Rev-erbA modulates the hypothalamic orexinergic system to influence pleasurable feeding behaviour in mice. *Addiction Biology*, 22, 411–422. https://doi.org/10.1111/adb.12339.

Flanagan, A., Bechtold, D.A., Pot, G.K., & Johnston, J.D. (2020). Chrono-nutrition: From molecular and neuronal mechanisms to human epidemiology and timed feeding patterns. *Journal of Neurochemistry*, 157(1), 53–72.

Garaulet, M., & Gómez-Abellán, P. (2014). Timing of food intake and obesity: A novel association. *Physiology & Behavior*, 134, 44–50.

Garaulet, M., Gomez-Abellan, P., Alburquerque-Bejar, J.J., Lee, Y.-C., Ordovás, J.M., & Scheer, F.A.J.L. (2013). Timing of food intake predicts weight loss effectiveness. *International Journal of Obesity*, 37(4), 604–611.

Gerda, K.P. (2021). Chrono-nutrition – an emerging, modifiable risk factor for chronic disease? *Nutrition Bulletin*, 46, 114–119.

Gibson, R. (2018). Working hours and cardiometabolic health – an emerging area of nutritional research. *Nutrition Bulletin*, 43(3), 255–261.

Gibson-Moore, H., & Chambers, L. (2019) Sleep matters: Can a good night's sleep help tackle the obesity crisis? *Nutrition Bulletin*, 44(2), 123–129.

Green, C.B., Takahashi, J.S., & Bass, J. (2008) The meter of metabolism. *Cell*, 134(5), 728–742.

Grill, H., & Hayes, M. (2012). Hindbrain neurons as an essential hub in the neuroanatomically distributed control of energy balance. *Cell Metabolism*, 16, 296–309. https://doi.org/10.1016/j.cmet.2012.06.015

Guilding, C., Hughes, A., Brown, T., Namvar, S., & Piggins, H. (2009). A riot of rhythms: Neuronal and glial circadian oscillators in the mediobasal hypothalamus. *Molecular Brain Research*, 2, 28. https://doi.org/10.1186/1756-6606-2-28

Herichová, I., Mravec, B., Stebelová, K., Križanová, O., Jurkovičová, D., Kvetňanský, R., & Zeman, M. (2006). Rhythmic clock gene expression in heart, kidney and some brain nuclei involved in blood pressure control in hypertensive TGR(mREN-2)27 rats. *Molecular and Cellular Biochemistry*, 296, 25–34.

Jakubowicz, D., Barnea, M., Wainstein, J., & Froy, O. (2013). High caloric intake at breakfast vs. dinner differentially influences weight loss of overweight and obese women. *Obesity*, 21(12), 2504–2512.

Johnston, J.D. (2014). Physiological responses to food intake throughout the day. *Nutrition Research Reviews*, 27(1), 107–118.

Kalra, S., & Kalra, P. (2004). NPY and cohorts in regulating appetite, obesity and metabolic syndrome: Beneficial effects of gene therapy. *Neuropeptides*, 38, 201–211.

Kalsbeek, A., Palm, I., La Fleur, S., Scheer, F., Perreau-Lenz, S., Ruiter, M., Kreier, F., Cailotto, C., & Buijs, R. (2006). SCN outputs and the hypothalamic balance of life. *Journal of Biological Rhythms*, 21, 458–469.

Kaneko, N., & Sawamoto, K. (2009). Adult neurogenesis and its alteration under pathological conditions. *Neuroscience Research*, 63, 155–164.

Koch, C. E., Begemann, K., Kiehn, J. T., Griewahn, L., Mauer, J., Hess, M. E., Moser, A., Schmid, S. M., Brüning, J. C., & Oster, H. (2020). Circadian regulation of hedonic appetite in mice by clocks in dopaminergic neurons of the VTA. *Nature Communication*, 11, 3071. https://doi.org/10.1038/s41467-020-16882-6

Lenard, N., & Berthoud, H. (2008). Central and peripheral regulation of food intake and physical activity: Pathways and genes. *Obesity*, 16, S11–S22.

Lynch, S., Johnston, J.D., & Robertson, M.D. (2021). Early versus late time-restricted feeding in adults at increased risk of developing type 2 diabetes: Is there an optimal time to eat for metabolic health? *Nutrition Bulletin*, 46(1), 69–76.

Martínez-Lozano, N., Tvarijonaviciute, A., Ríos, R., Barón, I., Scheer, F.A.J.L., & Garaulet, M. (2020). Late eating is associated with obesity, inflammatory markers and circadian-related disturbances in school-aged children. *Nutrients*, 12(9), 2881.

Mazri, F.H., Manaf, Z.A., Shahar, S., & Ludin, A.F.M. (2020). The association between chronotype and dietary pattern among adults: A scoping review. *International Journal of Environmental Research and Public Health*, 17(1), 68.

Merikanto, I., & Partonen, T. (2020). Increase in eveningness and insufficient sleep among adults in population-based crosssections from 2007 to 2017. *Sleep Medicine*, 75, 368–379.

Mistlberger, R., & Antle, M. (2011). Entrainment of circadian clocks in mammals by arousal and food. *Essays in Biochemistry*, 49, 119–136. https://doi.org/10.1042/bse0490119

Moon, S., Kang, J., Kim, S.H., Chung, H.S., Kim, Y.J., Yu, J.M. et al. (2020) Beneficial effects of time-restricted eating on metabolic diseases: A systemic review and meta-analysis. *Nutrients*, 12(5), 1267.

Morton, G., Meek, T., & Schwartz, M. (2014). Neurobiology of food intake in health and disease. *Nature Reviews Neuroscience*, 15, 367–378.

Murray, G., Allen, N., & Trinder, J. (2002). Mood and the circadian system: Investigation of a circadian component in positive affect. *Chronobiology International*, 19, 1151–1169.

Paul, S., Hanna, L., Harding, C., Hayter, E., Walmsley, L., Bechtold, D., & Brown, T. (2020). Output from VIP cells of the mammalian central clock regulates daily physiological rhythms. *Nature Communications*, 11, 1453. https://doi.org/10.1038/s41467-020-15277-x.

Pizinger, T.M., Aggarwal, B. & St-Onge, M.-P. (2018). Sleep extension in short sleepers: An evaluation of feasibility and effectiveness for weight management and cardiometabolic disease prevention. *Frontiers in Endocrinology*, 18(9), 392.

Pot, G.K., Almoosawi, S., & Stephen, A.M. (2016). Meal irregularity and cardio-metabolic consequences: Results from observational and intervention studies. *Proceedings of the Nutrition Society*, 75(4), 1–14.

Reutrakul, S., & Knutson, K.L. (2015). Consequences of circadian disruption on cardiometabolic health. *Sleep Medicine Clinics*, 10(4), 455–468.

Rivera-Estrada, D., Aguilar-Roblero, R., Alva-Sánchez, C., & Villanueva, I. (2018). The homeostatic feeding response to fasting is under chronostatic control. *Chronobiology International*, 35, 1680–1688. https://doi.org/10.1080/07420528.2018.1507036

Roenneberg, T., Kuehnle, T., Juda, M., Kantermann, T., Allebrandt, K., Gordijn, M. et al. (2007). Epidemiology of the human circadian clock. *Sleep Medicine Reviews*, 11(6), 429–438.

Ruddick-Collins, L.C., Johnston, J.D., Morgan, P.J., & Johnstone, A.M. (2018). The Big breakfast study: Chrono-nutrition influence on energy expenditure and bodyweight. *Nutrition Bulletin*, 43(2), 174–183.

Silver, R., LeSauter, J., Tresco, P., & Lehman, M. (1996). A diffusible coupling signal from the transplanted suprachiasmatic nucleus controlling circadian locomotor rhythms. *Nature*, 382, 810–813.

St-Onge, M.-P., Ard, J., Baskin, M.L., Chiuve, S.E., Johnson, H.M., Kris-Etherton, P. et al. (2017). Meal timing and frequency: Implications for cardiovascular disease prevention: A scientific statement from the American Heart Association. *Circulation*, 135(9), e96–e121.

Sun, X., Whitefield, S., Rusak, B., & Semba, K. (2001). Electrophysiological analysis of suprachiasmatic nucleus projections to the ventrolateral preoptic area in the rat. *European Journal of Neuroscience*, 14, 1257–1274. https://doi.org/10.1046/j.0953-816x.2001.0001755.x

Tahara, Y., & Shibata, S. (2013). Chronobiology and nutrition. *Neuroscience*, 253(3), 78–88.

Tan, K., Knight, Z., & Friedman, J. (2014). Ablation of AgRP neurons impairs adaption to restricted feeding. *Molecular Metabolism*, 3, 694–704. https://doi.org/10.1016/j.molmet.2014.07.002

Torres-Castillo, N., Martinez-Lopez, E., Vizmanos-Lamotte, B., & Garaulet, M. (2020). Healthy obese subjects differ in chronotype, sleep habits, and adipose tissue fatty acid composition from their non-healthy counterparts. *Nutrients*, 13(1), 119.

Van Cauter, E., Spiegel, K., Tasali, E., & Leproult, R. (2008). Metabolic consequences of sleep and sleep loss. *Sleep Medicine*, 9(Suppl 1), S23–S28.

Van Someren, E.J. (2000). Circadian rhythms and sleep in human aging. *Chronobiology International*, 17(3), 233–243.

Verwey, M., Dhir, S., & Amir, S. (2016). Circadian influences on dopamine circuits of the brain: Regulation of striatal rhythms of clock gene expression and implications for psychopathology and disease. *F1000 Research*, 5, 2062. https://doi.org/10.12688/f1000research.9180.1

Vincent, G.E., Jay, S.M., Sargent, C., Vandelanotte, C., Ridgers, N.D., & Ferguson, S.A. (2017). Improving cardiometabolic health with diet, physical activity, and breaking up sitting: What about sleep? *Frontiers in Physiology*, 8(8), 865.

Watts, A., Swanson, L., & Sanchez-Watts, G. (1987). Efferent projections of the suprachiasmatic nucleus: I. Studies using anterograde transport of Phaseolus vulgaris leucoagglutinin in the rat. *The Journal of Comparative Neurology*, 258, 204–229. https://doi.org/10.1002/cne.902580204

Williams, K., & Elmquist, J. (2012). From neuroanatomy to behavior: Central integration of peripheral signals regulating feeding behavior. *Nature Neuroscience*, 15, 1350–1355. https://doi.org/10.1038/nn.3217

Xiao, Q., Garaulet, M., & Scheer, F.A.J.L. (2019). Meal timing and obesity: Interactions with macronutrient intake and chronotype. *International Journal of Obesity*, 43, 1701–1711.

Zerón-Rugerio, M.F., Díez-Noguera, A., Izquierdo-Pulido, M., & Cambras, T. (2020). Higher eating frequency is associated with lower adiposity and robust circadian rhythms: A cross-sectional study. *The American Journal of Clinical Nutrition*, 113(1), 17–27.

Zhou, Q., Zhang, M., & Hu, D. (2019). Dose-response association between sleep duration and obesity risk: A systematic review and meta-analysis of prospective cohort studies. *Sleep and Breathing*, 23(4), 1035–1045.

19 Nutritional Approach to the Treatment of Metabolic Co-Morbidity

Ebenezer I. O. Ajayi, Olorunfemi R. Molehin,
Alaba A. Adebayo, Adeniyi S. Ohunayo, Mariam
A. Odebode, and Jacinta O. Okonkwo

19.1 INTRODUCTION

Aging and having a high body-mass index (BMI) have both risen to the top of the list of conditions associated with some type(s) of chronic metabolic disorder(s), such as obesity, diabetes, hypertension, liver abnormalities, cardiovascular disease, and metabolic syndrome, all of which commonly coexist (Schwarz *et al.*, 2018). Having a high body-mass index (BMI) (isolated/healthy obesity) does not totally indicate a morbid obesity condition, since fatal events of obesity have been reported to be mediated by other metabolic comorbid conditions (Ul-Haq *et al.*, 2012). Moreso, there are recent reports of individuals with normal BMIs diagnosed with morbid obesity while metabolically healthy individuals are confirmed with high BMIs (Ul-Haq *et al.*, 2012; Pujia *et al.*, 2022). Overall, obesity is indicated by higher BMI value (> 30 kg/m^2) that correlates with increased intra-abdominal fat and waist-length; it has been reported as a metabolic disorder that independently increases the risk of several metabolic comorbidities, impaired health, and death (Gisondi *et al.*, 2020; Branisteanu *et al.*, 2022). Globally, obesity has become a thorn in the side for health policy makers, physicians, and the public, considering the triple boom in its occurrence for the past five decades (NCD Risk Factor Collaboration, 2017; Pujia *et al.*, 2022). Within this period, the prevalence of severe obesity increased by 42% – equivalent to about 700 million adults (Hales *et al.*, 2020) – and the number of adults with obesity is projected to be 1.12 billion by 2030 (Kelly *et al.*, 2008; Pujia *et al.*, 2022). The recent and future surge in the prevalence of obesity represents those reported for other metabolic comorbidities (Forouhi *et al.*, 2018; Ojo, 2019; Branisteanu *et al.*, 2022). There is therefore an urgent need for a remedy to reverse and stop the trend worldwide.

There is growing evidence that behavior or modifiable lifestyle is central to other major genetic, physiological, and environmental factors that predispose people (aging and overweight) to chronic disease(s) and/or comorbidities (Ojo, 2019). Therefore, multidimensional approaches are required to manage or treat the metabolic comorbidities associated with these conditions, especially when diagnosed early. Nutrition (diet), which is a key player in behavior and/or lifestyle modification, can therefore be explored to increase the chances of treatment and/or management of several metabolic comorbidities. A study by the Global Burden of Disease Study on 188 countries reportedly associated diet with major morbidity and mortality in the world (Forouzanfar *et al.*, 2015). The effect of nutrition on weight and metabolic control in prevention, treatment, and/or management of obesity and consequent comorbidities has recently been established (Forouhi *et al.*, 2018). However, there are controversies and challenges relating to sustainability, individual-specific terms, and maintaining quality of health over the nutritional approach to treating comorbidities such as obesity. The nutritional approach to treatment of comorbidity requires a holistic consideration of factors such as efficiency, safety, affordability, nutritional value, long-term adherence, sustainability, and food preference.

DOI: 10.1201/9781003361497-21

19.2 COMMON METABOLIC CO-MORBIDITIES AND THEIR PATHOPHYSIOLOGY

Metabolic comorbidity, in this context, is a health-related condition consisting of one or more of the following morbidities associated with obesity, which, in most cases, coexist. Generally, severe obesity with proinflammatory cytokines and adipokines, if coupled with insulin resistance and some dysfunctions, heightens the risk of different metabolic comorbidities, including diabetes, hypertension, psoriasis/psoriatic arthritis, chronic cancer, liver abnormalities, atherogenic dyslipidemia, metabolic syndrome, and cardiovascular disease (Ul-Haq *et al.*, 2012; Gisondi *et al.*, 2018; Schwarz *et al.*, 2018; Yamazaki, 2021; Branisteanu *et al.*, 2022; Pujia *et al.*, 2022). Obesity is a phenomenon that is common with each morbid condition, which involves continuous (T-cell-mediated) release of inflammatory properties (such as adiponectin, leptin, IL-6, chemerin, TNF-A, fibrinogen, CRP, resistin, and PAI-1), plays major role in stimulating insulin resistance, vascular dysfunction, dysglycemia, and dyslipidemia, which enhance the onset of other metabolic comorbidities (Gottlieb *et al.*, 2008; Yamazaki, 2021; Branisteanu *et al.*, 2022).

19.2.1 OBESITY

Obesity is a chronic metabolic disease affecting a majority in the world. The level of BMI, measured by dividing the weight (kg) of an individual by their height (m^2), which indicates the amount of body fat, is a measure for obesity (Elmet *et al.*, 2019). Several factors such as modifiable lifestyle or behavior, genetics, physiology, and environment are associated with the morbidity (Ojo, 2019). Increased intra-abdominal fat (visceral adiposity) and waist-length and increased waist circumference are indications of obesity with a high risk of several metabolic comorbidities, like type 2 diabetes mellitus, hypertension, cardiovascular disease, stroke, sleep apnea, cancer, metabolic syndrome, atherogenic dyslipidemia, alcoholic steatohepatitis, osteoarthritis, and psoriasis, which, consequently, shorten life expectancy (Ul-Haq *et al.*, 2012; Gisondi *et al.*, 2020). Prevalence of severe obesity among adults is on the high side, resulting from consumption of a diet with excess calories (high sugar, fat, and salt), which is inverse with the rate of energy consumption, leading to an accumulation of energy in form of fat (Jensen and Skov, 2016). Pathophysiology of obesity and obesity-related comorbidity rely on a high level of serum fatty acids resulting from free fatty acids released through white adipocytes.

Studies have revealed the chances of side effects, like loss of therapeutic responsiveness to methotrexate, when treating obesity-related comorbidities with systemic and biological approaches. Moreover, during systemic therapy, obesity increased the level of cyclosporine, a lipophilic medication, in the serum, leading to aggravated nephrotoxicity in overweight or obese patients (Branisteanu *et al.*, 2022).

19.2.2 DIABETES

Diabetes is a metabolic disorder characterized by elevated level of sugar in the blood (hyperglycemia) due to insufficient release and activity of insulin in the body. A glycated hemoglobin (HbA1c) level of ≥ 48 mmol/mol for over 6-10 weeks, a plasma glucose concentration of ≥ 200 mg/dl, high fasting plasma-glucose level of ≥ 126 mg/dl, and a 2-hour post-load glucose level of ≥ 200 mg/dl are reliable symptoms of diabetes mellitus (Seino *et al.*, 2010). As an obesity-related comorbidity, diabetes mellitus serves as a risk factor for other metabolic comorbidities, like metabolic syndrome, cardiovascular events, liver impairment, and psoriasis (Radtke *et al.*, 2015). Excessive hepatic glucose release, insulin resistance in the liver and muscle tissue, and distorted pancreatic insulin secretion are the pathophysiological basis of diabetes mellitus (Branisteanu *et al.*, 2022). For instance, Brazelli *et al.* (2021) reported that a proinflammatory cytokine (TNF-A), which reduces the activity of tyrosine kinase of the insulin receptor, is an important pathogenetic factor linking type 2 diabetes and psoriasis.

19.2.3 Psoriasis

Psoriasis is an immune-mediated disease caused by inflammation, resulting from increasing kera-tinocyte (red plaques with silvery-white scales) on the skin (especially elbow, knees, and scalp) and other integumentary systems (Puig, 2017). Although it can affect individuals of any age and gender, psoriasis is dominant among those between 15 and 30 years of age (Jensen and Skov, 2016). Psoriasis is an inflammation characterized by the proliferation of subpopulations of Th-17, Th-22, and Th-1 cells and is mediated by T-cells, causing the lymphocytes and keratinocytes of the skin to release proinflammatory mediators (such as IL-1, IL-6, TNF-A, IFN-γ, IL-17, IL-22, IL-23, and VEGF) (Branisteanu et al., 2022). The mediators are capable of invading the systemic circulation to cause different inflammatory conditions (such as hypercoagulation, insulin resistance, increased oxidative stress, circulatory endothelial dysfunction, and increased angiogenesis), which exerts pro-atherogenic effects and also aids comorbidity conditions such as obesity (Von Stebut et al., 2020; Branisteanu et al., 2022). However, the pathophysiology of psoriasis is dependent on genetic factors and immune dysfunction coupled with environmental factors like medications, infections, and psychological stress. Furthermore, beneficial (reverse cholesterol-transport, antioxidant, and anti-inflammatory) properties attributed to high-density lipoprotein (HDL) cholesterol, through regulated dendritic cell, T-cell, and IL-12 functions, are affected (Yamazaki, 2021).

Although, insulin resistance/type 2 diabetes is mostly reported as a risk factor associated with psoriasis (Gottlieb et al., 2008), the most significant risk factor for the onset of several comorbidi-ties, including type 2 diabetes, is severe obesity (Jensen and Skov, 2016; Branisteanu et al., 2022).

19.2.4 Atherogenic Dyslipidemia

Atherogenic dyslipidemia is also a metabolic comorbidity caused by increased concentration of triglyceride and low-density lipoprotein cholesterol (LDL) in plasma and insufficient concentration of HDL cholesterol in serum (Branisteanu et al., 2022). Several studies have reported atherogenic dyslipidemia as associated with other metabolic comorbidities (Gottlieb and Dann, 2009; Ghafoor et al., 2015; Branisteanu et al., 2022). These altered plasma lipid concentrations were often observed in patients with atherogenic dyslipidemia when associated with comorbidities such as psoriasis, implicating the apolipoprotein E gene polymorphism, recorded for hyperlipidemia, observed in psoriasis (Ghafoor et al., 2015).

19.3 METABOLIC SYNDROME

Metabolic syndrome is a metabolic disorder consisting of such manifestations as visceral obesity, insulin resistance, dyslipidemia, and hypertension, making it a major risk factor for cardiovascular diseases (Schwarz et al., 2018). Having more than three of the following criteria – increased waist-length, high blood pressure ($\geq$ 130/85 mmHg), $\geq$ 5.6 mmol/l of fasting plasma glucose, $\geq$ 1.7 mmol/l of triglyceride, and < 1.0 mmol/l of HDL cholesterol in men (or < 1.3 mmol/l in women) – is an indi-cation of suspected metabolic syndrome for clinical diagnosis (Yamazaki, 2021). Elevated systemic inflammation, serving as the key pathophysiology of metabolic syndrome, like in other comorbidi-ties, relies on genetic components, immune dysfunction, environmental factors like smoking, and psychological conditions (Gisondi et al., 2018).

19.4 TRIPLE BURDEN OF OBESITY, DIABETES, AND HYPERTENSION

The rapid increase in the prevalence of obesity, diabetes, and hypertension together as a burden, labelled "triple burden", is a major challenge facing low- and middle-income countries (Mawaw et al., 2017). "Triple burden", in this context, is used to describe the comorbidity of hypertension, diabetes, and obesity, a term which is a level above the "double burden" that connotes coexistence of any two of the three comorbidities described by Al-Zubayer et al. (2021). Despite how threatening both double and triple burdens have relatively become to the global health quality and the attainment of sustainable developmental goals, research on the prevalence is quite scanty. Apparently, the concurrence of these comorbidities is the leading risk factor for non-communicable diseases, which have reportedly been responsible for 41 million deaths, projected to have risen to 52 million deaths worldwide by 2030 (Bigna and Noubiap, 2019; Vos et al., 2020; Al-Zubayer et al., 2021). Although, triple burden is associated with different risk factors, including biomedical, socio-demographic, occupational, anthropometric, and behavioral factors (Mawaw et al., 2017), including malnutrition, smoking, excessive alcohol, high salt and fat intake, among others, remain the leading risk factor (Lim et al., 2012; Mawaw et al., 2017). Furthermore, a recent study has reported that aged, female, married, wealthy, well-educated, and socio-economically high adults are highly vulnerable to non-communicable diseases associated with the triple burden, including cancer, chronic respiratory disease, and cardiovascular disease, among others (Al-Zubayer et al., 2021).

19.5 ROLE OF METABOLIC CO-MORBIDITY IN HEALTH-RELATED QUALITY OF LIFE

Beyond clinical events, quality of health encompasses physical, emotional, and psychological well-being, among others. Obesity is a metabolic morbid condition that is not only associated with and/or attracts several chronic comorbidities but also deteriorates the physical state (with increased intra-abdominal fat [visceral adiposity] and waist-length) of an individual. There is, though, growing evidence that high BMI, or overweightness, directly connotes neither a morbid obesity condition nor altered health quality. The major factor that plays the middle role, which automatically mediates a secondary condition (altered quality of health), is the development of morbidity and/or comorbidity conditions. However, several studies demonstrated that, as the health quality of individuals with metabolic comorbidity were affected, so were those of obese individuals without metabolic comorbidity (Garcia-Mandizabel et al., 2009; Castres et al., 2010; Ul-Haq et al., 2012). Similarly, some obese individuals (labeled "healthy obesity") do not develop these intermediate conditions, placing them at no risk of cardiometabolic events or metabolic comorbidity condition (Wildman, 2009), but their health quality did not improve through weight-loss therapy (Wildman, 2009; Velho et al., 2010). This is largely due to the fact that the studies categorically considered only obese individuals; and the risk of cardiometabolic conditions and impaired health were not previously known, in the clinical perspective, to be specific or not to obese individuals with metabolic comorbidity.

Historically, the risks of type 2 diabetes and cardiovascular diseases were lower for individuals with normal weight, and they enjoy good quality of health (Fortaine and Barofsky, 2001), but this has changed over time, as different studies have reported poor quality of health among individuals with a low BMI (Hoopman et al., 2007; Sach et al., 2007; Wee et al., 2008). Individuals with metabolic comorbidity were reported by Ul-Haq et al. (2012) with poor quality of health, compare to those without, irrespective of their BMI. Therefore, the consensus of the World Health Organization, which reported that the risk of cardiometabolic conditions attributed to obesity is mediated, significantly, by the onset of intermediate metabolic comorbidity such as hypertension, diabetes, and hypercholesterolemia (WHO, 2000), is consistent.

19.6 DIETARY INTERVENTION TO MANAGE/TREAT METABOLIC CO-MORBIDITY

Considering the role of modifiable lifestyle in the manifestation of these metabolic comorbidities, which stems from the effect of overweightness and/or high BMI attributed to obesity, a dietary approach that is efficient in losing or managing weight can be utilized in managing metabolic comorbidity (Schwarz et al., 2018). Apparently, the start of every chronic morbid condition largely depends on environmental and behavioral factors, especially unhealthy diet, which increases the chance of obesity, a central risk-factor for many other comorbidities. Hence, adoption of a healthy diet and/or weight-loss diet will minimize the risk of developing and combating developed chronic disease, respectively (Forouhi *et al.*, 2018; Ojo, 2019). However, effective nutritional approaches to treating/managing especially obesity-related comorbidity does not undermine knowing the associated morbidities, observing basic precautions, and adopting appropriate supporting therapies and monitoring.

The nutritional approaches that are adoptable for managing weight with the aim to treat or manage some chronic metabolic (especially obesity-related) comorbidity conditions can be categorized under: macronutrient restriction, energy restriction, and an energy-deficit dietary approach (Philpot and Johnson, 2019). Although several diets exhibit weight-loss effects, no single diet can be utilized universally to achieve weight loss. Affordability, sustainability, food preferences, culture, and existing comorbidity should therefore be critically considered when choosing a dietary approach.

19.7 DIETARY APPROACH BY RESTRICTION OF MACRONUTRIENTS

Controlling macronutrient constituents of diet is a nutritional approach that has been well studied and reported, with different outcomes on weight loss and quality of health. Ideally, the three primary macronutrients – carbohydrates, protein, and fat in a diet, respectively – yield 4 kilocalories (kcal), 4 kcal, and 9 kcal of energy per gram. Hence, deliberate alteration of these macronutrients in a diet, even in energy-matched diets, will affect the endocrine and changes the gut microbiomes, which, consequently, has an effect on energy storage in form of fat and body weight (Ludwig and Ebbeling, 2018).

19.7.1 Low-Fat Diet

Low-fat diets are made to strictly consist of just 20 to 35% fat, sometimes as low as ≤ 20% fat in "very-low-fat diet" or a bit ≥ 35% in "moderate-low-fat diet" (Makris and Foster, 2011). Diets modified to contain low fat (with highest energy yield) content have not only been reported for health-promoting and traditional cardioprotective potential; there is also an advocacy of weight loss for this diet (Ge *et al.*, 2020). Typically, a low-fat diet consists of some recommended foods to reduce, such as sodium, added sugar, saturated and trans-fats, refined grains, cholesterol, and alcohol; and foods to increase, such as low-fat dairy and protein foods, fruits, vegetables, whole grains, and oils (Makris and Foster, 2011).

19.7.2 Ornish (Very-Low-Fat) Diet

A typical example of a very-low-fat diet is the Ornish diet, which provides ≤ 20% fat, introduced by Dr. Dean Ornish in 1977 (Makris and Foster, 2011). The Ornish diet is a plant-based diet containing fruits, whole grains, beans, vegetables, and soy; and a relatively low amount of fat content, like fat dairy, egg, lean meats, and fish. Contrary to the low-fat diet plan, complex carbohydrates and a source of fibre are included in Ornish diet, a very-low-fat diet. The Ornish diet plan is best practiced as a lifestyle with resistance training, stress management, and exercise.

19.7.3 Mediterranean Low-Fat Diet

The Mediterranean diet is generally a plant-based diet, rich in fibre, with varying amounts of fat. Although some are reported with higher fat contents of about 47%, the Mediterranean low-fat diet plan containing about 35% fat is an example of a moderate-fat diet (Makris and Foster, 2011). High monounsaturated fatty acids (MUFA), antioxidants, omega-3 polyunsaturated fatty acid (n-3 PUFA), and micronutrients, and low saturated fat, glycemic load, and omega-6 polyunsaturated fatty acid (n-6 PUFA) are also typical attributes of a Mediterranean low-fat diet that enhance cardioprotective and health-promoting benefits (Esposito *et al.*, 2011).

Several meta-analyses and randomized studies have evaluated and demonstrated different efficacy, health effects, and sustainability of low-fat dietary approaches in relation to managing and/or
treating obesity and reducing risk factors for chronic metabolic comorbities (Makris and Foster,
2005; Svetkey *et al.*, 2008; Barnard *et al.*, 2009; Wing, 2010; Jenkins *et al.*, 2010; Makris and
Foster, 2011; Tobias *et al.*, 2015; Ge *et al.*, 2020). Overall, the Mediterranean low-fat diet plan has
been reported with better weight loss with long term results (especially when supported with energy
restriction and physical activity) and reduced risk of developing diabetes, metabolic syndrome, atherogenic dyslipidemia, and coronary heart disease (Shai *et al.*, 2008; Esposito *et al.*, 2011). However,
there is yet to be any established evidence to prove the superiority of this dietary approach over
other dietary interventions, due partly to several factors, including high attrition, low acceptability,
and poor adherence, among others (Jenkins *et al.*, 2010; Makris and Foster, 2011; Tobias *et al.*, 2015;
Ge *et al.*, 2020).

19.7.4 Low-Carbohydrate Diet

There is no distinct definition of the low-carbohydrate diet due to variation in the in-take of this macronutrient by location; hence, several versions of the low-carbohydrate exist. A low-carbohydrate
diet, as the name implies, is a plant-based diet that often consists of low (but gradually increasing)
carbohydrate (from whole grain, low glycemic vegetables), low glycemic index, high fibre, and relatively higher fat (about 60% fat) (from meat and fish) (Makris and Foster, 2011). The low-glycemic
index of this diet mediates in-take of adequate energy and nutrients, reducing insulin spikes (regulatory bursts) and blood glucose levels. This attribute (GI index), coupled with the nutritional quality
of low-carbohydrates, especially the high fat content, serves as the basis for a wide recommendation
of the dietary approach.

19.7.5 Atkins Diet

A typical example of a low-carbohydrate diet is the Atkins diet, introduced by Dr. Robert Atkins,
which does not have any restriction to fat and protein content. Furthermore, 20 to 35% of the energy
in the Atkins diet is from protein content, which contributes to increased total energy expenditure,
improved glycemic ratio, satiety, triglycerides, and HDL (Moon and Koh, 2020).

A previous study by Nordmann *et al.* (2006) could not observe significant difference in weight
loss effect between low-carbohydrate and low-fat dietary interventions, but significant reduction of
body weight, triglycerides, and fat, has been reported with low-carbohydrate diets compare to low-
fat diets (Mansoor *et al.*, 2016). Low glucose composition of the diet tends to trigger gluconeogen-
esis and insulin secretion, which stimulates lipolysis and glycemic index balance, which has been
demonstrated to improve obesity (on a short-term basis) and overall health and reduce risk of some
metabolic comorbidities, like diabetes and metabolic syndrome (Mansoor *et al.*, 2016; Wood *et al.*,
2016). Long-term sustainability of the low-carbohydrate dietary approach has not been established,
which could be attributed to concerns of cardiovascular disease-risk associated with increase LDL
through this approach. Moreso, the diet is disadvantaged by the adverse effect of its low fibre and
high fat content on gut microbiome and bowel health (Wood *et al.*, 2016). However, long-term, sustainable weight loss and health-promotion has been reportedly associated with a plant-based diet
consisting of relatively higher carbohydrates, low glycemic index, and resulting in lower satiety,
increased fat accumulation, and frequent insulin secretory bursts (Turner-McGrievy *et al.*, 2017).

19.7.6 High-Protein Diet

Diets containing more than 25% total energy or 1.6 g/kg body weight per day are considered as
high-protein diets. A typical high-protein diet contains low fat, which differentiates it from a low-
carbohydrate diet (Makris and Foster, 2011).

19.7.7 Paleolithic Diet

Paleolithic diet, a similar dietary pattern (involving a hunting and gathering lifestyle), adopted by the ancestors before agriculture, is a typical example of a high-protein diet. Although it varies according to geographical region with different climates and available food, the paleolithic diet is a plant-based diet consisting of legumes, vegetables, whole foods, fruits, seeds, meat, and fish (Cordain et al., 2005). The diet primarily consists of high protein (yielding 25% to 35% energy), moderate fat, and minimally processed carbohydrates (with low glycemic index) (O'keefe et al., 2010).

Significant weight loss and improved blood lipids and physical body structure with normal, lean body-mass; decreased waist circumference, intra-abdominal adipose tissue, and waist-to-hip ratio have been relatively associated with a high-protein diet over a low-fat diet in different studies (Makris and Foster, 2005; Wycherley et al., 2010; Anton et al., 2017). Although, overall, safety and long-term sustainability due to lack of adherence is still questionable, the paleolithic diet has been reported as promising in weight loss, improving insulin sensitivity, and reducing risk of comorbidities like diabetes, metabolic syndrome, and cardiovascular disease (Wycherley et al., 2010; Makris and Foster, 2011; Anton et al., 2017).

19.7.8 Vegetarian Diet

There has been an increase in the adoption rate of the vegetarian diet, which is often used to augment the efficiency of either macronutrient restriction or energy restriction dietary intervention in treating obesity and reducing the risk of other comorbidities. Among the popular vegetarian dietary approaches are the Vegan diet, which consists strictly of plant-based nutrients, without adding egg, meat, fish or dairy; the Lacto-Ovo diet, which contains eggs and dairy, together with the plant-based nutrients; and the Pescatarian diet, which consists of plants and fish (Huang et al., 2016).

A study demonstrated relatively significant weight loss with vegetarian diets, especially when augmented with energy restriction, over nonvegetarian diets and vegetarian diets without energy restriction. Better efficiency of Vegan diets over Lacto-Ovo diets in weight loss is also established (Huang et al., 2016).

19.8 DIETARY APPROACH BY TIME-BASED ENERGY RESTRICTION

Calorie restriction based on reduced energy intake is another dietary mechanism that has been reportedly effective in weight reduction and promotion of health-related quality of life as well as stimulation of factors that reduce the risk of chronic metabolic comorbidity. Several systemic benefits, such as increased insulin sensitivity, reduced oxidative stress, reduced inflammatory markers, decreased mitochondrial free radical production, which contribute to the control of glucose and blood pressure and reduce risk of hypertension and cardiovascular disease, have been associated with a calorie-restriction dietary approach (Merry, 2004; Scheer et al., 2009; Catenacci et al., 2016; Dong et al., 2020). Calorie restriction has also been reported with the potential of slowing down the progress of neurodegenerative diseases like Parkinson's and Alzheimer's disease (Calabrese et al., 2008) and changing the pace of aging by modulating Sirtuin1 (SIRT1) in adipose tissue, which reduces fat storage and resets hormonal levels (Martin et al., 2006).

19.8.1 Intermittent Fasting

Intermittent fasting is a dietary approach that depends on calorie restriction based on fasting periods, without any macronutrient restriction. The fasting periods may be on alternate days or restricted eating times, when eating will be at a stipulated time only (Dong et al., 2020). Intermittent fasting stimulates the optimization of circadian rhythm and ketogenesis, which consequently reduces the risk of several metabolic comorbidities (Scheer et al., 2009).

Studies have demonstrated a long-term effect of intermittent fasting with an energy-restriction approach on weight loss and control over metabolic comorbidities like obesity, metabolic syndrome, diabetes, hypertension, and cardiovascular disease. This can be attributed to the fact that adherence and compliance to the dietary plan is highly sustainable, especially when mild calorie restriction is adopted with changes in feeding frequency (Dong *et al.*, 2020).

19.8.2 DIETARY APPROACH BY CALORIE-DEFICIT

The principle behind weight loss and health promotion by the calorie-deficit approach is based on creating a negative energy deficit through physiological adaptation to reduced energy expenditure due to restricted carbohydrate and fat content of the diet (Parretti *et al.*, 2016).

19.8.3 LOW-CALORIE DIET AND VERY-LOW-CALORIE DIET

Low-calorie diets with 1,000 to 1,500 kcal/day and very-low-calorie diets consisting of ≤ 800 kcal/day are major examples of calorie deficit dietary approaches, which rely on "calories-in-calories-out" principle. Very-low-calorie diets with varying compositions of energy (600 to 800 kcal/day), carbohydrate (< 30 to 50 g/day) and appropriate protein intake (0.8 to 1.2g/day) per ideal body weight (kg), also called "very-low-calorie ketogenic diet" (VLCKD), can be used for short periods of time before transiting to a low-calorie diet (Parretti *et al.*, 2016).

In a recent study, very-low-calorie diets, augmented with behavioral programs, were reported to result in significant weight loss and improved blood pressure, total cholesterol, and triglycerides over a short period of 2 years without changes in LDL and HDL levels (Castellana *et al.*, 2021). It is quite disadvantageous that long-term sustainability of weight loss and quality of health by the low-calorie diet is not guaranteed; and adoption of a very-low-calorie diet requires medical supervision.

19.9 MEAL REPLACEMENTS

A dietary approach that involves replacement of one or more meals to create negative energy deficit has gained popularity in the recent times due to its convenience. Although the calorie content of such food is under/overestimated, several commercial products with varying cost are available to achieve this dietary plan.

A recent review study comparatively reported average weight loss ranging from -2.2 to -6.13 kg with meal the replacement approach over other dietary approaches that required support alone (Astbury *et al.*, 2019). Long-term sustainability of weight loss with meal replacement is not, however, attainable, partly due to physiological adaptations that reduce energy expenditure (Astbury *et al.*, 2019).

19.10 MOLECULAR MECHANISM UNDERLYING THE DIETARY INTERVENTION IN MANAGEMENT/TREATMENT OF METABOLIC CO-MORBIDITY

Consumption of animal-based diets and plant-based diets both have nutritional benefits. Many nutritionists believe that cutting down on animal-based diets while increasing the intake of plant-based foods is fundamental for healthy living. Animal-based products such as processed meats and kinds of beef have been associated with the risk of developing cancer; nevertheless, ingestion of plant-based foods does not necessarily mean there are no pieces of evidence of health hazards. However, diets rich in plant products such as vegetables, fruits, and some grains are healthy to take from a nutritional point of view. Such plant-based products have high fibre composition and low energy density, contributing to the potential of preventing cardiovascular diseases and proper management of body weight (Castro-Barquero *et al.*, 2020). The recent scientific evidence available has shown the relationship between metabolic comorbidity and dietary habits. Researchers have shown many times how dietary patterns could influence healthy living; for example, the Mediterranean diet, which is attributed to people residing in the Mediterranean sea basin, is rich in plant-based products, characterized by frequent intake of vegetables, fruits, nuts, legumes, and various plant extracts, has shown a great deal of promise by preventing health problems of metabolic comorbidity (Franquesa *et al.*, 2019). Diet pattern is gradually becoming a prominent mechanism for treating diseases. A diet full of vegetables, whole grains, low-fat or fat-free dairy products, fruits, and legumes intake, while, at the same time, reducing the intake of red meat and sugar-sweetened beverages, is a dietary approach to stop hypertension while also capable of reducing the incidences of many tragic diseases (Castro-Barquero *et al.*, 2020). Reduction of total carbohydrate intake in diets practically implies a self-imposed restriction on sugar, starchy foods, ultra-processed foods, and refined grains and has been studied to be a good dietary lifestyle. Individuals with a high intake of carbohydrates have been studied to have an increased likelihood to develop comorbidities (Liu *et al.*, 2019). Low carbohydrate diets such as the ketogenic diet are characterized by a reduction in the daily carbohydrate intake (less than 10% daily) and have some therapeutic role in controlling obesity and overweightness (Castro-Barquero *et al.*, 2020). Aside from controlling the intake of carbohydrates, low-fat diets have also been explored to monitor obesity in adults. Dietary interventions based on low-fat or fat-free intake have been significantly explored to reduce the chances of metabolic syndrome.

Dietary interventions to reduce comorbidity diseases are also aimed at ensuring that diet and food taken provide health benefits beyond providing basic nutritional requirements. Functional foods are capable of providing health benefits beyond basic nutrition because they play an important role in the management of metabolic comorbidity. Functional foods have been found to have the potential in regulating body weight and maintaining normal blood pressure while controlling blood lipid and glucose levels. Function foods such as ginger, red pepper, and green tea have a thermogenesis effect where the body heat production increases; functional foods such as curcumin have anti-inflammatory potentials, while cinnamon could increase insulin sensitivity (El Shebini *et al.*, 2018). Fruits such as apple, garlic, and fish are rich in pectin, allium sativum, and omega-3 fatty acids, respectively. Fortified foods with specific nutrients are also types of functional foods that can house elements such as iron, calcium, and zinc, all in fortified forms. Fermented foods are also functional foods because they are rich in pro- and prebiotics (Soliman, 2020)

19.11   CONCLUSION

Owing to poor modifiable lifestyle, some metabolic disorders like obesity develop from mild and reversible health situations like high BMI and increase the risk of several other metabolic comorbidities, impairing health-related quality of life and death. Nutritional approaches involving diets for weight loss are therefore a promising therapy. Overall, intermittent fasting with a mild energy restriction has proven to be more effective in long-term weight loss. This can be attributed to its flexibility, affordability, and sustainability in relation to adherence and compliance with little or no support. Meanwhile, regardless of the dietary approach, plant-based diets that offer a moderate level of glycemic index take the lead among sources of macronutrients.

REFERENCES

Al-Zubayer, M. A., Ahammed, B., Sarder, M. A., Kundu, S., Majumder, U. K., Islam, S. M. S. 2021. Double and triple burden of non-communicable diseases and its determinants among adults in Bangladesh: Evidence from a recent demographic and health survey. *Int J Clin Pract.*, e14613.

Anton, S. D., Hida, A., Heekin, K., Sowalsky, K., Karabetian, C., Mutchie, H., Leeuwenburgh, C., Manini, T. M., Barnett T. E. 2017. Effects of popular diets without specific calorie targets on weight loss outcomes: Systematic review of findings from clinical trials. *Nutrients.* **9**(8).

Astbury, N. M., Piernas, C., Hartmann-Boyce, J., Lapworth, S., Aveyard, P., Jebb, S. A. 2019. A systematic review and meta-analysis of the effectiveness of meal replacements for weight loss. *Obes Rev.*, **20**(4): 569–587.

Barnard, N. D., Gloede, L., Cohen, J., Jenkins, D. J., Turner-McGrievy, G., Green, A. A., Ferdowsian, H. 2009. A low-fat vegan diet elicits greater macronutrient changes, but is comparable in adherence and acceptability, compared with a more conventional diabetes diet among individuals with type 2 diabetes. *J. Am. Diet. Assoc.*, **109**(2): 263–272.

Bigna, J. J., Noubiap, J. J. 2019. The rising burden of non-communicable diseases in sub-Saharan Africa. *Lancet Global Health*, **7**(10): e1295–e1296.

Branisteanu, D. E., Pirvulescu, R. A., Spinu, A. E., Porumb, E. A., Cojocaru, M., Nicolescu, A. C., Branisteanu, D. C., Branisteanu, C. I., Dimitriu, A., Alexa, A. I., Toader, M. P. 2022. Metabolic comorbidities of psoriasis (review). *Exp. Ther. Med*, **23**: 179–186.

Brazzelli, V., Maffioli, P., Bolcato, V., Ciolfi, C., D'Angelo, A., Tinelli, C., Derosa, G. 2021. Psoriasis and diabetes, a dangerous association: Evaluation of insulin resistance, lipid abnormalities, and cardio-vascular risk biomarkers. *Front Med.* (Lausanne) **8**: 605691–605706.

Calabrese, V., Cornelius, C., Mancuso, C., Pennisi, G., Calafato, S., Bellia, F., Bates, T. E., Giuffrida Stella, A. M., Schapira, T., Dinkova Kostova, A. T., Rizzarelli, E. 2008. Cellular stress response: A novel target for chemoprevention and nutritional neuroprotection in aging, neurodegenerative disorders and longevity. *Neurochem Res.* **33**(12): 2444–2471.

Castellana, M., Biacchi, E., Procino, F., Casanueva, F. F., Trimboli, P. (2021). Very-low-calorie ketogenic diet for the management of obesity, overweight and related disorders. *Minerva Endocrinol* (Torino). **46**(2): 161–167.

Castres, I., Folope, V., Dechelotte, P., Tourny-Chollet, C., Lemaitre, F. (2010). Quality of life and obesity class relationships. *Int. J. Sports Med.*, **31**: 773–778.

Castro-Barquero, S., Ruiz-León, A. M., Sierra-Pérez, M., Estruch, R., Casas, R. 2020. Dietary strategies for metabolic syndrome: A comprehensive review. *Nutrients*, **12**(10): 2983.

Catenacci, V. A., Pan, Z., Ostendorf, D., Brannon, S., Gozansky, W. S., Mattson, M. P., Martin, B., MacLean, P. S., Melanson, E. L., Troy-Donahoo, W. A. 2016. Randomized pilot study comparing zero-calorie alternate-day fasting to daily caloric restriction in adults with obesity. *Obesity* (Silver Spring). **24**(9): 1874–1883.

Cordain, L., Eaton, S. B., Sebastian, A., Mann, N., Lindeberg, S., Watkins, B. A., O'Keefe, J. H., Brand-Miller, J. 2005. Origins and evolution of the Western diet: Health implications for the 21st century. *Am. J. Clin. Nutr.*, **81**(2): 341–354.

Dong, T. A., Sandesara, P. B., Dhindsa, D. S., Mehta, A., Arneson, L. C., Dollar, A. L., Taub, P. R., Sperling, L. S. 2020. Intermittent fasting: A heart healthy dietary pattern? *Am. J. Med.*, **133**(8): 901–907.

El Shebini, S., Moaty, M. I., Fouad, S., Ahmed, N. H., Tapozada, S. T. 2018. Obesity related metabolic disorders and risk of renal disease: Impact of hypocaloric diet and Avena sativa supplement. *Maced. J. Med. Sci.*, **6**(8): 1376–1381

Elmets, C. A., Leonardi, C. L., Davis, D. M., Gelfand, J. M., Lichten, J., Mehta, N. N., Armstrong, A. W., Connor, C., Cordoro, K. M., Elewski, B. E. 2019. Joint AAD-NPF guidelines of care for the management and treatment of psoriasis with awareness and attention to comorbidities. *J. Am. Acad. Dermatol.*, **80**: 1073-1113.

Esposito, K., Kastorini, C. M., Panagiotakos, D. B., Giugliano, D. 2011. Mediterranean diet and weight loss: Meta-analysis of randomized controlled trials. *Metab. Syndr. Relat. Disord.*, **9**(1): 1–12. [PubMed: 20973675]

Fontaine, K. R., Barofsky, I. 2001. Obesity and health-related quality of life. *Obes. Rev.*, **2**: 173–182.

Forouhi, N. G., Krauss, R. M., Taubes, G., Willet, W. 2018. Dietary fat and cardiometabolic health: Evidence, controversies, and consensus for guidance. *BMJ.*, **361**: k2139.

Forouzanfar, M. H., Alexander, L., Anderson, H. R. 2015. GBD 2013 risk factors collaborators: Global, regional, and national comparative risk assessment of 79 behavioural, environmental and occupational, and metabolic risks or clusters of risks in 188 countries, 1990–2013: A systematic analysis for the global burden of disease study. *Lancet*, **386**: 2287–323.

Franquesa, M., Pujol-Busquets, G., García-Fernández, E., Rico, L., Shamirian-Pulido, L., Aguilar-Martínez, A., Medina, F. X., Serra-Majem, L., Bach-Faig, A. Mediterranean Diet and Cardiodiabesity. 2019. A systematic review through evidence-based answers to key clinical questions. *Nutrients*, **11**: 655.

Garcia-Mendizabal, M. J., Carrasco, J. M., Perez-Gomez, B., Aragones, N., Guallar-Castillon, P., Rodriguez-Artalejo, F. 2009. Role of educational level in the relationship between body mass index (BMI) and health-related quality of life (HRQL) among rural Spanish women. *BMC Public Health*, **9**: 120.

Ge, L., Sadeghirad, B., Ball, G. D. C., da Costa, B. R., Hitchcock, C. L., Svendrovski, A., Kiflen, R., Quadri, K., Kwon, H. Y., Karamouzian, M., Adams-Webber, T., Ahmed, W., Damanhoury, S., Zeraatkar, D., Nikolakopoulou, A., Tsuyuki, R. T., Tian, J., Yang, K., Guyatt, G. H., Johnston, B. C. 2020. Comparison of dietary macronutrient patterns of 14 popular named dietary programmes for weight and cardiovascular risk factor reduction in adults: Systematic review and network meta-analysis of randomised trials. *BMJ.*, **369**: m696.

Ghafoor, R., Rashid, A., Anwar, M. I. 2015. Dyslipidemia and psoriasis: A case control study. *J. Coll. Physicians Surg. Pak.*, **25**: 324-327.

Gisondi, P., Bellinato, F., Girolomoni, G., Albanesi, C. 2020. Pathogenesis of chronic plaque psoriasis and its intersection with cardio-metabolic comorbidities. *Front. Pharmacol.*, **11**: 117.

Gisondi, P., Fostini, A. C., Fossà, I., Girolomoni, G., Targher, G. 2018. Psoriasis and the metabolic syndrome. *Clin. Dermatol.*, **36**: 21-28.

Gottlieb, A. B., Chao, C., Dann, F. 2008. Psoriasis comorbidities. *J. Dermatolog. Treat.*, **19**: 5-21.

Gottlieb, A. B., Dann, F. 2009. Comorbidities in patients with psoriasis. *Am J Med.*, **122**: 1150. e1-1150.e9.

Hales, C. M., Carroll, M. D., Fryar, C. D., Ogden, C. L. 2020. Prevalence of obesity and severe obesity among adults: United States, 2017–2018. *NCHS Data Brief.*, **360**: 1–8.

Hopman, W. M., Berger, C., Joseph, L., Barr, S. I., Gao, Y., Prior, J. C. 2007. The association between body mass index and health-related quality of life: Data from CaMos, a stratified population study. *Qual. Life. Res.*, **16**: 1595–1603.

Huang, R. Y., Huang, C. C., Hu, F. B., Chavarro, J. E. 2016. Vegetarian diets and weight reduction: A meta-analysis of randomized controlled trials. *J. Gen. Intern. Med.* **31**(1): 109–116.

Jenkins, D. J., Chiavaroli, L., Wong, J. M., Kendall, C., Lewis, G. F., Vidgen, E., Connelly, P. W., Leiter, L. A., Josse, R. G., Lamarche, B. 2010. Adding monounsaturated fatty acids to a dietary portfolio of cholesterol lowering foods in hypercholesterolemia. *CMAJ.*, **182**: 1961–1967. [PubMed: 21041432]

Jensen, P., Skov, L. 2016: Psoriasis and obesity. *Dermatology*, **232**: 633-639.

Kelly, T., Yang, W., Chen, C. S., Reynolds, K., He, J. 2008. Global burden of obesity in 2005 and projections to 2030. *Int. J. Obes.*, **32**: 1431–1437.

Lim, S. S., Vos, T., Flexman, A. D., Daniei, G., Shibuya, K. and Adair-Rohani, H. 2012. A comparative risk assessment of burden of disease and injury attributable to 67 risk factors and risk factor clusters in 21 regions, 1990–2010: A systemic analysis for the global burden of disease study 2010. *Lancet*, **380**(9859): 2224–2260.

Liu, Y. S., Wu, Q. J., Xia, Y., Zhang, J. Y., Jiang, Y. T., Chang, Q., Zhao, Y. H. Carbohydrate intake and risk of metabolic syndrome. 2019. A dose-response meta-analysis of observational studies. *Nutr. Metab. Cardiovasc. Dis.*, **29**: 1288–1298.

Ludwig, D. S., Ebbeling, C. B. 2018. The carbohydrate-insulin model of obesity: Beyond "calories in, calories out". *JAMA Intern Med.*, **178**(8): 1098–1103.

Makris, A., Foster, G. D. 2011. Dietary approaches to the treatment of obesity. *Psychiatr. Clin. North Am.*, **34**(4): 813–827.

Makris, A. P., Foster, G. D. 2005. Dietary approaches to the treatment of obesity. *Psychiatr. Clin. North Am.*, **28**(1): 117–139, viii–ix. [PubMed: 15733615]

Mansoor, N., Vinknes, K. J., Veierød, M. B., Retterstøl, K. 2016. Effects of low-carbohydrate diets v. low-fat diets on body weight and cardiovascular risk factors: A meta-analysis of randomised controlled trials. *Br. J. Nutr.*, **115**(3): 466–479.

Martin, B., Mattson, M. P., Maudsley, S. 2006. Caloric restriction and intermittent fasting: Two potential diets for successful brain aging. *Ageing Res. Rev.* **5**(3): 332–353.

Mawaw, P. M., Yav, T., Mukuku, O., Lukanka, O., Kazadi, P. M., Tambwe, D., Omba, J., Kakoma, J. Bangs, M. J., Luboya, O. N. 2017. Prevalence of obesity, diabetes mellitus, hypertension and associated risk factors in a mining workforce, democratic Republic of Congo. *Pan African Medical Journal*, **28**: 282.

Merry, B. J. 2004. Oxidative stress and mitochondrial function with aging – the effects of calorie restriction. *Aging Cell.* **3**(1): 7–12.

Moon, J., Koh, G. 2020. Clinical evidence and mechanisms of high-protein diet-induced weight loss. *J. Obes. Metab. Syndr.*, **29**(3): 166–173.

NCD Risk Factor Collaboration (NCD-RisC). 2017. Worldwide trends in bodymass index, underweight, overweight, and obesity from 1975 to 2016: A pooled analysis of 2416 population-based measurement studies in 128·9 million children, adolescents, and adults. *Lancet.* **390**: 2627–2642. doi: 10.1016/S0140-6736(17)32129-3

Nordmann, A. J., Nordmann, A., Briel, M., Keller, U., Yancy, W. S. Jr., Brehm, B. J., Bucher, H. C. 2006. Effects of low-carbohydrate vs low-fat diets on weight loss and cardiovascular risk factors: A meta-analysis of randomized controlled trials. *Arch. Intern. Med.*, **166**: 285–293. [PubMed: 16476868]

Ojo, O. 2019. Nutrition and chronic conditions. *Nutrients*, **11**: 459–464.

O'Keefe, J. H., Vogel, R., Lavie, C. J. and Cordain, L. 2010. Achieving hunter-gatherer fitness in the 21(st) century: Back to the future. *Am. J. Med.*, 123(12): 1082–1086.

Parretti, H. M., Jebb, S. A., Johns, D. J., Lewis, A. L., Christian-Brown, A. M., Aveyard, P. 2016. Clinical effectiveness of very-low-energy diets in the management of weight loss: A systematic review and meta-analysis of randomized controlled trials. *Obes. Rev.*, **17**(3): 225–234.

Philpot, U., Johnson, M. I. 2019. Diet therapy in the management of chronic pain: Better diet less pain? *Pain Manag.*, **9**(4): 335–338.

Puig, L. 2017. Cardiometabolic comorbidities in psoriasis and psoriatic arthritis. *Int J Mol Sci.*, **19**: 58–63.

Pujia, R., Tarsitano, M. G., Arturi, F., De-Lorenzo, A., Lenzi, A., Pujia, A., Montalcini, T. 2022. Advances in phenotyping obesity and in its dietary and pharmacological treatment: A narrative review. *Front. Nutr.*, **9**: 804719.

Radtke, M. A., Mrowietz, U., Feuerhahn, J., Härter, M., von Kiedrowski, R., Nast, A., Reich, K., Strömer, K., Wohlrab, J., Augustin, M. 2015. Early detection of comorbidity in psoriasis: Recommendations of the national conference on healthcare in psoriasis. *J. Dtsch. Dermatol. Ges.*, **13**: 674-690.

Sach, T. H., Barton, G. R., Doherty, M., Muir, K. R., Jenkinson, C., Avery, A. J. 2007. The relationship between body mass index and health-related quality of life: Comparing the EQ-5D, EuroQol VAS and SF-6D. *Int. J. Obes.*, **31**: 189–196.

Scheer, F. A., Hilton, M. F., Mantzoros, C. S., Shea, S. A. 2009. Adverse metabolic and cardiovascular consequences of circadian misalignment. *Proc. Natl. Acad. Sci. U S A.,* **106**(11): 4453–4458.

Schwarza, A., Billetera, A. T., Scheurlena, K. M., Blüherb, M., Müller-Stich, B. P. 2018. Comorbidities as an indication for metabolic surgery. *Visceral Medicine*, **34**: 381–387.

Seino, Y., Nanjo, K., Tajima, N., Kadowaki, T., Kashiwagi, A., Araki, E., Ito, C., Inagaki, N. and Iwamoto, Y. 2010. Report of the committee on the classification and diagnostic criteria of diabetes mellitus. *J. Diabetes Investig.*, **1**: 212-228.

Shai, I., Schwarzfuchs, D., Henkin, Y., Shahar, D. R., Witkow, S., Greenberg, I., Golan, R., Fraser, D., Bolotin, A., Vardi, H., Tangi-Rozental, O., Zuk-Ramot, R., Sarusi, B., Brickner, D., Schwartz, Z., Sheiner, E., Marko, R., Katorza, E., Thiery, J., Fiedler, G. M., Blüher, M., Stumvoll, M., Stampfer, M. J. 2008. Dietary intervention randomized controlled trial (DIRECT) group. Weight loss with a low carbohydrate, Mediterranean, or low-fat diet. *N. Engl. J. Med.*, **359**: 229–241.

Soliman, S. F. 2020. Metabolic syndrome: Impact of dietary therapy. In J. Khan, P. Hsieh (Eds.), *Cellular Metabolism and Related Disorders*. IntechOpen. https://doi.org/10.5772/intechopen.90835

Svetkey, L. P., Stevens, V. J., Brantley, P. J., Appel, L. J., Hollis, J. F., Loria, C. M., Vollmer, W. M., Gullion, C. M., Funk, K., Smith, P., Samuel-Hodge, C., Myers, V., Lien, L. F., Laferriere, D., Kennedy, B., Jerome, G. J., Heinith, F., Harsha, D. W., Evans, P., Erlinger, T. P., Dalcin, A. T., Coughlin, J., Charleston, J., Champagne, C. M., Bauck, A., Ard, J. D., Aicher, K. 2008. Weight loss maintenance collaborative research group. Comparison of strategies for sustaining weight loss: The weight loss maintenance randomized controlled trial. *JAMA.*, **299**: 1139–1148.

Tobias, D. K., Chen, M., Manson, J. E., Ludwig, D. S., Willett, W., Hu, F. B. 2015. Effect of low-fat diet interventions versus other diet interventions on long-term weight change in adults: A systematic review and meta-analysis. *Lancet Diabetes Endocrinol.*, **3**(12): 968–979.

Turner-McGrievy, G., Mandes, T., Crimarco, A. 2017. A plant-based diet for overweight and obesity prevention and treatment. *J. Geriatr. Cardiol.*, **14**(5): 369–374.

Ul-Haq, Z., Mackay, D. F. Fenwick, E., Pell, J. P. 2012. Impact of metabolic comorbidity on the association between body mass index and health-related quality of life: A Scotland-wide cross-sectional study of 5,608 participants. *BMC Public Health*, **12**: 143–150.

Velho, S., Paccaud, F., Waeber, G., Vollenweider, P., Marques-Vidal, P. 2010. Metabolically healthy obesity: Different prevalences using different criteria. *Eur. J. Clin. Nutr.*, **64**: 1043–1051.

Von Stebut, E., Boehncke, W. H., Ghoreschi, K., Gori, T., Kaya, Z., Thaci, D., Schäffler, A. 2020. IL-17A in psoriasis and beyond: Cardiovascular and metabolic implications. *Front. Immunol.*, **10**: 3096.

Vos, T., Lim, S. S., Abbafati, C. 2020. Global burden of 369 diseases and injuries in 204 countries and territories, 1990–2019: A systematic analysis for the global burden of disease study 2019. *Lancet.* **396**(10258): 1204–1222.

Wee, H. L., Cheung, Y. B., Loke, W. C., Tan, C. B., Chow, M. H., Li, S. C. 2008. The association of body mass index with health-related quality of life: An exploratory study in a multiethnic Asian population. *Value Health*, **11**: 105–114.

Wildman, R. P. 2009. Healthy obesity. *Curr. Opin. Clin. Nutr. Metabo. Care*, **12**: 438–443.

Wing, R. R. 2010. Look AHEAD research group: Long-term effects of a lifestyle intervention on weight and cardiovascular risk factors in individuals with type 2 diabetes mellitus: Four-year results of the Look AHEAD trial. *Arch. Intern. Med.*, **170**: 1566–1575.

Wood, T. R., Hansen, R., Sigurðsson, A. F., Jóhannsson, G. F. 2016. The cardiovascular risk reduction benefits of a low-carbohydrate diet outweigh the potential increase in LDL-cholesterol. *Br. J. Nutr.*, **115**(6): 1126–1128.

World Health Organization. 2000. *Obesity: Preventing and managing the global epidemic: Report of a WHO consultation.* WHO.

Wycherley, T. P., Noakes, M., Clifton, P. M., Cleanthous, X., Keogh, J. B., Brinkworth, G. D. 2010. A high-protein diet with resistance exercise training improves weight loss and body composition in overweight and obese patients with type 2 diabetes. *Diabetes Care*, **33**: 969–976.

Yamazaki, F. 2021. Psoriasis: Comorbidities. *J. Dermatol.*, **48**: 732–740

Index

Note: Page numbers in *italics* indicate a figure and page numbers in **bold** indicate a table on the corresponding page. Page numbers followed by "n" with numbers refer to notes.

For Product Safety Concerns and Information please contact our EU
representative GPSR@taylorandfrancis.com
Taylor & Francis Verlag GmbH, Kaufingerstraße 24, 80331 München, Germany